IS YOUR BODY BABY FRIENDLY?

IS YOUR BODY BABY FRIENDLY?

"Unexplained"
Infertility,
Miscarriage
& IVF Failure

Explained.

Alan E. Beer, M.D.

with Julia Kantecki and Jane Reed

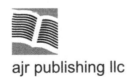

ajr publishing llc

Is Your Body Baby Friendly?
Revised Edition

Copyright © 2019 by Alan E. Beer, M.D., Julia Kantecki & Jane Reed
(Originally published in 2006)

ALL RIGHTS RESERVED

For permission to reproduce selections from this book contact:
jkantecki@gmail.com

Published by AJR Publishing

Cover image provided by Sheila Alice Brandon
"Portrait of Julia Kantecki and Baby Thomas" Acrylic, 2004
Special thanks to Kristina Lerman for providing the back cover photo of Dr Beer.

ISBN: 0-9785078-0-0
Printed in the United States of America

Except as permitted under the United States Copyright Act of 1976, no part of this publication may be reproduced or distributed in any form or by any means, or stored in a database or retrieval system, without prior written permission of the publisher.

This book is for informational purposes only; it is not intended to replace medical advice or to be a substitute for a physician. The material within this book should be used in cooperation with your own physician to help deal with your personal health problems. All efforts have been made to ensure the accuracy of the information contained in this book as of the date published. However, as medical information can change rapidly, it is strongly recommended that you discuss all health matters and concerns with your physician before embarking on new diagnostic or treatment strategies. The authors and the publisher expressly disclaim responsibility for any adverse effects arising from the use or application of the information herein.

Dedicated to Dr Rupert E. Billingham, PhD, DSc,
my mentor, collaborator and dear friend.

Alan E. Beer

"The purpose of science is to change belief! If you believe that infertility, IVF failure, recurrent miscarriages, prematurity, and low birthweight are 'God's will', which is not testable scientifically, you will never try to find effective treatment."

Sir Peter Medawar (Nobel laureate)

CONTENTS

Forewords by Christo Zouves, M.D., Professor Gamal Matthias and
Jeffrey Braverman M.D..iii
Preface...ix
Introducing Alan E. Beer, M.D..xi
Introduction by Julia Kantecki...xiii
The Birth of an Idea..xxiii
Miscarriage: A Silent Epidemic..xxvii

1.	Reproductive Immunology: Helping to Explain the"Unexplained........25
2.	Defining Reproductive Failure 29
3.	Recurring Nightmares. 37
4.	The Immune System...49
5.	Being Too Genetically Similar...61
6.	Blood clotting Disorders..65
7.	Immunity to Pregnancy...79
8.	Antibodies to Sperm..83
9.	High Natural Killer Cell Levels...87
10.	Antibodies to Hormones and Neurotransmitters.........................107
11.	Hope for Older Mothers-to-Be 129
12.	Immune Problems and Pregnancy..135
13.	Comprehensive Immune Testing..143
14.	Immunotherapies..157
15.	Immunotherapy: Rejected by a Body of Opinion.........................181
16.	Critics of Reproductive Immunology.......................................189
17	Trials on Trial...221
18.	"Hope" by Alan E Beer...233

Addendum...259
I.   Fertility under Fire...261
II.   The Legacy of a Toxic Pregnancy...271
III.   The Toxins Eating at Our Health...275
IV.   "Natural Immunotherapy For Life" by Zita West.......................279
Post scripts..301
Notes..309
Glossary.. 445
Resources...455
Index..499

ii

Christo Zouves, M.D.

Zouves Fertility Center, Foster City, California, USA

Reproductive failure and repeated pregnancy loss is devastating for the patients involved, emotionally, physically and financially. It can mean the loss of valuable ovarian time for the patient and frustration and disappointment for the practitioners involved. There is always a reason for pregnancy loss and this book very eloquently lays out the standard testing.

Dr Alan Beer then examines and categorizes what can be done in the so called unexplained and by inference, "hopeless," cases. Once the usual factors like chromosomal abnormalities, uterine defects, infections and the hormonal milieu have been excluded, this book speaks to a group of patients who still have unexplained loss.

The immune system is at the center of who we are. It protects us against infections and abnormal cells that can in some cases become malignant. Many patients with cancers previously labeled terminal and untreatable are now being treated by inducing a favorable immune response to markers derived from the actual tumors themselves.

It amazes me how long it has taken fertility practitioners to make the connection between recurrent reproductive failure and the immune mechanism of attack, given the fact that the implanting embryo is genetically different from the mother or carrier. Something almost magical happens to prevent rejection of this graft in the vast majority of pregnancies. But for a small group of patients, this does not happen and we are left with immune attack and thrombosis, which either prevents implantation or causes loss or inadequate intrauterine nutrition.

It is now 12 years since the book was first published and this revised edition includes new treatments that have been added as well changes brought about by advances in our understanding of immunology.

Dr Alan Beer devoted his life to the investigation and treatment of recurrent failed treatment and pregnancy loss. I had the privilege of knowing him and treating patients with him for almost 15 years. In this book, he seeks rational explanations and lays out modalities of treatment, which have helped thousands of patients who previously had been given no hope, to receive the precious gift of Parenthood.

Professor Gamal Matthias

Sydney Reproductive Immunology, Sydney, Australia

I am delighted to contribute to the second edition of "Is Your Body Baby Friendly?" by Dr Alan Beer, Julia Kantecki and Jane Reed. This book provides both useful information and practical clinical management in the challenging area of unexplained repeated implantation failure and recurrent miscarriages.

Dr Alan Beer was an eminent pioneer in this field. His passion and extensive knowledge were unparalleled. He dedicated his life and career to research and to help patients from across the globe with pregnancy losses. It was my privilege and honour to have had him as a teacher, mentor and colleague.

For decades voluminous research has been carried out to try to answer basic questions. How, in a normal pregnancy, do two genetically different individuals coexist? How is the embryo allowed to implant and the placenta permitted to keep growing without challenge from the maternal immune system? What makes the embryo/fetus so immune privileged? Why do excellent quality embryos repeatedly fail to implant?

There are so many interacting mechanisms and pathways that work to achieve a state of maternal immune tolerance allowing the fetus to thrive and develop. Unfortunately, defects can can occur in these stages, resulting in implantation failure, miscarriage or obstetric complications such as fetal growth restriction, premature labour, preeclampsia or stillbirth.

Today we have significantly expanded our knowledge at the cell, tissue and laboratory level. Our understanding of the processes and mechanisms of maternal immune tolerance of the fetus is constantly growing. However, it has been our challenge to transform all of this information and knowledge into management strategies to assist women whose bodies are "non baby friendly."

The evidence for the role of immunologic and immune/genetic factors in implantation and placentation is strong. One of biggest hurdles in research and treatment is the heterogenic (multiple genetic combinations of materials from the man and woman) nature of the problem. It makes standardization of research and immune treatment a big challenge.

As repeated pregnancy losses and implantation failures are a highly heterogeneous and diverse condition it is logical and vital that a workable classification is utilized to divide it into groups to facilitate clinical management and research. Dr Alan Beer designed the first such classification, which is covered in these pages. He provides a systematic, practical and an insightful approach in this regard. It is a step towards standardization that should hopefully be followed by other steps such as formulating a consistent methodology for testing.

In fertility centers and miscarriage clinics today, over 70% of repeated implantation failures and approximately 50% of repeated miscarriages remain labelled "unexplained" or "idiopathic." Women experiencing these outcomes are usually grouped together in the in the "too hard to treat" basket. They suffer terribly, both emotionally, physically and financially. Yet they are simply advised to keep trying again, keep doing more IVF cycles until they give up. Chipping away at this "unexplained" group by better diagnostics to discover the causes is vital if we are to provide patients with management plans and proper advice.

Perhaps some readers would be interested in the history and controversy surrounding reproductive immonology and its therapies. The disbelievers consider this field to be "on the fringe," unorthodox, unproven and without merit. What everyone should focus on is it is the outcome that matters.

Genetics and immune pathways are interrelated. Traditional approaches to genetic screening have targeted individuals at high risk based on a clinical history, family history and ethnicity. More recently there have been moves towards screening for the more common disorders in the broader reproductive population. Changes in genomic technology now mean that hundreds of genetically inherited disorders can be idenified. This is beneficial in patients with repeated pregnancy losses.

There is also no doubt the egg quality is very important. However, it is an error to focus on just the eggs rather than considering the interactions of the genetics of the mother and the father and their whole immune/genetic and immune system relationship.

Undoubtedly this book has achieved its goal in focusing on helping its readers to understand the main issues surrounding this challenging and constantly developing scientific area.

It is a summary of the futuristic vision of Dr Alan Beer and the editors are congratulated on their diligence and industry and on a job well done.

Foreword by Jeffrey Braverman, M.D.

Braverman IVF and Reproductive Immunology, New York

I remember my entrance into the world of Reproductive Immunology over 25 years ago. I like everyone else at the time, I was seeing so many women with unexplained miscarriage. Their trips to the local RE yielded no results. Later, as I was looking for answers I found the ground breaking work of Dr Beer in his book. I began to understand that the immune system played a part in these unexplained miscarriages and thought he was brilliant for connecting these two fields.

I read his book from cover to cover and asked myself how could I improve on what he had already done. Dr Beer started my journey into what I believe was the next step in understanding and treating this group of women.

We needed to learn all the fields of immunology, since they appeared to all be related to not only implantation failure and pregnancy loss, but also to late pregnancy complications such as pre term labor, fetal growth restriction, preeclampsia, stillbirth and even autism. To this end, our center has organized a team of research specialists to seek and gain in depth knowledge of the critical fields of allergy immunology, autoimmune disease immunology, cancer immunology, transplant immunology and the immunology of inflammation.

This has led us to develop one of the most expansive immunology profiles available anywhere in the world, giving us a clear insight yet into the workings of the reproductive immune system. We have found that by closely identifying immune problems we can diagnose and treat unexplained poor embryo quality and early diminished ovarian reserve that presents as a low anti-Müllerian hormone level, (the hormone given off by developing follicles) in women under the age of 40. Our immunology data has also helped us to begin to explain the strong association of immune issues in those with pregnancy failure and endometriosis.

An abnormal immune response is also a leading cause of failure to conceive both naturally and with assisted reproductive technology. When these issues are treated, many times I have seen my patients avoid IVF and become pregnant on their own.

Over the last five years, 70% of our patients in all age groups combined, with a history of at least five miscarriages had a successful pregnancy using their own egg as defined by a live birth. 95% of these patients had at least one documented chromosomally normal loss.

Since we have instituted this multidisciplinary approach we have had great success in some of the most difficult cases that found no answers in the general RE facilities. Many in fact, have now begun to refer their complicated cases to a dedicated center for reproductive immunology, which indicates that this field is now considered to be a separate specialty. I envisage that it will soon become standard practice for ob/gyns and fertility doctors to refer patients with unexplained infertility, IVF failure and recurrent loss for more advanced care.

PREFACE

Infertility, recurrent pregnancy loss and IVF failure are not a matter of chance. Your immune response may be the cause.

The worst feeling for most women, after the physical pain of miscarriage and the emotional anguish of a failed embryo transfer have long passed, is that of sheer hopelessness. With no answers to be found and no prospect of achieving a healthy pregnancy many sink into total depression. Living without hope is a soul destroying existence. The months and then the years pass by. Time may heal, but the doubts and questions remain; Why did it happen? What went wrong? Was it my fault? What if I had done this, eaten that or avoided the other…

Having investigated the subject for more than 25 years, the late Dr Alan E. Beer discovered that there are solid, quantifiable explanations for previously "unexplained" infertility, IVF (in vitro fertilization) failure and pregnancy loss.

During his lifetime he treated over 7,000 couples and through his pioneering program achieved a pregnancy success rate of more than 85% within three natural cycles or IVF attempts. Today fertility centers that follow his protocols, or modified versions thereof, are seeing similar results.

Averaging just over 36 years old, Dr Beer's patients could be considered the "no hopers" of the reproductive populace, having endured around four failed IVF cycles or pregnancy losses that had previously been written off as "idiopathic" (a fancy word for "unexplained") by mainstream medical practitioners. These were not young women with minor problems, but the battle weary survivors of years of infertility treatments who had tried every conventional and alternative therapy. Yet they achieved success with Dr Beer's program, using treatments to moderate their immune response.

Dr Beer's patients were often self referred, having discovered him through a combination of frustration and determination, refusing to accept that no one could explain why they were unable to have a baby. In a way, they too have become pioneers, forging a path through new medical territories to make the journey easier for others like myself today. Some have shared their stories here to assist others who are stuck in a hopeless void of unanswered questions.

Dr Beer has identified several types of immune problem that can cause pregnancy loss, IVF failure and infertility. The logic behind these theories is explained. The way the immune system works and how imbalances within it affect pregnancy outcome is also addressed. It is then revealed how such immune dysfunction can be solved by temporarily regulating the immune response to make the woman's body more "baby friendly."

The information in this book will put many minds at rest by providing answers to the unanswered questions that plague those who are going through, or have suffered reproductive failure. As Dr Beer once said, "The only way to live with infertility and loss is to fill your mind with facts. You need to discover what the problems are and find out if they have a reasonably good chance of being treated. Otherwise you sentence yourself to an endless punishment of self blame, sadness, loss of hope and doubt."

In these pages you will find evidence based facts concerning a serious human health concern that has so far been shrouded in mystery and confusion. Never before has so much scientific knowledge about pregnancy failure and the immune system been made publicly available and presented in a way that can be generally understood.

This book represents the work and the views of Dr Beer, whose contributions have led to significant developments in the field of reproductive immunology, which is still one of the most rapidly expanding areas of biomedical science. New cutting edge treatments are just becoming available within mainstream medicine and critics of this area of science are becoming increasingly silenced by the sheer weight of supportive evidence and growing smaller in number by the year.

For whatever the arguments and controversies, there is one fact that nobody can dispute, Dr Beer succeeded where others failed enabled thousands of women all over the world to realize a previously impossible dream: to love and hold a baby of their own.

Julia   Kantecki

i

Introducing Alan E. Beer, M.D.

Dr Alan Beer was a world renowned physician and scientist who spent much of his academic life analyzing the relationship between the immune system and reproductive health. In the latter part of his career he dedicated himself to helping couples with infertility, IVF or implantation failure and recurrent miscarriage.

In 1962 he received his medical degree from Indiana University School of Medicine. This was followed by a residency in Immunology and Genetics and a fellowship in Obstetrics and Gynecology at the University of Pennsylvania. It was here that he became fascinated by genetics and immunology and conducted experiments that were to lead to a major breakthrough in the treatment of reproductive failure. He noticed that when related males and females were mated to produce an inbred strain, the pregnancies were often rejected and the female soon became infertile. This phenomenon made him wonder about possible explanations for infertility in humans.

In 1971 Dr Beer was board certified by the American Board of Obstetrics and Gynecology. He then became a faculty member of the University of Pennsylvania and later of the University of Texas Southwestern Medical School at Dallas and the University of Michigan. An appointment as Chairman of Obstetrics and Gynecology at the University of Michigan Medical School followed in 1979.

It was here that he treated a couple with seven miscarriages. By then, Dr Beer was convinced of the significance of natural killer cells in pregnancy and had devised a pioneering form of therapy to control their activity. Within a year, his first "immune patient" had delivered a healthy boy.

Dr Beer joined the Chicago Medical School in 1987, where he accepted a joint appointment as Professor of Obstetrics and Gynecology and Professor of Microbiology and Immunology. He subsequently established the School's Reproductive Immunology Clinic where he continued to specialize in treating couples that had repeatedly failed with conventional approaches to infertility and miscarriage and in the majority of cases, he made it possible for them to have babies.

In 1988 he extended his care to those undergoing assisted reproduction (IVF) and treated a couple who had failed to carry to term after

20 IVF attempts. Within a year the woman delivered healthy twins. From then on Dr Beer saw every IVF couple, no matter how difficult their case "as long as there was hope."

While continuing to handle an ever growing patient caseload, Dr Beer contributed to many books, monographs and scientific articles concerning the impact of the immune system on fertility and presented his findings at national and international medical conferences in Australia, Europe and South America.

He believed that it was only by sharing knowledge with scientists from allied and interrelated fields that progress in the study of the immunological and genetic aspects of the reproductive process could be advanced.

For this reason, he was always keen to promote cooperation between laboratories involved in experimental and clinical studies. And it is for this reason that this book reflects the advances in this field of immunology from a global perspective in order to provide the most current information that is available for those in need. Recurrent miscarriage and recurrent IVF failure can be analyzed, explained and treated. Pregnancy failure is not "God's will" or " Just one of those things."

In addition to his role as Chairman of the National Institute of Health Study Section on Human Embryology and Development, Dr Beer served as Editor-in-Chief of the *Journal of Reproductive Immunology* and was a founding member and past President of the American Society for Reproductive Immunology.

In 2003, Dr Beer established The Alan E. Beer Center for Repro-ductive Immunology and Genetics for the evaluation and treatment of couples with immune related problems.

Since Dr Beer's death in 2006, the center has been headed by Dr Raphael Stricker who advocated the same kind of approach as the facility's founder. In January 2019, Dr Stricker announced that due to his heavy workload at his other clinic specializing in the treatment of Lyme disease, he must now relinquish this role. The center is currently in negotiations with possible successors who specialize in reproductive immunology and are familiar with Dr Beer's program.

INTRODUCTION

"We don't know why it didn't work.– everything looked perfect"

By Julia Kantecki

The nurse on the phone just delivered the news of my third negative pregnancy result. I was filled with disbelief, confusion, anger and disappointment. Here I was at the age of 40 with time having virtually run out according to all the statistics, with yet another "unexplained" IVF failure behind me. I was walking around my local shopping mall at the time, holding my cell phone and looking for a place to cry. There wasn't a lot more I could do.

My quest to have a baby via IVF was born of necessity as my husband had undergone a vasectomy over 20 years ago. Early in our relationship, he'd asked me if I wanted children and my honest answer was "one day." I was 29. Little did I know that my years of peak fertility had passed me by five years ago.

A career in copywriting and a demanding job as a marketing director took care of another nine years. Then at the age of 38 I woke up to the realization that if I didn't try to conceive soon I might never have a baby. The thought of it left me feeling so miserable that I went to see my family doctor to ask for some counseling or medication, whatever there was, to ease the weight of depression. He was surprised I hadn't considered assisted reproduction and gave me the name of a fertility clinic about 30 miles away. My husband already had two grown up boys and had recently become a grandfather at the age of 52. He was looking forward to retirement, so I was grateful that he was open to IVF and the responsibility of another child.

My appointment with the fertility doctor was a day of anticipation and excitement. Even though I was approaching 40 I still had a reasonable chance of success, although the doctor said from now on it was "downhill all the way" and I was probably just "borderline" as far as fertility went.

I took the doctor's notes home, showed his scribbled diagrams of the sperm extraction procedure to my husband and then proceeded to read every book I could find about IVF and pregnancy after the age of 35. It seemed that my major problem would be egg quality which declined with age. I might also produce fewer eggs and perhaps need an egg donor. A simile that seemed to keep cropping up was of IVF being like a rollercoaster. I subconsciously braced myself for a wild and uncontrollable journey into the unknown.

It was shocking to discover how little I knew about my fertility. I had assumed that because my mother had given birth to five children with ease, her last at the age of 40, I had also inherited her magnetic ability to conceive. Having taken contraceptive pills since the age of 18 to avoid instant pregnancy I was sure my uterus was bursting with hormones and ready to grab onto any stray sperm that came its way. Little did I know what my body actually held in store.

The spring of 2001 was an exciting and happy time with the prospect of a baby on the horizon. The pregnancy success rates at my clinic were comparatively good at about 35% per cycle for women aged 35 to 39. The nurses were sweet and soft spoken and I was soothed and reassured by their compassion and looked forward to my visits. The complicated drug regime was a challenge, the injections were a necessary evil and my periods became a monthly obsession.

In June, my husband underwent a procedure to extract semen via his testicles. His sperm was frozen and then thawed to test its motility to see if would be of sufficient quality to inject into my eggs. He was sure that he would deliver a good sample as apparently his first wife could get pregnant just by looking at him.

The results were not good. The embryologist explained that after the freeze/thaw process, there was not much movement in any of the samples, "just a slight twitch of the tail," so they would need to extract a fresh sample on the day of my egg harvest. The follow up consultation with the fertility doctor didn't give us much cause to celebrate either. My blood tests had shown a follicle-stimulating hormone (FSH) level of

7.4, which was "normal," although the doctor added, "We see these readings all the time, but when it comes to egg collection, a woman in her early 30s can have the egg quality of a woman in her 40s.-In some of these cases, the eggs are totally gone, or of very poor quality." The message seemed to be "don't build up your hopes."

I started my first IVF cycle in August 2001, three months before my 40th birthday. Amazingly my aging ovaries produced 15 eggs. These were injected with sperm and 13 fertilized. The doctor decided that just two embryos should be transferred. One was four celled with no fragmentation which the nurse declared was "absolutely beautiful," saying, "we don't see many like that."

Two paranoid weeks later, during which I recorded every imaginable potential symptom of pregnancy, my HCG hormone level came in at zero. Not even a hint of a pregnancy. I hadn't drunk coffee or touched red wine. I'd walked the dogs every day, eaten broccoli and generally tried hard to be in good shape.

After two days of abject misery I signed up for emergency acupuncture and hypnotherapy. I had to do something. The Chinese acupuncturist looked at my tongue and checked my pulse and decided that my body needed to be rebalanced. She prescribed some herbs that looked like chopped tree bark which I boiled and drank as a tea. The noxious brown soup was undrinkable, so she gave me ground up herbs which I added to milkshakes and gulped down quickly. The mixture was so disgusting it had to be doing some good.

Our appointment for the post mortem would hopefully give us an insight into what could have possibly gone wrong. "Well," the doctor sighed, "We can't explain it. Everything looked perfect. There was no reason for this to happen. It just goes that way sometimes. All your hormones were fine, perhaps the egg quality could have been better, but I feel that you still stand a very good chance of success."

We left the clinic deflated and somber. I had convinced myself that the transfer itself had been traumatic and that my uterus had contracted and repelled the embryos. I needed a reason why this hadn't worked. Dealing with unknowns was too hard to bear.

Waiting outside the ultrasound room during the preparations for our second attempt, I got chatting to another woman. This was her sixth cycle. I remember her saying that IVF was "just a numbers game." Something in my head told me she was wrong and although I didn't know why, I said, "No, I think there are reasons for what happens. It can't just be about luck."

My next transfer was carried out by the doctor himself, not a nurse. I didn't feel a thing. It all went smoothly and three embryos were transferred. The result this time was "a hint of pregnancy" with a partial implantation that had raised my HCG level just off zero to 5.4. A further cycle with the transfer of three good embryos also resulted in a negative.

My husband and I cried, talked it over and tried to find some hope at the bottom of our pit of despair. My baby dream was slipping away and I was scared now. I was fearful of loss and worried about shriveling into menopause and a childless future. Once again, I sought informa-tion, an explanation, anything to help point us in the right direction. Once again there were no answers to be found.

The doctor at the fertility clinic was genuinely concerned and very sympathetic but he couldn't tell me why I wasn't getting pregnant. He looked at my file, pondered the results of the stimulation, assessed my hormone levels again and decided that there was no reason for any of the three failed cycles. He said there were no signs of age related problems and I should think about going for transfer number four.

A nurse then told me that one woman had sixteen IVF attempts before she was successful. I was horrified. No way was I going through another possible four or five egg recoveries, endless injections, blood tests and hormone jangling drugs. I couldn't face it. So I decided to look for answers myself. I'd read every book and tried everything: organic food, chemical free cleaning products, acupuncture, Chinese herbs, regular exercise, massage, hypnotherapy and prayer. There was nothing else to do but consider the possibility that something about my body was just not baby friendly.

"The good news is you have a problem"

The Internet had been a constant source of support during the past year. I'd joined a discussion board and regularly posted updates on the minutiae of my IVF focused life. The Internet also provided me with access to the world's fertility centers and the latest research.

My first thoughts were to look for the best success rates. My mother lived in Lake Bluff, north of Chicago so it made sense to try a clinic over there. My investigations led me to the Finch University of Health Sciences, which offered a unique program of in depth blood testing for autoimmune issues. As I had mild arthritis in my fingers, which is an immune system problem, I wondered if this could be a factor in my inability to conceive. It seemed a tenuous link, but worth investigating, if only to rule it out.

An appointment was scheduled with Joanne Kwak-Kim, M.D. who had recently taken over from Dr Beer as Director of the Reproductive Medicine Program at Finch University (now the Rosalind Franklin University Health Clinics). Dr Kwak-Kim had been sent my notes from my fertility clinic in the U.K.

After explaining what they did at the center she said that on the basis of my results it was likely I had immune issues which were causing my body to attack the embryos just as it would a foreign object or cancer cells. In fact, she said just two IVF failures were an indicator of a possible immune reaction.

Numerous blood samples were taken from my husband and myself. We had no idea what kind of results to expect. Deep down I was looking for evidence to support my inner belief that there was nothing wrong with me and all we had to do was try again.

We returned a week later and a senior nurse explained the pile of test results to us. "Well Julia," she began brightly, "It's good news. You have a problem, several in fact, but we know how to get round them so don't worry." The stack of reports in her lap provided an incredibly detailed insight into the workings of my body. Apparently, my blood contained abnormally high levels of natural killer cells and harmful antibodies that made implantation virtually impossible. In addition, my husband and I shared HLA-DQ alpha numbers (specific codes of DNA) and two that matched exactly was bad news. It all meant that my immune system needed to be suppressed so that it didn't automatically kill off another embryo. This could be done, I was told, using a low dose form of a corticosteroid that is normally prescribed for transplant patients to help their body accept a new organ.

A test for factor V (five) Leiden was also "heterozygous positive" meaning I had inherited the gene from one of my parents. This Germanic sounding condition is quite common among the white western population and is associated with an increased susceptibility to blood clotting and strokes. I made a mental note to buy a pair of compression socks for my flight back to the U.K.

The MTHFR (another type of gene mutation) test was also heterozygous positive. This meant I had "an error of folate metabolism" and an increased chance of developing hardened arteries and thrombosis. It also indicated that I was at greater risk of miscarriage or having a baby with neural tube defects. I was prescribed a high strength B vitamin pill containing folic acid.

The conclusion of an hour long ultrasound scan in which the condition of my uterus and the blood flow were monitored brought further perturbing news. I knew I had poor circulation to the extremities of my body (cold hands, feet and nose) but apparently this also continued internally with "sparse" blood flow. In all, my uterus only managed a score of 14 out of 21, which put me the category of being only 60% capable of holding a pregnancy. I may have looked okay on the outside, but inside I had virtually seized up.

Suddenly I was overwhelmed with technical explanations for my years of IVF failure. From being completely in the dark I was totally bedazzled by a torrent of scientific data that virtually ruled out the possibility of me ever becoming pregnant through IVF or even naturally in the past for that matter. The nurse was quite definite when I asked her to clarify the findings. "No, you could never have gotten pregnant *ever* without treatment," she repeated.

To say this was a revelation is an understatement. It was a complete bombshell and a total reversal of all my preconceptions. I did not take after my highly fertile mother after all. My body was a hostile, sluggish non baby friendly environment. So serious were the implications of one of the results that I was urged to inform my family about the factor V Leiden blood clotting problem as it's a genetic trait. I was also advised to take steps to reduce the risks of stroke and deep vein thrombosis by taking low dose soluble aspirin every night for the rest of my life.

Still, the nurse insisted this was all very good news, and wait for it, my chance of success with the right medication was now 85%. "Well maybe 80%," she reconsidered, "because of your age." There was a moment's silence. I could hardly believe what I was hearing. This was totally incredible news. Then my skeptical head took over within a matter of seconds and I decided that it was best not to get excited. It all sounded far too good to be true.

INTRODUCTION

Dr Kwak-Kim sent a letter to my clinic in the U.K. detailing the findings of the immune evaluation and her recommendations for treatment. The solution to what seemed highly complex issues was remarkably straightforward. For my next cycle of planned conception my protocol was – to the word – as follows:

1. Take one baby aspirin (81 mg) daily.
2. Begin progesterone vaginal suppositories, with a minimum of 100 mg twice a day or a higher dose (at your doctor's discretion) 48 hours after ovulation or within 48 hours of embryo transfer and continue through 16 weeks of pregnancy. Discontinue if the pregnancy test is negative.
3. Begin heparin injections of 5,000 units twice daily on day 6 of the cycle of planned conception and continue throughout pregnancy until instructed to stop.
4. Take 500 mg calcium twice a day.
5. Take one Folgard RX2.2 daily.
6. Take 5 mg prednisone twice a day 48 hours after ovulation. Increase prednisone to 10 mg twice a day at the time of a positive pregnancy test.

The next step was to obtain these medications from my doctor at the medical center in my small hometown of Doncaster in the North of England. My fertility doctor had already sent my general practitioner a polite letter asking for his help, so I wasn't expecting any problems.

I sat in his office while he studied a copy of the instructions from Chicago. Finally he shook his head and sighed deeply. "I can't prescribe these drugs. They're too unorthodox I'm afraid. These medications are not normally associated with pregnancy. If I were to prescribe them it would be like trying to fly a Jumbo jet. I could read the manual and understand in principal how it worked but it wouldn't mean that I could fly it."

His obtuse reply came as something of a surprise. I had expected him to show a slight degree of admiration for the transatlantic efforts I had made in obtaining an explanation for my inability to get pregnant. I made a final plea as I was desperate and he finally relented and gave me a prescription for a week's supply of blood thinning injections to give me time to source it elsewhere. I am sure he was very relieved that he never saw me again.

I ordered the Folgard and prednisone and had them delivered to my mother in the U.S. who forwarded them to me and obtained the heparin (Clexane) privately through my fertility clinic.

Dr Kwak-Kim had been quite clear about her preference for a fresh transfer rather than a frozen one. She also told me that taking Folgard throughout the cycle would improve the quality of my eggs. This was news to me as I had been led to believe that women were born with a finite number of eggs, the quality and quantity of which degenerated with every passing year.

Although I still had five embryos "in the freezer" I went through another stimulated cycle and 14 eggs were retrieved, ten of which fertilized. Five were left to mature and two days later the best three were transferred: two four celled embryos and one with three.

Two weeks later the dreaded phone call to the clinic was made and to my total disbelief and delight, I learned that the result was positive! To avoid invasive testing for Down's syndrome, I had a screening scan at 12 weeks and blood samples were sent for analysis. Fantastic news! The chances of Down's syndrome were 1 in 3,300 and 1 in 41,000 for Edward's syndrome. At last, I felt truly, healthily pregnant and cele-brated by buying a crib and a stroller.

Over the next few months, my intake of prednisone was tapered down to avoid the problems of suddenly coming off the drug although I hadn't experienced any side effects. Being pregnant I was now under the care of a hospital consultant. He assured me the dose was very low and didn't cross the placenta so it would have no effect on the baby.

The daily Clexane injections continued and every two weeks I reported to my consultant for a check up. and he would write me another prescription. During one of these visits a nurse told me that this anticoagulant drug was commonly given to women who had previously miscarried. Yet my doctor had still refused to prescribe it!

Successive scans revealed a good sized baby with a strong, regular heartbeat. The baby was also a "he." As I was categorized as an older mother the consultant felt sure that I would have a C-section, so I didn't really pay much attention to finding out about other ways of giving birth.

A few weeks prior to the anticipated delivery date, I was told to stop taking the Clexane in case they had to carry out an emergency operation to deliver the baby. My due date came and went and I was scheduled for the C- section two days later.

On the morning of surgery my waters broke and I was given drugs to induce the birth. Twelve hours later, following an hour of intense and exhausting pushing, our highly prized little boy was born.

After the delivery a midwife commented on the strange look of my placenta and wanted to pass it round so everyone could feel how gritty it was. My mother and husband both declined the offer. In fact, the midwife said it looked as if it was inside out.

I was later told the placenta can look like this in women with immune problems. The grittiness is caused by excessive calcification. Luckily the baby's health had not been compromised but with slightly more intensive immunotherapy this potentially dangerous situation might have been prevented.

I subsequently learned that my protocol with Dr Kwak-Kim was relatively conservative as immune treatments go. For more aggressive therapies patients often sought the help of the founder of the clinic's reproductive immunology program and the main instigator of its revolutionary testing procedures and treatments, Dr Alan Beer.

IS YOUR BODY BABY FRIENDLY?

The Birth of an Idea

While I was trying to find out more about my immune problems I was conversing with other women via a Yahoo website called "Reproductive Immunology Support." Having been used to talking about straightforward IVF issues for the previous couple of years, this was like venturing into a completely different world where everyone spoke "immune language" and had complicated discussions about "cytokine ratios," "NK cell assays," and "NK flares."

Some of the group's members sounded more like medical experts than patients. Many had suffered a succession of losses and IVF failures or worse, stillbirth. Some had seen their marriages disintegrate, while others were being treated for depression. Among this community of driven, courageous women there was a sense of relief at being in a place where they could post a question and receive a logical answer backed up with medical data and case studies.

These women were focused, determined, cool and thorough, not a gullible group of hormonally challenged women as some critics of this treatment have implied. Years of being let down by doctors who refused to think beyond the rigid boundaries of current practice had made them cynical. Dealing with insurance companies and making legitimate but unorthodox requests for cover had made them firm and pragmatic. Sentimentality had been replaced by clarity and objectivity. This was a group of fighters and researchers.

The group's founder, and the source of this invaluable help was an exceptional woman named Jane Reed who had had four children with Dr Beer's help. She seemed to be able to operate her life online in a parallel universe with its own separate time zone. How she managed to spend the hours giving advice and replying to the many posts that came in every day as well as looking after her large family amazed me.

Typical of her morale boosting replies was a response to a new member who was at a low ebb. Jane wrote, "Sorry you are going through all these feelings of fatigue and loneliness with this immune journey. One thing I say for certain, you are not alone. Fear, apprehension and isolation: these are emotions we all feel, especially when we are first starting along this long, scary immune path. In fact, I don't

xxiii

think a single one of us did not feel overwhelmed by the medications, the costs and the "strangeness" of it all when we first began this journey, especially when local doctors do not always agree. But that's what this group is here for: to provide education, companionship and support, connected in spirit through the miracle of cyberspace."

The group's members had often suggested that someone should write a book about Dr Beer and his work so that more women could benefit from his treatments. As if further prompts were needed two media reports signaled that it was time to bring this medical science into the wider public domain.

The first story appeared early in 2003 and concerned a 42 year-old British woman named Annette Quinlan. Her tragic history involved a succession of 19 miscarriages. She lost her first baby at seven weeks and after seven more miscarriages she was referred to the Liverpool Women's Hospital where it was discovered she had a very high number of aggressive natural killer cells in her uterus. Annette was given steroids to suppress her immune system. However, she continued to miscarry, at which point she nearly gave up. Yet she still kept undergoing tests, believing that it might help other women in the same position even if it didn't work for her. Finally, after 14 years, her perseverance was rewarded with the birth of a girl.

A couple of weeks later another national U.K. newspaper ran the front page headline "Parenting: The simple £15 'cure' for miscarriage: A new theory about the body's immune system could help prevent thousands of women losing babies." The report featured a TV producer named Gillian Strachan who had endured six miscarriages before giving birth to a baby boy.

Gillian had started trying to conceive in her late 30s but again, every pregnancy had ended in loss. She had hair clippings analyzed for mineral deficiencies and saw a dietician to make sure she was eating properly. None of the doctors seemed to be able to help. It was eventually discovered that she suffered from a blood clotting disorder. However, she was not given the blood thinning treatment she needed until she was in the sixth week of pregnancy, the point at which she usually lost the baby.

In late 2001, she heard a radio report about a physician in Chicago named Dr Alan Beer, who had discovered that natural killer cells might play a role in miscarriage, and contacted him by tracing his details on the Internet. She learned how the immune system works in pregnancy and how it can also work against it. According to Dr Beer she needed a program of immunotherapy in order to see a live birth.

Gillian Strachan described the reaction to the idea by her doctor in England as totally dismissive saying, "It was as if I'd told him I thought Father Christmas was going to bring me a baby."

Undeterred, she contacted a fertility specialist with knowledge of immune issues in pregnancy, Dr Hassan Shehata, (now the Medical Director and Founder of the Centre for Reproductive Immunology and Pregnancy Miscarriage Clinic in Surrey, England). Tests showed she had a high natural killer (NK) cell count, for which he prescribed immune suppressing steroids. Within months she was pregnant and went on to deliver a healthy baby.

Asked for his opinion on the medical profession's skepticism about immune testing, Dr Shehata says, "It is unfortunate that women are still struggling to get their doctor to listen to them because of a supposed lack of clinical evidence. Some doctors' attitudes are very bad. They treat these women as if they are not intelligent enough to know anything. These women have done their research and are often more knowledgeable than the doctors. Losing one chromosomally normal baby after another is not a matter of bad luck as these poor women are often told. We now understand that in some instances the mother's immune system can turn on itself and damage her own pregnancies. With "reproductive immunology" and other established therapies, a much greater proportion of women can be successfully treated. Even women in their late 30s and early 40s who have suffered several miscarriages consecutively without any apparent reason are able to carry their pregnancies to full term.

On the subject of Dr Beer, he says. "Personally, I think he is a great pioneer." "My interest in the subject started after I studied his original work. Having researched the subject myself for many years I am convinced that there is a link between the immune system, infertility and miscarriage."

IS YOUR BODY BABY FRIENDLY?

Miscarriage: A Silent Epidemic

A few months after the birth of my baby, my cousin came to stay. One evening she proudly announced that she and my brother were expecting their first child. We opened the champagne and toasted the wonderful news and she drank soda water. A few days later during dinner, she said she felt something wasn't right and rushed upstairs to the bathroom. Half an hour later, she crept back downstairs crying and asked if her husband could come and talk to her. We left them alone in the living room. Finally, they both emerged, distraught and drained and told us what had happened.

She had been 11 weeks pregnant and virtually out of the first trimester danger zone but had been bleeding occasionally over the past three weeks. Her doctor had told her not to worry as this was quite common. Now she was sure there was something seriously wrong as the amount of blood was increasing. They decided not to risk staying another night and traveled home to arrange for an ultrasound the next morning.

The scan revealed their fetus had died. There was a choice between waiting for it to be expelled naturally or having a D&C (dilation and curettage, where the cervix is dilated and an instrument called a curette is used to remove fetal tissue from the womb). A week later, nothing had happened so they went ahead with the D&C.

So many happy thoughts and optimistic plans are attached to the words "We're having a baby." Now all theirs were gone. Instead of anticipating their pregnancy with carefree hope they were worried that the same thing would happen again.

In fact, a study by a team of psychologists in Australia says that the grief experienced by couples after a miscarriage is severely underestimated by health professionals. The report, published in the *British Journal of Medical Psychology* reveals that women experience feelings of loss on a daily basis up to four months later. One of the main reasons for their unsettled state is the lack of closure. The "not knowing why" of losing a baby has a profound psychological effect on both partners with self blame adding to an already stressful and emotionally devastating time.

Many women reported feeling responsible for the miscarriage in some way, telling the researchers it might be due to them working too hard, drinking coffee, having some wine or enjoying themselves on vacation during the early months of pregnancy. Others looked back on their lives, blaming an earlier abortion or the use of contraceptives for their inability to carry a baby to full term.

I knew how much I had cried for my failed IVF attempts and those perfect embryos that had been destroyed by my own body. Although my pregnancies hadn't even reached the implantation stage I blamed myself, simply because there was nothing and nobody else to blame. Each time I wondered whether I had done something to kill our future baby. Was it because I had vacuumed the house when I should have been lying in bed, drank that glass of wine or got stressed over some unimportant work matter…?

After reading Dr Beer's Q&A replies, with his words resounding in my head, "A woman's body is overbuilt for reproductive success," I wondered just how many pregnancies failed in the early stages and why so many couples found it so difficult to become parents.

My immune problems had been identified relatively early in my IVF journey. If I had tried to become pregnant without suppressing my immune system and taking blood thinning injections, the chances are I would never have conceived, or would have suffered one miscarriage after another. Why was it that some women just didn't seem to have a baby friendly body?

Early pregnancy losses are so frequent that they are virtually considered the norm. In his 2003 book on miscarriage, Dr Henry Lerner describes them as, "Spontaneous, frequent and normal reproductive events." Indeed, the figures from the miscarriage societies of the U.K. and U.S. make depressing reading. Miscarriages occur in approximately 10 to 25% of all pregnancies. In around 75% of cases the cause is never established as the majority of women are not tested after miscarrying. After a single loss, there is usually no advice given other than to "try again."

As chromosomal defects are more likely to affect older women, the American College of Obstetrics and Gynecologists recommends testing after a second loss especially for those over the age of 35. However, most doctors will still write off a first or second miscarriage as "unexplained" and won't consider investigative action until at least three consecutive pregnancies have been lost.

This is not an approach Dr Beer agreed with. In fact, he believed that *any* lost pregnancy could be indicative of problems to come. He warned, "When a baby dies something is wrong, and it is my strong feeling that first losses should be tested. There is absolutely no need to wait for three consecutive losses before seeking help. Waiting for three has no science to underpin it in my database. It's like having to get pneumonia three times before asking for a doctor's attention. Any time there is a first biopsy of any part of the body it is examined immediately and seriously. Yet when a baby miscarries, it is not considered an issue. This is wrong."

The following advice taken from the website www.womenshealth.co.uk conveys the generally accepted view: "More than a quarter of all pregnancies end in miscarriage...The majority of these losses occur in the first trimester between weeks one and 13. Early after implantation (i.e., before a pregnancy is clinically recognized) the rate of pregnancy loss is about 30%. It is possible that as many as 50% of these are just due to bad luck...Most early miscarriages remain unexplained. About 1 in 36 women will have two miscarriages due to nothing more than chance."

Leaving aside the statistics themselves, let's just agree that they are high, there is a real problem here. The words "unexplained," "nothing more than chance" and "bad luck" are not consistent with the medical terminology that is used to describe the majority of health disorders. This lottery language makes losing a baby sound like an accidental catastrophe, an indiscriminate and random act like being struck by lightning or hit by a bus. Why when we are dealing with the loss of a life and the utter devastation this creates, is the use of such words acceptable in modern medical practice? Beyond this, why does there seem to be little interest in finding out what exactly could be causing so many pregnancies to fail?

One woman recalling the events surrounding her miscarriage commented, "I wish when we lost our first baby, we could have had quick and easy testing that told us what went wrong. Then we could have done something that would have prevented it from happening again. But that's not the way it works. Sometimes the only way to know there is a problem for sure is to lose another baby. I hate that and am troubled by the practice."

Even after conventional testing there is still a large knowledge gap when it comes to providing a diagnosis. It is clear that the medical profession, perhaps restricted by financial constraints and recommended procedures, is limited in providing real solutions for women in need of help.

For example, a guide entitled *"What Causes Miscarriage?"* supplied by the St. Mary's Hospital in London claimed, "Many cases of recurrent miscarriage will remain unexplained even after detailed investigations have been performed."

The American College of Obstetricians and Gynecologists says that the inundation of widely varying studies and guidelines has led some women and physicians to turn to "alternative therapies or unproven hypotheses." The Royal College of Obstetricians and Gynecologists, (now under the leadership of Professor Lesley Regan) which sets guidelines for public reproductive healthcare in the U.K. even went as far as to make the following statement: "...the use of empirical treatment in women with unexplained recurrent miscarriage is unnecessary and should be resisted."

Implantation failure and miscarriage caused by immune problems is largely preventable. This message must be conveyed to couples who are losing their babies or are unable to conceive. This is why, despite an inordinate amount of casework, a hectic travel schedule and the demands of setting up a new laboratory, Dr Beer made time to help with this book to provide explanations where there have previously been none.

"You have nothing to fear. If there is a problem, we will know. If there is not a problem, we will rejoice. The most important thing is to know that what is wrong with you is not your fault. It has a specific cause and understanding that cause fully brings with it the power to persist and move onward, even though the fear of failure will never leave you."

Alan E. Beer, M.D.

IS YOUR BODY BABY FRIENDLY?

1

Reproductive Immunology:
Helping to Explain the "Unexplained"

By Alan E. Beer, M.D.

Trying and failing to have a baby is a soul destroying experience. I have seen the damage it causes to the spirit, to relationships – and to hope itself. Women who have suffered the emotional torment of infertility, miscarriage or IVF failure often feel isolated and bitter. Eventually these women refuse to be optimistic, become emotionally hardened and believe that no one knows anything about their situation or can help them. They lose trust in their body, get pregnant and wonder every day if that pregnancy will fail like the rest. The only thing that can rid them of this feeling is to prove to themselves that their body is indeed made to have babies.

For years now, doctors have dealt with recurrent miscarriages saying, "It's God's will" and "The body knows when a baby needs to be rejected." Others simply believe that it is just bad lack when miscarriages occur. It is also bad luck when you get cancer, pneumonia or HIV, yet no thinking doctor would ever consider writing a thesis on "bad luck" as a serious diagnosis. When everything that the medical community sanctions as proper work up has failed, these doctors send their patients off to IVF thinking this may help – even though infertility is not their problem.

For those who cannot conceive, their IVF failures are once again mostly written off as bad luck. The couple will be encouraged to try another cycle, use donor eggs or embryos. Holding on to the belief that their luck will change at some point, some of these poor couples can end up spending their life savings or borrowing huge amounts only to go through more unsuccessful attempts.

When they have tried everything and failed, they become sad, dejected, mistrusting and don't believe that anyone can help them.

This is what I hate the most; it's like a kind of rust on a person's internal "hope machine" that just keeps on eating it away and eventually destroys the human spirit. Every day I meet emotionally bruised and burnt out women looking for proper explanations for their failures, and most of all, for help. This enormous, unfulfilled demand has strengthened my resolve to understand the immune processes within the body that prevent normal, outwardly healthy women from conceiving or carrying a child to term.

In the 1980s, it became clear to me that products of an activated immune system could damage the placenta and cause miscarriage, as well as damaging the embryo and causing implantation failure. Natural killer cells, which help to keep the body from developing cancer, can overpopulate the uterus or exist at too high levels within the bloodstream. These cells then go overboard, killing the embryo or interfering with the endocrine system that produces the hormones essential for pregnancy. This response can often be associated with complications for both the mother and her baby if the pregnancy continues without immunosuppressive treatment.

My research has also taught me, among many other things, that there are couples who are an unlucky genetic match, who produce embryos that are misinterpreted by the immune system as foreign objects, or even cancer cells. The problem eventually worsens, making the uterus behave like a den of lions, and every pregnancy attempt fails. This occurs even when beautiful embryos are produced in the test tube following IVF. Effectively, women become serial killers of their own babies.

If autoimmunity is damaging the baby, the same autoimmunity can damage the thyroid gland, the insulin producing cells of the pancreas and the serotonin producing cells which live all over the body. Yes, infertility can make you truly biologically crazy. I am not being cute or insincere. It is time we took the infertile woman and the woman losing pregnancies seriously, as these conditions can certainly be hazardous to the health of the individual.

So we are not just talking about a "quick fix" to the immune system to get pregnant, but making sure that the patient understands her condition for the sake of her own wellbeing long term. With specialized testing, it is possible to identify the underlying disorders that are preventing pregnancy from happening. Appropriate therapies to initiate the correct immunosuppressive response can then be provided.

Unfortunately, if you mention these ideas to your doctor you must still be prepared for them to laugh at you and not take you seriously. Yet these same doctors would take autoimmunity seriously if it affected your thyroid gland, insulin producing cells and joints. It's only infertility and recurrent losses that they consider have no biological causes outside of those that can be treated with fertility drugs. I can make statements like this because no one in the world has more experience in treating older women with three or more failures than I do.

I long for the day when couples will stop suffering the abuse of three or more implantation failures or recurrent losses before someone acknowledges there may be an immune problem that requires treatment. Pregnancy risk assessment is advocated in many areas of medicine. We must now add "immune risk assessment" to find the unfortunate people who end up spending a fortune in money, time and emotion, and get nothing in return. I strongly believe that we can identify these couples even before a first IVF failure. The reproductive system is incredibly overbuilt for success and when it fails, something is surely wrong.

My research has shown there are five categories of immune problem that can cause infertility, IVF failure and pregnancy loss. In over 25 years, I have treated over 7,000 patients – and more than 7,000 babies have been born within my program. Virtually nine out of ten of my patients have conceived within three natural cycles or IVF attempts. I have come across many inspirational stories in the course of my work and a small handful of these are featured in this book.

Half of the couples who contact me for immune evaluation do so independently, without referral from their doctor or fertility expert, sometimes traveling thousands of miles for treatment. In cases where immunological problems can be diagnosed, most do become pregnant, resulting in a child born partly out of their determination to find answers. These people are gradually clearing the path for others to follow and making the journey easier for those who have traveled a long way and may be running out of strength to keep on trying. I do not see myself as one who knows all the answers. However, I do hold my experience as almost sacred to me. For I have acquired it from patients like many of you who are reading this.

I know that even when all hope is gone, all tears are used and all discussions of your problem with spouse, family and friends have been tabled, there is a great chance that you too can complete your family. It would be immoral of me to say or write these words if I had not learned the truth from patients like many of you. Truly, I say again, the reproductive system is overbuilt for success and given the chance, most of you can prove this to yourselves.

2

Defining Reproductive Failure

The emptiness of a failed IVF cycle, months of trying and failing to conceive and the raw emotional and physical pain of losing a baby... Whatever path the reproductive failure takes, it always ends with the same question: "Why?"

The generally accepted reasons for reproductive failure are:

1. Chromosomal abnormalities
2. Abnormal uterine or cervical anatomy
3. Hormonal imbalances
4. Infection and illness
5. Environmental factors
6. Immune system problems

These definitions may appear to be quite separate and distinct, but virtually all of them can relate directly or indirectly to abnormal immune system activity. Indeed, Dr Beer anticipated that immune dysfunction would eventually prove to be a component in most commonly recognized causes of miscarriage as well as infertility and IVF failure. To understand how these links are possible, it is necessary to consider each of the categories in more detail.

Chromosomal and genetic abnormalities

Miscarriages due to chromosomal and/or other genetic anomalies often occur before ten weeks of gestation. Such problems are often caused by random errors that cells make during cell division. When the inherited instructions stored in the DNA are altered so they do not function properly, cellular mutations occur. This problem is mainly associated with advancing age, although it can also be influenced by mutagenic environmental agents that have the ability to damage genes and chromosomes.

Within the category of chromosomal anomalies, there are two basic kinds of defect: structural and numerical. During fertilization, two sets of 23 chromosomes combine to create the full quota of 46 chromosomes. In some instances, when the chromosome number within the sperm or egg halves from 46 to 23 (meiosis) an extra chromosome is accidentally retained (trisomy). The resulting embryo will then contain 47 chromosomes and will either abort in the first or second trimester, or produce a baby with congenital abnormalities. Trisomies are more often associated with "advanced maternal age" (i.e., women over 35 years old) and occur in approximately one in 660 births.

Such embryos can also be subjected to the effects of an aggressive immune response in the early stages of development, as Dr Beer observed. In his opinion, "If there is an immune problem we find that it is directed against the normal *and* genetically abnormal embryos. To say the pregnancy loss is due to the chromosomal problems does not entirely rule out an immune etiology (cause or origin of a disease).

I have studied paraffin blocks that contained tissue from the first pregnancy that was lost by couples who came to me after their fourth or fifth miscarriage. Blood tests revealed immune problems at that time and it was very surprising to find the same immune problems in the placenta of the first pregnancy that was lost. It did not matter if the baby was genetically normal or abnormal."

Studies have shown that approximately half of all embryos are chromosomally abnormal in women undergoing IVF and in non-recurrent spontaneous abortions around 66% are defective.

This means that 40 to 50% of miscarriages involve healthy, normal fetuses. If immune problems are causing their losses the majority of these women can be successfully treated.

Anatomical abnormalities

Cervical disorders are associated with approximately 15 to 20% of all pregnancy losses during the second trimester. If the cervix is weak it may start to widen and open too early. There are several reasons for this, including multiple D&C procedures or an extreme inflammatory immune response.

Cervical problems can also be associated with fetal exposure to diethylstilbestrol (DES). This drug was commonly used as a treatment to prevent miscarriage from the 1940s to the early 1970s. It was banned for use during pregnancy in the U.S. in 1971 after it was discovered that it promoted a rare form of vaginal cancer, and that approximately half of DES exposed female offspring had uterine abnormalities and a third of these were infertile.

Researchers have since observed certain alterations in the immune systems of DES exposed women. Dr Beer noticed that many of these alterations were the inherited autoimmunities that originally caused their mother's tendency to miscarry. He once said, "I have found that daughters of mothers who took DES often experience the same immune problems as their mother, which in those days, caused infertility and miscarriage and DES was the treatment. DES daughters with proper immune treatment do just as well in becoming mothers as non DES daughters."

Some women who miscarry repeatedly have an irregularly shaped uterus that may impair fetal growth. For example, a septate uterus, where the two sections of tissue that normally fuse together to form the uterus only fuse at the bottom, means that blood flow to certain areas is minimal and as the pregnancy progresses there is a lack of nutrition to the baby.

Other abnormalities include a bicornuate (double) uterus, a uni-cornuate uterus (an unusually small uterus) and a T-shaped uterus. However, in Dr Beer's opinion, "a T-shaped uterus is not a significant factor in causing miscarriages. It is the underlying inherited auto-immunities that are associated with such problems that need to be resolved."

Large uterine fibroids can affect implantation for a small number of women. Dr Beer only recommended removal when they occupied a large area and protruded into the uterine cavity, affecting blood flow.

Hormonal (endocrinal) imbalances

Progesterone prepares the lining of the uterus to receive a fertilized egg during the second half of the menstrual cycle. Low progesterone levels can signal that follicle-stimulating hormone (FSH) levels are too high indicating poor quality ovulation or inadequate corpus luteum development (the structure that develops from an ovarian follicle after the release of an egg). Insufficient amounts of progesterone may also mean the woman is producing antibodies to this vital hormone.

Pregnancy can also be stalled if there is a low level of thyroxin being produced from the thyroid gland. This can happen when antithyroid antibodies are being produced in the case of thyroid disease. In addition, the high levels of natural killer cells associated with this illness can play a direct role in implantation failure. However, this natural killer cell diagnosis is often missed in a standard hormone work up.

Infection and illness

Pathogens can also activate the immune system. Examples of these include the Epstein Barr virus, herpes virus type 6 and cytomegalovirus (CMV) another type of herpes virus. Dr Beer has found that adult-onset chicken pox and the Epstein Barr virus are among the worst offenders in causing immunologic infertility.

There are also proven links between some illnesses and recurrent miscarriage. For example, severe kidney disease (especially when coupled with high blood pressure), German measles, thyroid disease, uncontrolled diabetes and heart disease can all act to create conditions within the body that are not conducive to a healthy pregnancy.

Other triggers of potentially harmful immune activity include infections caused by bacteria such as mycoplasma and chlamydia and by fungi like candida. Toxoplasma gondii (an organism found in cat feces and raw meat) also activates the immune system and carries a risk for pregnancy as does food poisoning caused by the bacteria salmonella, E.coli and listeria. Pregnant women with chronic gum disease during the second trimester are also up to seven times more likely to give birth prematurely.

Chlamydia is the most common sexually transmitted disease in the United States and Europe. This infection of the uterus can damage the lining of the fallopian tubes which increases the risk of a tubal or ectopic pregnancy and spontaneous abortion. One in a hundred pregnancies is ectopic (when the fertilized egg implants outside the cavity of the womb, usually in one of the fallopian tubes).

Gonorrhea and syphilis are also known to be associated with first trimester pregnancy losses, while infections that directly involve the reproductive organs, such as an abscess in the ovary, can cause extensive tissue damage and in severe cases, may lead to irreversible infertility.

Environmental factors

Environmental factors have been associated with unusually large clusters of birth abnormalities. For example, limb deformities seen in babies born in the 1960s were related to the anti morning sickness drug Thalidomide.

In the U.K, the 50% increase in hypospadias (the malplacement of the urinary outlet of the penis) has been linked to "gender bending" reproductive toxins like petrochemical compounds and dioxins. Boys with hypospadias also have a curved penis, problems urinating and undescended testicles In the U.S. about 5 boys out of every 1,000 have hypospadias, making it one of the most common birth defects there is.

Some chemicals can also interfere with implantation and fertility. Criteria that determine how damaging toxins are include their ability to cross the placenta, timing and length of exposure, and if they can be stored in maternal body tissue. In animal studies, some toxic chemicals have even been shown to alter the structure of genes and chromosomes. Their disruption to the hormonal balance has also been linked to fetal distress, premature labor and genital defects. These issues, as well as personal lifestyle choices that can have an adverse effect on fertility and pregnancy outcomes are discussed in more detail in the Addendum.

Immune system problems

As well as providing defense against infection the immune system plays a key role in autoimmune disease, cancer, the aging process, pregnancy, infertility and miscarriage. An immune system problem may be suspected in cases of unexplained infertility or repeated implantation failure with IVF. Premature birth, intrauterine growth retardation, early rupture of the membranes, distress on delivery, or a history of miscarriages can all indicate a possible immune etiology (set of causes) that is harmful to pregnancy.

Dr Beer has identified several kinds of immune problem which often exist in combination. Essentially, women with immune problems in one category will most likely have problems in another. Beginning with the least serious, they are summarized as follows:

Blood clotting problems

The production of antibodies to phospholipids (the fatty molecules on the surface of a cell) has been identified as a cause of miscarriage. Anti-phospholipid antibodies (APAs) can make the blood clot more easily, thereby choking off the blood supply to the embryo. Hereditary blood disorders such as factor V Leiden and protein S and protein C deficiencies can also contribute to the tendency of the blood to clot too fast, a disorder known as "thrombophilia."

Autoimmune diseases such as endometriosis, systemic lupus erythematosus (SLE), rheumatoid arthritis or Crohn's disease coupled with IVF failure (especially multiple failures) can also trigger the production of APAs.

Because there are so many inherited or acquired conditions that can produce blood clotting disorders, thrombophilia is a very common factor in pregnancy loss.

An immune reaction to the baby

Women with this problem make antibodies to DNA components in the embryo or to the pregnancy tissue that surrounds it. These antibodies form first in the blood and later graduate to the lymphatic system and the tissue. After repeated losses, antibodies to DNA components can develop into antibodies that occupy organs such as the uterus and cause local inflammation that are likely to contribute to further miscarriages.

Both partners produce antibodies to sperm

Infertile women often produce their own brand of antibodies to antibody covered sperm produced by the male. As a result, the sperm become stuck in the cervical mucus and conception is not possible. Immune treatment, combined with IVF using intracytoplasmic sperm injection (ICSI) where an embryo is created by injecting the sperm directly into the egg, is needed to achieve pregnancy in these cases.

An abnormally aggressive immune response

Reproductive failure can result if certain types of immune cells increase in number and activity. These cells include:

Natural killer (NK) cells
NK cells reside in the blood and in the uterus (uNKs). Above a certain level, they can cause infertility and pregnancy loss. Sometimes the cytokines (cell signalling molecules that influence immune responses) they release create conditions in which the woman's eggs can become fragmented, resulting in poor quality embryos with cells that divide slowly or not at all.

Antibodies to hormones
NK cells can indirectly induce the production of harmful antibodies to the hormones that are required for a pregnancy to develop safely: estradiol, progesterone and human chorionic gonadotropin (HCG). Reduced levels of these hormones are associated with insufficient

uterine lining development, luteal phase defects, poor stimulation during IVF and slowly rising HCG levels when pregnant.

Antibodies to neurotransmitters
These antibodies also target "feel good" neurotransmitters (including serotonin, endorphin and enkephalin). Their activities can render the ovaries resistant to stimulation, inhibit lining development, interfere with the muscle development of the uterus and prevent blood flow to these areas at the time of implantation.

3

Recurring Nightmares

Recurrent IVF Failure

"About half of my patient population comprises healthy couples who make beautiful embryos in the test tube. But when these embryos are transferred to the uterus they just 'wither on the vine.' The average individual I see has been through IVF three times, has spent a lot of money, feels angry and let down by the medical community and is looking for answers.

Having studied immune mediated implantation failure over 25 years, I believe no one in the world has more data on this subject. The incidence of Category 1 and Category 5 immune problems [tissue type compatibility plus an abnormally high NK cell count/hyperactivity] is 60% for those who have failed their second IVF. For women failing their fifth IVF there is 100% incidence of excessive NK cell numbers and/or activity. Effective treatments are available to deal with this. I truly believe that in a perfect world, IVF successes should equal 50% parenthood per cycle. This is the figure I quote for women who have failed three cycles prior to seeing me."

Alan E. Beer, M.D.

Infertility is a distressing, defeating and draining experience. Month after month goes by and despite eliminating junk food, taking vitamins, meditating, going organic, doing yoga and "all the right things" nothing happens. Each partner silently blames the other and wonders if they are doing something to reduce their chances of being parents.

Studies have reported that many couples consider infertility to be at least as, or more stressful than divorce or the death of a loved one, with up to half of infertile women feeling depressed and anxious. Defined as the inability to conceive after a year (including those trying for a second child) infertility now affects 25% of couples in developing countries.

For those with normal fertility levels, the maximum conception rate is between 20 and 25% per month. After two years of failing to conceive approximately 5% of couples will have virtually no chance of becoming pregnant naturally and for many of these couples IVF may seem to be their only hope of success. However, the likelihood of a positive outcome depends on what kinds of tests and treatments they're given. When Dr Beer was working in association with fertility clinics offering immunological testing, the success rate for the next cycle was around 50 to 60%. Without this intervention the success rate was low. Only one in every five to ten embryos would develop into an ongoing pregnancy.

On average only half of all embryos are chromosomally normal. It is likely that of the 50% of good quality embryos, many are "wasted" on failed cycles caused by the same immune mechanisms that led to the problem of recurrent miscarriage.

Dr Beer noted that women who were diagnosed with "unexplained infertility" before their first IVF attempt had a high incidence of immune problems that resulted in implantation failure or miscarriage. After their third IVF failure, a high percentage of these women were found to have overactive natural killer cells. Even so, many fertility doctors still attribute these failed cycles to poor quality embryos or a lack of necessary hormones.

Some doctors may suggest preimplantation genetic diagnosis (PGD) to weed out chromosomally abnormal embryos. But it's statistically unlikely this is the cause of their recurrent failures.

Dr Beer says, "I have never seen one patient whose repeated implantation failures were solely due to chromosomal factors. Testing for genetic problems is another thing fertility clinics offer when they don't know what's wrong."

Repeated IVF failure takes its toll physically, emotionally and financially. Yet many couples still persevere despite feeling confused, powerless, victimized and angry about their lack of success.

If they don't conceive after five or more attempts, donor eggs, donor embyos, adoption or trying again are suggested. When donor eggs or donor sperm are used, pre-existing immune problems make it more likely that even this option will also result in failure. As Dr Beer explained, "Even with donor eggs, the resultant embryos will not succeed, just as they did not using their own eggs. I have learned this from studying women with untreated autoimmunities who had donor egg pregnancies. These eventually failed also."

Immune problems that cause infertility and implantation failure are even more severe than those associated with miscarriage. For couples like these, Dr Beer an NK cell assay (a type of blood test), cytokine testing and other blood tests (detailed in Chapter 13) would be required before the appropriate protocol is devised.

Whenever possible Dr Beer advised that couples tried to conceive with immunotherapy for two cycles before returning to their fertility center for IVF. Many of the men and women previously diagnosed as infertile discovered they didn't need IVF at all. In Dr Beer's experience, "Of my patients who had never been pregnant and failed three IVF cycles, 30% ended up getting pregnant on their own when treated immunologically."

Recurrent Miscarriage

"As much as 40% of unexplained infertility may be the result of immune problems, as are as many as 80% of 'unexplained' pregnancy losses. Unfortunately for couples with immunological problems, their chances of recurrent loss increase with each successive pregnancy."

Carolyn B. Coulam, M.D. and Nancy P. Hemenway,
"Immunology May Be Key to Pregnancy Loss"

The term "recurrent miscarriage" is used when a woman miscarries twice in a row before 20 weeks' gestation. In the past, authorities have recommended this term be used for three or more consecutive miscarriages. However, there is now a tendency to classify them as recurrent after just two, with approximately 1 in 25 couples fitting this category. Most obstetricians/gynecologists (Ob/Gyns) or reproductive endocrinologists (REs) tend to attribute these miscarriages to "bad luck" and will say that the baby was probably abnormal.

The American College of Obstetricians and Gynecologists claims in its May 2016 patient guide that "about 65% of women with unexplained recurrent pregnancy loss have a successful next pregnancy." In fact, it is now known that women who lose a chromosomally normal baby are at a *greater* risk of a recurrence. Moreover, the likelihood that the fetuses being lost are chromosomally normal increases with the number of miscarriages the woman experiences.

In an analysis of clinical trials, it has been found that the risk of miscarriage in a first pregnancy is 11 to 13%. In a pregnancy immediately following that loss, the risk of miscarriage is 13 to 17%. But the risk to a third pregnancy after two successive losses nearly triples to 38%. Professor David Clark at McMaster University in Ontario, Canada goes even further, saying that in a subset of recurrent miscarriage patients the risk is nearer 100%.

As far as genetic causes for recurrent losses are concerned the incidence of significant parental chromosome rearrangements may actually be quite small. For example, one study found that just 3.6% of 500 couples with recurrent miscarriage had such problems.

Dr Beer has also experienced a similarly low rate of occurrence in a similar patient population, declaring, "I have seen very few chromosomal abnormalities in women experiencing repeat implantation failure or pregnancy loss, certainly nowhere near the 50% level that is regularly quoted." According to his records, 75% of women who have had three or more previous losses have autoimmune problems that are associated with reproductive failure. As an additional concern, he has also observed that miscarriage is not just a benign process, it usually indicates an underlying health condition associated with autoimmune disease and may even aggravate or cause such problems.

When immune system dysfunction has been identified, the chance of carrying a baby to term without immunotherapy after three miscarriages is 30%, after four miscarriages 25% and after five miscarriages 5%. Furthermore, if the pregnancy does continue without proper therapy, the baby is automatically at greater risk of premature birth and/or other potentially fatal pregnancy complications.

Stillbirth

"It's easy to say that a defect in the umbilical cord might have starved the baby of oxygen. Of women I have studied with unexplained stillborn babies, 86% had immune problems that attacked the placenta, which I believe caused their fetal demise."

Alan E. Beer, M.D.

Even in the 21st century, stillbirth is an unacceptably common event. Classed as the loss of a baby after the 20th week of pregnancy, the incidence of stillbirth is estimated to affect 1% of pregnancies in the US. It is estimated that 14% of deaths occurring during labor and delivery and 86% before labor begins. A baby born via IVF is also around twice as likely to be stillborn and twice as likely to die within its first month of life when compared to one that is naturally conceived.

In over a third of all cases, the cause of fetal demise is never established despite genetic testing and an autopsy of the baby and the placenta. These shocking statistics are accompanied by the unimaginable suffering and anguish of the parents. The incident will usually remain painfully unresolved, along with the fear that it could happen again.

The obvious physical problems associated with stillbirth are clearly categorized but the reasons for these fatal complications are not generally understood. However, once again, immune dysfunction can play a key role in many of the following critical events:

Placental problems: Preeclampsia, or pregnancy induced hypertension, increases the risk of stillbirth and placental abruption (early separation of the placenta from the wall of the uterus) Symptoms include increasing blood pressure, kidney problems and blood proteins in the urine.

Worldwide this condition affects between 5 and 10% of all pregnancies and is associated with approximately 4,500,000 growth restricted babies (12% of whom die within the first month) and between 40,000 and 60,000 maternal deaths every year.

Birth defects: Chromosomal disorders are present in approximately 25% of stillbirths.

Growth restriction: Babies that fail to grow properly are at risk of dying from asphyxia before or during birth. In most cases, the causes of intrauterine growth restriction are classified as "unknown."

Infections: Between 10 and 25% of stillbirths are caused by an infection that may go unnoticed by the mother. Infections that occur between 24 and 27 weeks of gestation can cause infant death through direct fetal contact, placental damage or severe maternal illness. Bacteria and viruses associated with stillbirth include E.coli, rubella, Group B streptococci, CMV, syphilis and herpes.

Other causes: Stillbirth can result from umbilical cord problems, trauma, maternal diabetes, high blood pressure, Rh blood type incompatibility (where maternal antibodies cross the placenta and destroy fetal red blood cells) and gestation that exceeds 42 weeks.

Subclinical immune disorders that involve an untreated inflammatory immune response are rarely cited as a cause of stillbirth. Yet, as Dr Beer and others have discovered, this is probably the most significant factor in the majority of preterm or early infant deaths.

The Conventional Approach to Diagnosis

For those who repeatedly fail with IVF, often nothing is done to determine the cause. A few of the more progressive IVF clinics may suggest immune evaluation for the couple, but the usual suggested choices are donor eggs or embryos, surrogacy or adoption.

Most hospitals and specialist miscarriage clinics provide a basic set of tests and physical examinations for women who have experienced two or three miscarriages. Their medical history, past pregnancies and/or abortions, lifestyle (including diet, stress, smoking, alcohol, caffeine consumption and drug use) and work environment is taken into account. A complete physical check up, uterine ultrasound and pelvic examination is usually recommended.

During the pelvic examination, swabs are collected for cultures to detect the presence of chlamydia and other infections. A pap smear may also be carried out to ensure there is no evidence of uterine or cervical cancer.

Diagnostic procedures currently include the following:

Transvaginal ultrasound: This involves the use of a non invasive device, which enables the operator to view the ovaries, the ovarian follicles, the uterus and the fallopian tubes to see, for example, if scar tissue, polyps or fibroids could be impeding the chances of pregnancy.

Saline sonogram: Like the transvaginal ultrasound, the saline sonogram is used to evaluate the reproductive organs and identify growths or other abnormalities.

Endometrial biopsy: A sample of the tissue from the uterus is extracted and studied under a microscope. In conventional testing, hormonal problems affecting the uterine lining are diagnosed this way. This test is usually performed between day 21 and day 24 of the cycle. The biopsy takes a few seconds and involves minimal discomfort.

Hysterosalpingography (HSG): An X-ray of the uterus and fallopian tubes is taken after the organs have been injected with a small amount of dye. It is then possible to see if the tubes are open or damaged and whether the uterine cavity is normal. An HSG is scheduled between the 5th and 12th day, or between the time of bleeding and ovulation.

Hysteroscopy: A hysteroscope (a thin, telescopic device) is inserted through the vagina and cervix and into the uterus. Hysteroscopy provides a view of fibroids, scar tissue, polyps and anatomical defects inside the uterine cavity.

Laparoscopy: Here a laparoscope, another small telescopic probe with a light at the end, is used to view the ovaries, fallopian tubes, and outer wall of the uterus. The procedure allows the detection of adhesions (scar tissue), fibroids, endometriosis, and other structures that may cause tubal blockages. It can sometimes show if chlamydia is present, which can later be confirmed by a culture sample.

Blood and tissue tests: In addition, some or all of the following may be performed:

- Basic blood tests to detect problems with hormone levels
- Blood tests for bacterial or viral infections including sexually transmitted diseases
- Blood tests for thyroid function
- Blood tests to detect antisperm antibodies (and perhaps other related antibodies)
- Blood tests for blood clotting issues
- Chromosomal testing of both partners
- Chromosomal testing of tissue from the miscarriage

Despite these investigations, many cases of recurrent miscarriage will still remain unexplained. In fact, the largest category of diagnosis after chromosomal problems is that of "unknown."

Conventional Immune Testing

There is some confusion about the level of testing that constitutes a complete immune work up. Many women are convinced by their doctors that they have had complete immune evaluations, but in reality provide no more than superficial screening for immunological issues. With such preliminary testing, few, if any significant immune system problems will be identified. This can divert the couple away from comprehensive immunological testing and away from effective treatments.

If they are very lucky, couples suffering repeated IVF failures or miscarriages might be referred to a reproductive immunologist who will work with their fertility center, Ob/Gyn or RE to provide a comprehensive immune work up. This will involve a more extensive panel of blood tests and perhaps an endometrial biopsy. However, for most women, it is more likely that their doctor will assure them that a standard panel of blood tests and a basic ultrasound will suffice.

The American College of Obstetricians and Gynecologists (ACOG) and the Royal College of Obstetricians and Gynecologists (RCOG), who determine professional guidelines, currently suggest only a limited selection of tests for couples experiencing recurrent miscarriage:

- Blood karyotyping (genetic analysis) of both partners
- Cytogenetic (chromosomal analysis) of the products of conception
- Ultrasound/hysteroscopy to assess uterine anatomy
- A limited number of antiphospholipid syndrome tests "in the setting of three or more unexplained spontaneous abortions before the 10th week of gestation or after a single unexplained loss of a morphologically normal fetus at or beyond 10 weeks of gestation."

The RCOG also recommends:

- Screening for factor V Leiden (a blood clotting disorder)
- Screening for viruses and bacteria

A local hospital may carry out tissue analysis on the fetus to determine if there is an obvious immunological reason for the miscarriage but these tests cover very few of the markers for immune problems and do not include the Natural Killer Cell Assay (an "assay" is a quantative analysis) or testing for tissue type compatibility between partners, for example. The ACOG and the RCOG also advise against screening for diabetes, thyroid disease and antithyroid antibodies. The relatively narrow set of options that they do endorse means the results of hospital investigations are often inconclusive.

In most instances, it is up to the couple to seek the advice of a specialist reproductive immunologist who will work with their local healthcare provider to help them achieve a successful pregnancy based on the outcome of a comprehensive immunological assessment.

Perhaps the most significant of all the blood tests is one devised by Dr Beer himself: the Natural Killer Cell Assay. Any variation above normal levels can predict future pregnancy loss, whether the woman is preparing for an IVF cycle or trying to conceive naturally. This and several other important tests are explained in more detail in Chapter 13.

Comprehensive Immune Testing
Who Needs It?

It is important that immunological disorders are identified early, as there can be serious implications for the health of both the mother and baby if these disorders are left untreated during pregnancy.

Dr Beer discovered that patients who test positive for immune issues tend to fall into distinct groups and have experienced any number of the following:

General Health Problems:

Previous immune problems (e.g., rheumatoid arthritis, psoriasis Raynaud's syndrome or lupus)
A thyroid condition
Insulin resistance
A family history of stroke, heart problems or autoimmune disease
Chlamydia
A history of depression or severe postnatal depression
Fibromyalgia
Chronic fatigue syndrome
Food intolerances/allergies

Fertility and/or Reproductive Problems:

Unexplained infertility
Poor egg production from a stimulated IVF cycle (less than six eggs)
One blighted ovum
Three miscarriages or IVF failures before the age of 35
Two miscarriages or IVF failures after the age of 35
Miscarriage of a normal baby without a known cause
Endometriosis or any kind of pelvic inflammation
The birth of one or more children followed by miscarriage or infertility (referred to as secondary infertility)

Problems in a Previous Pregnancy:

Unexplained uterine bleeding in pregnancy (especially in the first trimester)
Cervical incompetence
Preterm labor
Premature rupture of the membranes
Preeclampsia
Retarded fetal growth

4

The Immune System

"The immune system is highly complex and some of its mechanisms are still the subject of intense debate. Although significant progress has been made there is still much to learn. I do not claim to know everything there is to know, but I do understand from studying immune responses and pregnancy for over 25 years that there is a strong link between overaggressive immune activity and poor reproductive outcome.

It is important that those who are experiencing such problems try to understand a little more about the way the immune system works and realize how and why it can impact upon a pregnancy."

Alan E. Beer, M.D.

Our Internal Armed Forces

All day long, the body is under attack from toxins and infections (pathogens). The immune system fights hard to kill off these invaders with its army of immune cells and an arsenal of chemical weaponry. Quite simply, without this defensive firepower we would die.

The first obstacle an invader must get past is a physical one: the skin. Oil, tears, saliva, perspiration and mucus all act as chemical weapons as a first line of defense against the enemy. Anything that ends up in the stomach is usually dissolved by hydrochloric acid. Despite all this, some pathogens do manage to invade the body. This is when the immune system activates its forces for immediate direct combat, or if the threat is more dangerous, starts the lengthy preparations for all out war.

Armies of white blood cells (also called leukocytes) handle routine operations. One set provides ground cover and frontline troops. Another set is kept in reserve for more challenging missions. Their main task is to distinguish between "self" and "non self" substances. Both sets of armies have their own unique strengths. Some have firepower and some do not. Some are programmed to kill while for others the prime objective is surveillance and intelligence.

The ground troops handle all threats the same way, delivering a non-specific or "innate" immune response. For serious assaults, the special task forces of the B and T cells are brought in. Their objective is to deliver a specific or "adaptive" immune response, based largely on the information that is reported back to them from the frontline fighting divisions.

Biological substances that are capable of activating innate and adaptive immune reactions are called antigens. Foreign antigens are proteins encoded with genes of a virus, bacterium or mutant gene (e.g., cancer). As the body's own cells also contain antigens, the immune system has to learn to identify which are dangerous and which are not. Cells that contain foreign antigens are considered a threat and are targeted for destruction. Unfortunately, this can sometimes include the antigens of embryonic cells.

Cells with a Stomach for War

When a foreign invader enters the body, the alarm is raised by the most versatile white blood cells of the frontline forces, the macrophages. One of their jobs is to act as sentinels, sending out intelligence to other divisions via chemicals known as cytokines. First to the scene are the neutrophils which make up around 70% of the white blood cells. Other macrophages eventually arrive about three or four hours later. These cells literally "eat" the enemy and any bits that are left over are put on display so the other immune cells can identify what they have killed.

These remnants are loaded onto molecules on their cell's surface called Major Histocompatibility Complex (MHC), otherwise known as tissue compatibility molecules. They are then compared with "good" antigens that make up a person's tissue type, called Human Leukocyte Antigens (HLAs). By displaying pieces of forensic evidence alongside the HLAs it can be determined if other immune cells need to be sent out to find the rest of the invaders and destroy them.

We all inherit the genes for HLA "self" molecules from our parents (i.e., half from the father and half from the mother). HLA-DQ molecules are found on lymphoid and other cells and are important when matching organs for transplantation and for determining whether or not a pregnancy will be accepted.

Lines of Communication – Cytokines

All the cells of the immune system produce chemical messengers that alert various fighting forces to the field of action. These chains of information are made from proteins called cytokines. When cytokines provide a messaging service between white blood cells, they are also known as interleukins (IL). Interferons (IFN) are another group of cytokines that literally "interfere" with viral growth to fight infection.

Some cytokines limit the growth of cells and inflammatory responses while others do the opposite and cause inflammation. These pro-inflammatory cytokines send the armies of the immune system out to destroy targets such as cancer cells and in some circumstances, those of the developing embryo.

Armed with Chemical Weapons and Explosives – The Natural Killer Cells

Among the immune system's most aggressive fighting divisions are the natural killer cells, otherwise called NK cells. NK cells circulate the body looking out for cancerous or virus infected cells, anything that fits the category of "altered self." They then inject them with an enzyme that makes the cell voluntarily implode, a process known as apoptosis. This ensures that any hazardous enzymes and chemicals stay inside the walls of the dying cell and are not released into the surrounding tissue.

NK cells are also major manufacturers of cytokines themselves, including a deadly variety called tumor necrosis factor alpha (TNF-alpha) which kills cancer cells. Unfortunately, unregulated TNF-alpha can have a disastrous effect on every stage of reproduction, from egg quality and implantation to fetal growth and survival. So although NK cells are mostly a force for the good in regulating cell growth and protecting the body from tumors, they can also play a major role in infertility, IVF failure and miscarriage.

The Special Task Forces of the Adaptive Immune System

The best armed forces in the world have military elites, which are better equipped and trained than the average soldier. Among immune cells, these special task forces are the lymphocytes of the adaptive immune system. They comprise two main divisions: B cells (produced in the Bone marrow) and T cells (produced in the Thymus gland next to the heart). These cells not only track and identify their targets; they also keep records of all infiltrators. In other words, they have an immunological memory (although this can start to fade with time, which is one reason why older people become more prone to disease).

B and T cells have receptor molecules that allow them to recognize and respond to their specific targets; pathogens such as viruses are at the top of their hit list. Some can be too aggressive for the innate immune system's frontline forces to deal with single handedly. This is when a specific, targeted immune response is needed.

The adaptive immune response involves complex strategic planning before the combined firepower of its immune cells is unleashed. This planning stage can take days or even weeks to complete, during which time the body will probably suffer from illness. The reason for the delay is that when it does happen, the attack will be hard hitting and decisive. If this onslaught is accidentally directed at the wrong target, for example, the body it is supposed to be defending, the results can be catastrophic. Such immune dysfunction can also be associated with infertility or pregnancy loss. This is why the NK cells, in addition to the B and T cells, are the subject of intensive research in the field of reproductive immunology.

Identifying Their Individual Ranks

All the B and T cells are coded according to the type of receptors they have on their surface and which antigens cluster onto them. These surface markers, known as clusters of differentiation (CD), define the cell's function. Their numbers start from CD1 and are now in the hundreds. A "minus" sign means the cell lacks the marker, while a "plus" sign means the cell contains the marker. This means there are many ways that a cell can be named. For example, a natural killer cell is called CD56+ because it has the 56 marker. The same cell can also be called CD56+/16- because it has a 56 marker but not the 16 marker.

T-Helper Cells (CD4)

When there is evidence of major threat to the body's health the T-helper cells will send out a barrage of chemical messages (lymphokines) to the B cells telling them to make antibodies. T-helper 1 cells (Th1 cells) can also activate additional fighting forces, including the macrophages, NK cells and other T cells. A second type of T-helper cell (Th2 cells) acts to restrain them. So in effect, Th1 are the aggressors and Th2 the pacifiers of the immune system. The balance between them affects how well the body accepts an organ transplant, overcomes disease and carries a pregnancy to term. Their influence is so great that the Th1/Th2 relationship is the focus of most medical efforts when treating major disorders of the immune system, including infertility, pregnancy complications and miscarriage.

Th1 – The Aggressors

In a Th1 immune response, cytokines are released which can lead to inflammation and antiviral responses. Cytokines such as IL-1, IL-2, TNF-alpha, TNF-beta and interferon-gamma prompt the T cells of command control to direct cell mediated responses. Th1 cells also encourage the B cells to produce antibodies, activate the macrophages, NK cells and other cytotoxic lymphocytes, and stimulate delayed type hypersensitivities.

When Th1 cells become overly aggressive, they can start going for the wrong targets, leading to the development of "tissue specific" health problems. Examples of Th1 driven conditions include multiple sclerosis, type 1 diabetes, rheumatoid arthritis, vitiligo, certain forms of alopecia, Crohn's disease, psoriasis and organ transplant rejection. Repetitive spontaneous abortions and implantation failures are also Th1 mediated events.

Th2 – The Pacifiers

The cytokines generated by Th2 cells help calm the actions of the T cells and allow the body to accept foreign cells. Th2 cells therefore play a vital role in successfully integrating tissue into the body, for example in the case of an organ transplant or a pregnancy. However, when they over suppress the Th1 cells, this can leave the body vulnerable to infection and tumors.

Th2 cells make interleukins (cytokines) IL-4, IL-5, IL-6, IL-10 and IL-13 that encourage antibody responses including the special "blocking antibodies" that help to ensure a successful pregnancy.

Tracking the Enemy with Antibodies

When a B cell is alerted to the presence of an antigen, it transforms, with the aid of a T-helper cell, into a rapidly multiplying clone of itself. Some B cells take the process a step further and produce antibodies. Despite their image as fighting force, antibodies don't actually kill anything.

Antibodies are small pieces of protein equipped with biologic "tracking" devices that can target one specific antigen. This enables other cells in the immune system to attack invading or foreign cells and leave normal, healthy tissue intact. It can take up to three days for the antibodies to be mobilized because equipping them is an energy draining and complex task, so they are only sent on missions through the bloodstream and other body fluids when the threat is serious.

Antibodies belong to a group of blood proteins called immunoglobulins. Each B cell has immunoglobulin (Ig) molecules on its surface. A huge number of different antibodies are needed because there are so many different types of antigens. Without reserves of preprepared antibodies, dangerous antigens can get a head start and inflict damage to the body. In situations like this, outside assistance can be provided by a course of antibiotics. This is effective in the short term but can create another problem when antigens start adapting to resist the effect of these drugs.

Unfortunately, as in all wars, mistakes can occur. Occasionally, antibodies attach themselves to the wrong targets, through poor communications or inadequate preparation. This can provoke a torrent of "friendly fire" against parts of the body the immune cells are supposed to be defending. The devastating consequence of all this misguided activity is autoimmune disease.

Autoimmune Disease

An autoimmune tendency or disease occurs when a defect in the body's immune system leads to the production of "auto" antibodies targeted against the body's own organs or tissues. This happens when rogue T cells start objecting to the presence of normal cells, or their components. Certain human genetic profiles, viral infection, hormones and environmental toxins are some of the factors that can cause this sudden shift of behavior.

Accompanying this antibody onslaught is an overproduction of pro-inflammatory cytokines that prompts the NK cells, macrophages, neutrophils and T cells to go in for the kill. Most common targets include the connective tissues such as cartilage, bone and tendons as well as nerves, red blood cells, blood vessels, the thyroid or pancreas, muscles, joints and skin.

Rheumatoid arthritis is the result of an attack by the NK cells during which TNF-alpha is released into the linings of the joints. In insulin dependent diabetes, the insulin producing islet cells of the pancreas are targeted. In Myasthenia Gravis, the connections between nerves and muscles are affected. Indeed, as the understanding of the immune system grows, it is becoming clear that some variety of autoimmune disease exists for almost every function of the body.

One of the factors that make some people more likely to develop autoimmunity is genetic and relates to their HLA tissue types. For example, a mutation in the gene that controls the release of cytokines can mean that too many inflammatory molecules are produced. Genes can also determine how the T cells distinguish between "self" and "non self" cells. What is inherited is not one specific gene that causes a defect in the immune response, but several genes that increase a person's susceptibility to autoimmunity. This is one reason why family members can have a high incidence of the same antibodies but different autoimmune conditions. For example, the grandmother may have rheumatoid arthritis, her daughter may have diabetes and her grand-daughter may have thyroid disease.

As only 30 to 50% of identical twins develop the same autoimmune disease, other factors are involved, notably environmental, hormonal or viral elements. For instance, there are viruses that look very similar to the coverings around the nerves and parts of the brain, called the myelin sheath. When the immune system attacks this virus, it can cause multiple sclerosis. Another strain of streptococcal bacteria is known to trigger an attack on the valves of the heart leading to rheumatic fever.

Autoimmune diseases often occur during a woman's childbearing years. They are also more prevalent in women than in men because of differences between their immune systems. Women tend to produce more autoantibodies than men, which could be why organs donated by women are more likely to be rejected and why women who receive transplants are less likely to survive. Paradoxically, some Th1-driven autoimmune diseases such as Crohn's and rheumatoid arthritis can improve during pregnancy but will flare up again after delivery. Others actually worsen during pregnancy, which also indicates that hormones play an important role in moderating the immune response.

Despite its high incidence - one in 12 women and one in 20 men in the U.S. will develop some sort of autoimmune disease in their lifetime - autoimmunity remains a relatively neglected area of medical research. Many autoimmune diseases only become clinically evident after considerable tissue damage has occurred, making it difficult to establish a developmental pattern for the condition or identify how it began. Consequently, autoimmunity is still one of the least understood categories of illness today. For some women the only indication they have autoantibodies may be seemingly unrelated factors, such as the inability to conceive and aching joints or recurrent miscarriage and thyroid problems. Many women with subclinical autoimmunity have only their infertility as evidence that something might be wrong.

There is currently no cure for autoimmunity and most drugs are aimed at reducing its symptoms. However, some effective treatment approaches are possible. Hormones can be replaced, for example, when the thyroid gland has been damaged. Immuno-suppressive drugs and therapies can also moderate the immune system's aggressive tendencies long enough for the body to heal and for pregnancy to be achieved.

The Baby Resistant Body:
How the Immune System Can
Sabotage Fertility

"The immune system is balanced between a Th1 (autoimmune) and Th2 (pregnancy or suppressive) response. Most people have a balanced system. Women with implantation failure or recurrent pregnancy losses are unbalanced. They are too Th1 activated with the autoimmune 'bad guys' that produce TNF-alpha, interferon-gamma and interleukin-2.

Immune system abnormalities that compromise fertility or threaten the life of the fetus are relatively easy to identify and treat. In my opinion, there is no reason why women with such problems should not receive proper evaluation and therapy to achieve a more baby friendly balance."

Alan E. Beer, M.D.

In a normal pregnancy, a woman's body accommodates what is essentially a foreign body that should be destroyed by her immune system. In fact, when the embryo first implants, the surrounding tissue looks inflamed, as if it was dealing with an infection. However, immunological adaptations usually take place to protect the baby from attack.

During the "window of implantation" (when the uterus is most receptive to accepting the embryo), pregnancy specific proteins are released into the mother's blood. A series of changes then takes place in the uterus that enables the embryo to survive and promotes the development of the placenta.

Estrogen and progesterone are released by the ovaries. Estrogen is needed first, followed by progesterone and then a combination of both. Progesterone is required throughout pregnancy to maintain a baby-friendly uterine environment. It also induces a "pre-receptive state" that is responsive to the estrogen. If the woman produces antibodies to these hormones, the pregnancy is likely to fail without appropriate treatment.

Although T and B cells are excluded from the implantation site, macrophages and NK cells are welcomed to a degree. They are instructed by hormones from the uterus to release cytokines that promote implantation and fetal development. Interleukin-1, produced by the macrophages, helps to soften the uterine tissue and create a local inflammatory response that brings in blood vessels to the placenta. Nitric oxide from the NK cells and a neurotransmitter called serotonin relax the uterine arteries. All of these actions are essential for the creation of good blood supplies to the developing baby.

In women who constantly miscarry or cannot conceive the immune system does not modify in this way. Instead, it wages war against the embryo as it attempts to implant, or gradually cuts off its life support systems later on during pregnancy. When TNF-alpha cytokine ratios are too high, they can stop the placental cells from dividing. Cytokines such as TNF-alpha and interferon-gamma are also capable of activating the blood clotting system. This can cause the shutdown of the small blood vessels that supply the critical nutrients and oxygen needed by an implanting embryo.

Dr Beer treated thousands of women whose levels of circulating NK cells and/or TNF-alpha cytokines were extremely high, who had unexplained infertility, failed many times with IVF or kept losing their babies. Abnormal, inflammatory immune activity is also responsible for other adverse pregnancy complications.

For example, in preeclampsia a strong maternal inflammatory response against the pregnancy tissue causes inflammation, which damages the placenta and the mother's blood vessels. The subsequent lack of blood flow through the placenta (which can be reduced to between 30 and 50% of normal levels) can lead to restricted fetal growth or premature delivery. With such limited blood and oxygen supply, the process of labor can prove too arduous for some babies and can even result in stillbirth.

Women who have suffered such traumas may show no signs of obvious autoimmunity or they may be in the first stages of developing autoimmune disease. To find out if an over aggressive immune tendency is affecting the chances of a healthy pregnancy, Dr Beer devised a series of tests called the "Reproductive Immunophenotype" which determines the quantities of eight of the most important white blood cell types including NK cells. This is just a small part of a general panel of blood tests or "assays" that are used to diagnose and treat the immune problems that can prevent a pregnancy from continuing.

There is still much debate about whether there is a direct link between subclinical autoimmune dysfunction and reproductive failure, yet there is convincing evidence that such a relationship exists (which is presented in Chapter 15). For many couples though, their often heart-rending experiences will still be labeled "idiopathic" another word for "unexplained."

According to Dr Beer, there are several identifiable categories of immune problem associated with infertility, IVF failure and loss. These categories do not exist in isolation but interconnect in a way that perpetuates the vicious circle of autoimmunity and loss. For example, without treatment a woman with a blood clotting disorder may suffer miscarriages that trigger other adverse immune reactions. This cascade of responses can also generate other autoantibodies, which may further reduce the chances of a successful pregnancy.

As it will become clear in the following pages, these categories do not just predict the likelihood of reproductive failure, they also predict the onset of disease.

IS YOUR BODY BABY FRIENDLY?

5

Being Too Genetically Similar

"While kidney, bone marrow and heart transplants survive best when the donor is similar to the recipient, the opposite occurs in pregnancy. When husband and wife share tissue proteins that are too similar, the pregnant mother will not produce 'blocking antibodies' that protect the fetus from being attacked by her immune system."

Alan E. Beer, M.D.

The saying "opposites attract" has particular relevance in the case of human reproduction, as couples with completely different DNA types are at a distinct advantage. It is thought that the preference for couples who are genetically incompatible to mate successfully developed over the generations to prevent inbreeding and improve resistance to disease. Unfortunately, for some couples, their genetic similarity makes it very difficult to achieve a successful pregnancy.

Studies have also shown that there is a significant increase in genetic compatibility between couples with unexplained infertility and recurrent miscarriage. To explain how these problems arise, we have to look at the immunological relationships between cells from the father, the mother and the embryo during the earliest stages of pregnancy.

A baby develops from a single cell that is created when an egg is fertilized by a single sperm. It then undergoes a process called cleavage until up to 150 cells have been formed and the egg's original outer membrane, called the zona pellucida, starts to break down. At this point, the embryo is referred to as a blastocyst. The outermost cells of the blastocyst develop into the trophoblast. Trophoblast cells attach the embryo to the wall of the uterus by dividing into two layers, the chorion and the placenta. Trophoblast cells therefore maintain placental contact with maternal tissue through which nutrient exchange occurs. When the genetically dissimilar tissue and cells of the embryo come into contact with maternal tissue and cells, the site is known as "the feto-maternal interface." It is here that maternal immune recognition of the trophoblast must occur so that a protective immune response is initiated. Lack of recognition can lead to "unexplained" IVF failure and miscarriage.

Most cells of the body have proteins on their surfaces called human leukocyte antigens (HLA) which are the essential distinguishing characteristics of cell and tissue types. These antigens also act like antennae, distinguishing between "self" and "non self" cells in order to identify foreign invaders like germs, viruses or cancer cells. When a woman becomes pregnant, her body must tolerate an embryo that expresses an unfamiliar HLA protein molecule from the father as well as her own "self" molecule.

The placenta contains paternal proteins, and paternal genes play a part in governing its invasion and growth, yet somehow it must escape the mother's anti tumor immune defense mechanisms. (In fact, there are many similarities between the behaviors of invasive placental cells and invasive cancer cells.)

The embryonic trophoblast is able to avoid destruction in the following ways. First, the classical HLA molecules (the ones that are matched for transplant purposes) are not expressed on the pregnancy trophoblast at all, so the risk of rejection is reduced. Second, to help keep the pregnancy safe, "non-classical" HLA-G molecules are expressed which work to help turn off the aggressive immune response, shifting the mother's Th1:Th2 balance towards Th2 dominance.

For example, HLA-G molecules are able to make activated CD8 cells self destruct, switch natural killer cell receptors from "on" to "off," stimulate the macrophages to produce Th2 protective cytokines and encourage the production of T regulatory cells (which regulate the other T cells so they don't behave in an inflammatory manner). All of these actions contribute towards the creation of a baby friendly immune response. Without HLA-G in an excessive Th1 cytokine environment, the placenta may not develop and there is less chance the embryo will implant.

A protective immune response from the mother is also more likely when there is a distinct genetic difference between her own cells and those of the developing embryo. This difference helps avoid the problem of lack of recognition of the pregnancy by the mother's immune system.

A DQ alpha antigen is coded by a specific area of DNA. If the mother and baby share a genetic DQ alpha match, the mother's immune system can be aggravated in such a way that it does not recognize the HLA-G as being a pregnancy, but instead treats the invasion of foreign cells as some form of "altered self" or cancer.

In this situation, the mother's pregnancy tolerance signal system will become muted, T regulatory cell activity will be diminished, NK cells will not be switched off and a non baby friendly cytotoxic Th1 immune response will predominate.

Dr Beer described the process saying, "Certain couples are matched for DNA and during pregnancy the embryo is mistaken for a cancer cell and natural killer cell activity increases the more a couple tries."

Moreover, in the case of recurrent miscarriage, there is a 10 to 15% chance that the mother will also develop new antibodies to the fatty molecules on the cells of the baby that miscarried. These antibodies are targeted against phospholipids and in many cases the woman's reproductive problems will escalate to include other categories of immune problem.

Couples at risk of producing a baby with poor HLA-G response in pregnancy can be identified with the Lymphocyte Antibody Detection assay (LAD or "Crossmatch") test. This test determines whether or not a woman is producing enough blocking antibodies to her partner's lymphocytes. If her blocking antibody levels are low then the couple is at higher risk of producing a pregnancy that induces an inadequate HLA-G signaling response.

If the results of the LAD test are poor, preconception immunization with white blood cells from the male partner, known as Lymphocyte Immunization Therapy (LIT), is often recommended.

LIT can encourage a proper blocking antibody and suppressive response to the baby's HLA-G signal the next time the woman is pregnant. This is known as "alloimmunity" as it involves an immune reaction to "non self" cells.

For certain recurrent miscarriage patient groups with chromosomally normal embryos, the use of LIT alone has been shown to increase the livebirth rate to between 75% and nearly 100%. For those with more severe immune problems, preliminary data indicate that a combination of both LIT and intravenous immunoglobulin G (IVIG) therapy is effective.

6

Blood Clotting Disorders

"In a normal pregnancy the mother's ability to produce blood clots in the uterus and placenta is suppressed and the blood flows freely to the baby. Some mothers have a condition called thrombophilia where this clotting of the blood is not suppressed. This can cause many things to go wrong, including implantation failure, miscarriage, preeclampsia and even unexplained fetal death. Doctors are prone to counsel patients saying 'it will be better next time' or 'these complications occur for no good reason.' This is simply bad advice and poor judgment. Once diagnosed, this disorder can be treated and healthy, normally grown babies can be born."

Alan E. Beer, M.D.

Mention the word thrombophilia and most people think of deep vein thrombosis, where a blood clot that forms in the leg travels to other parts of the body. Thrombophilia ("thrombus" means clot and "philia" means a liking for) in the context of this category of reproductive immune problem is associated with blood clotting, not in the veins of the body, but in the smallest arteries and blood vessels, essentially the very lifelines that support the developing fetus.

Pregnancy is a time when the blood is hypercoagulable or prothrombotic, meaning it has a tendency to clot. This is thought to be due to an evolutionary trait to stop women from dying in childbirth. Unfortunately, a proportion of women with recurrent miscarriages are in a prothrombotic state even when they are not pregnant. Alternatively, they may carry genes that make it even more likely for blood clots to happen.

Blood flow, or principally the lack of it, is one of the most important issues associated with chronic disease and is a prime consideration when addressing the problems of implantation failure, early pregnancy loss and recurrent miscarriage. Indeed, thrombophilia is found in approximately two thirds of women with unexplained pregnancy loss.

Many women have absolutely no idea they have a blood clotting disorder and that it may be a major factor in their inability to conceive or successfully gestate a baby. Thrombophilia, both inherited and acquired, is very common and is associated with the following conditions:

- Preeclampsia
- Intrauterine fetal death
- Poor fetal growth
- Low amniotic fluid level
- Subchorionic hemorrhages or hematomas
- Placental abruption
- Toxemia of pregnancy
- HELLP syndrome (**H**emolysis, **E**levated **L**iver enzymes, and **L**ow **P**latelets, a severe form of preeclampsia)
- Premature labor (often called incompetent cervix syndrome)
- Miscarriage
- Pregnancy induced hypertension (high blood pressure of pregnancy)
- Preterm birth
- Stillbirth

Risks to the mother may include:

- Stroke
- Thrombophlebitis (blood clots in the veins or the arteries that can occur during pregnancy)
- Deep vein thrombosis
- Autoimmune thrombocytopenia (low platelet count)
- Anemia (low red blood cell count)
- A blood clot in the lung (pulmonary embolism)
- A blood clot in the brain
- TIAs (transient ischemic attacks or "mini strokes")

Phospholipids:
Building the Baby's Life Support System

Every human, animal and plant cell is surrounded by a cell membrane which houses the biological components that are needed for the cell's survival. Cell membranes are made up of a double layer of phospholipid molecules. The outward facing layers contain phosphate and the two fatty inner layers between them contain lipids. (Imagine two pieces of buttered bread, with both buttered layers joined together in the middle.) This enables the cell to both take in and repel water. Because of this unique semi permeable molecular structure, cell membranes play an essential role in embryonic growth and survival.

Of the six types of phospholipid molecules, cardiolipin, serine, ethanolamine, phosphatidic acid, inositol and glycerol, the most important at the time of fertilization and implantation are serine and ethanolamine. These molecules have adhesive properties that allow cells to fuse together and help the embryo to attach firmly and grow deeply into the lining of the uterus. The phospholipid ethanolamine also acts like "glue" on the sperm, enabling it to attach firmly to the egg in the process of fertilization. Any kind of immune response that prevents these phospholipids from binding to these sites of activity can severely impede a woman's chances of conceiving or carrying a baby to term.

For example, anti-ethanolamine antibodies effectively "de-glue" the sperm so although they get to the egg they do not stick. One way to bypass this is to put the sperm directly into the uterus via intrauterine insemination, so the sperm can reach the fallopian tube before they are deactivated.

Antibodies directed towards phospholipids also have the effect of making the blood clot too fast. When these cell membrane molecules are targeted, the chances of a successful pregnancy stands at less than 10%. Anticoagulant medication can increase the livebirth rate to approximately 70%. As it is often the case that these antibodies are a symptom of a broader immune etiology, this success rate can be increased with the addition of other therapies.

The Antibodies That Can Switch the Baby's Life Support System Off

"I think any woman with a history of infertility or recurrent pregnancy losses, or a family history of stroke, heart problems or autoimmune disease should be tested for antiphospholipid antibodies. Many women experiencing infertility or miscarriages have antibodies to the phospholipids serine and ethanolamine and as a result, they have immunities that prevent implantation or cause miscarriages. Not all doctors agree with this opinion, but I know it to be true. I get every one else's failures."

Alan E. Beer, M.D.

Antibodies to phospholipid molecules prevent the structural transformations vital for implantation from taking place. They can also trigger an immune reaction that damages the inside of the blood vessel walls. This encourages blood cells to stick to the site of the injury and form blood clots or "micro thrombi" in the tiny blood vessels of the placenta, making it unable to attach itself firmly to the uterus. Thus, the baby will be starved of nutrients and in effect 'wither on the vine.'

The production of antibodies to phospholipids can be activated when there is damage to the endothelial cells that line the blood and lymph vessels. In Dr Beer's opinion, "Any kind of tissue trauma, caused by bacteria, toxins or heat for example, can invoke cell death or cell injury which can lead to the production of antibodies to phospholipids. I have also been able to show that a serious infection can elevate or induce antiphospholipid antibodies. These antibodies disrupt cell functions, thereby increasing the clotting speed of the blood and causing pregnancies to fail early. Once antiphospholipid antibodies develop, in my opinion they are likely to stay with you the rest of your life. The only thing that can erase or reduce them is a successful pregnancy."

When cell damage occurs, phospholipids that are normally sited on the inner layer of the cell's membrane flip to the outside. Proteins then bind to these phospholipids. These proteins are the antigens that trigger the immune response. Autoantibodies are then directed against these proteins (mainly a protein named beta-2-glycoprotein-I). This stops the phospholipids from being able to bind to their usual sites of activity.

Once there is inflammation, scarring, narrowing or any other irregularities in the blood vessels, blood has a tendency to clot too fast. As its viscosity increases, blood flow is reduced throughout the body, elevating the risk of thrombi forming in the vessels. These are the characteristics of an autoimmune condition known as "acquired thrombophilia," in other words, we are not born with it.

What appear to be minor blood vessel problems can then sow the seeds for more serious complications such as strokes and heart attacks as well as recurrent spontaneous abortions, catastrophic events that are associated with the "Antiphospholipid Syndrome." Approximately 70% of people diagnosed with antiphospholipid syndrome are female.

A positive test result for one or more kinds of antiphospholipid antibody (APA) indicates there is an immune response that can contribute to miscarriage. Up to 30% of women who repeatedly miscarry or are infertile, test positive for antiphospholipid antibodies. The percentage is even higher for women who have failed three or more IVF cycles.

Furthermore, it is estimated that with every IVF failure or miscarriage, there is a 10% chance that the woman will develop an antibody to a phospholipid molecule. In other words, each pregnancy failure can increase the chances of another one happening. This vicious circle of immune response illustrates that APAs are not only the cause of pregnancy loss, but can become a consequence of it.

The problems associated with these antibodies usually strike very early, or during the first trimester of pregnancy. Implantation failure in IVF can occur when the first pregnancy tissue to be formed, the trophoblast, is destroyed by APAs, which are also thought to interfere with cell division of the embryo. Should the pregnancy progress beyond this stage, these antibodies will make its survival extremely difficult. A typical example of their effect in miscarriage is a fetal heartbeat that is seen at six to seven weeks but then stops between eight and ten weeks.

The majority of losses of chromosomally normal fetuses among women with high levels of APAs occur within the first 12 weeks. In 10 to 15% of pregnancies in women with blood clotting tendencies, fetal death occurs after 20 weeks of gestation. The baby is often lost when the placenta separates from the uterine wall too early, a process known as placental abruption. Damage to the placenta can also stop the fetus from thriving, so the baby is either small at birth or stillborn. All these problems can arise from a lack of free flowing blood and subsequent clotting in the microscopic vessels (called "villi") of the placenta. Yet this is one of the most easily treatable causes of miscarriage.

Awareness of the condition is growing as more women in the public eye undergo IVF or have trouble with their pregnancies. For example, the TV actress Courteney Cox disclosed in an interview that antiphospholipid antibodies had prevented her from carrying a baby to term. For years, she had struggled to maintain her pregnancies and suffered several miscarriages. After receiving the appropriate treatment, her third IVF cycle progressed successfully and she gave birth to a daughter at the age of 39.

It is important to emphasize that the presence of APAs can also be an indicator of other immune conditions. A large review was carried out by the American Society for Reproductive Immunology (ASRI) to define a condition known as the "Reproductive Autoimmune Failure Syndrome" where APAs are just one among several markers that point to an activated immune system.

Significantly elevated levels of natural killer cells have been found in women with antibodies to phospholipids. For example, around 15% of people with systemic lupus erythematosus have antiphospholipid syndrome.

This immune imbalance can only be detected through a comprehensive panel of tests and will require additional treatment. Yet many doctors still conclude that when APAs are present they are the sole reason for the pregnancy loss and will only prescribe anticoagulants. However, the woman could still lose her baby because her abnormally heightened immune response was not addressed.

More on the Sticky Subject of
The Antiphospholipid Syndrome

The Antiphospholipid Syndrome (APS) a.k.a Hughes Syndrome, was first described in 1983 by Dr Graham Hughes who observed the link between this immune mediated blood clotting disorder and autoimmune disease, fetal loss and other thrombotic events.

APS is defined by the presence of antiphospholipid antibodies (namely lupus anticoagulant or anticardiolipin antibodies) in addition to thrombosis or a history of miscarriage. It is seen mainly in women under the age of 50 who experience their first thrombotic event in their 20s or 30s.

This syndrome is associated with approximately 20% of all cases of DVT and up to 40% of strokes in young people. It can also lead to brain hemorrhages, renal vein and artery thrombosis and pulmonary hypertension. Its other common manifestations include poor circulation, migraines, eye diseases and transient memory loss ("brain fog").

The incidence of APS in the general population could be as high as one or two in a hundred, making it one of the important "new" diseases of the late twentieth century. It is therefore highly recommended that any woman who is having difficulties conceiving or who is suffering recurrent pregnancy loss should look at her family's history to see if a common thread of autoimmunity or thrombophilia emerges.

In a study of those who tested positive for APAs, many relatives were found to have other autoimmune diseases such as rheumatoid arthritis, lupus, Sjögren's syndrome, alopecia, Crohn's disease, multiple sclerosis, low platelets (ITP), thyroid disease, type 1 diabetes and scleroderma. In other words, antiphospholipid antibodies can be associated with one disease process in one family member and a different illness in another. A third of family members with elevated levels of APAs were related to someone with the same problem. A further third tested positive for antinuclear antibodies and several of these relatives were diagnosed with rheumatic autoimmune conditions. Many women with endometriosis will also test positive for antiphospholipid antibodies.

Virginia Ladd, President of the American Autoimmune Related Diseases Association (AARDA) has speculated on this link, saying, "It may be premature to say, but APAs may end up being one of the common threads that ties together all of the seemingly unrelated 80 known autoimmune diseases."

To add to their incidence rate, the development of APAs has been associated with viral infections such as measles, chicken pox, syphilis, hepatitis C and HIV, and they are known appear temporarily when certain medications are used (e.g. hydralazine and phenytoin). Exposure to heavy metals, chemicals, allergens, physical trauma and vaccinations can also play a role in immune mediated coagulation.

Other factors that may aggravate the condition include severe burns, gum disease, smoking, pregnancy, hypertension, obesity, dehydration, immobility (e.g., air travel or bed rest), or an inherited genetic defect that impairs the ability of the blood to clot. The more risk factors an individual is exposed to, the more susceptible they are to experiencing the potentially life threatening effects of this syndrome.

Pregnancy itself is a considerable risk factor. Indeed, women in their 20s and 30s are four to five times more likely to develop deep vein thrombosis or pulmonary embolism (where a blood clot reaches the lung) if they are pregnant, undergoing IVF, or taking contraceptive pills, as all these situations can raise levels of estrogen in the body. Too much estrogen can disrupt the function of the endothelial cells. When the blood clots more easily, the blood vessels can become constricted and cause high blood pressure.

Women with blood coagulation disorders are therefore more prone to developing a potentially fatal form of preeclampsia known as HELLP syndrome. Here, the blood pressure is so high it makes the kidneys swell and leak, releasing protein into the urine.

During pregnancy the uterus expands and pelvic blood circulation slows down, which can also increase the chance of developing deep vein thrombosis or pulmonary embolism. However, the risk is many times greater for women with clotting disorders such as APS. Pulmonary embolism is now the leading cause of maternal death in the United States. In fact, recent studies have revealed that more than half of pregnant women who develop a pulmonary embolus (or similar disorder) have preexisting blood clotting problems that in the majority of cases had remained undiagnosed.

Premature strokes, heart attacks and recurrent miscarriages can be avoided with simple tests and the appropriate treatment. It is so important to realize that infertility and repeated miscarriages are not just about the inability to produce a baby. The immune system dysfuntions that cause these events are ultimately extremely damaging to the woman's health and will limit her lifespan if they remain untreated.

Inherited Thrombophilia

"Women who carry the genes for inherited thrombophilia are between 8 and 40 times at greater risk of having a stroke, heart attack, blood clot or pregnancy loss than women without the genes. It is a gift to know that you have these mutations because then they can be treated and you do not have to suffer these dangerous complications."

Alan E. Beer, M.D.

In Europe over the centuries, men who were wounded in battle would bleed to death unless their blood clotted quickly. Blood loss through childbirth, diet and disease resulted in the genetic dominance of those with coagulation defects as they were equipped to survive. Because we now live at least twice as long as our distant ancestors and have better medical care, this rapid blood clotting ability is no longer the evolutionnary advantage it once was, actually, it's quite the opposite.

The blood clotting process involves a complex cascade of about 30 interacting proteins and platelets. The cascade starts when a protein called "tissue factor" is exposed to the bloodstream and is activated via a cut or other injury. Tissue factor generates thrombin, a blood clotting enzyme. Thrombin causes platelets to clump together and reacts with fibrin, to produce the clot. It also encourages coagulation by activating various blood clotting proteins. Two of these are factor V and factor VIII. Certain gene defects can adversely influence the speed of the coagulation cascade: too slow and the outcome is hemophilia, too fast and the result is thrombophilia.

As many as 1 in 20 people have inherited a predisposition to developing blood clots or thrombophilia. Add to this the risk factors associated with APS and you can see why these conditions affect about 15% of people in the United States and kill more Americans than breast cancer, AIDS and car accidents combined. Indeed, thrombosis is one of the most common causes of death worldwide.

Inherited thrombophilia is a major cause of fetal loss and complications at all stages of pregnancy and particularly affects those who carry genes for more than one condition. Yet the majority of people is unaware of these health issues. Indeed, even as recently as the 1990s, doctors graduating from medical school had no knowledge of inherited blood clotting disorders.

Today, laboratory testing has made it possible to identify a genetic cause in up to half of patients with venous thromboembolism, the most common of these causes are described here.

Factor V Leiden

"The Leiden factor V gene mutation in pregnant untreated women is associated with a high rate of complications, which in some cases can be life threatening. Couples are strongly encouraged by me to have testing before attempting to conceive and certainly during early pregnancy if not tested previously. Testing for acquired and inherited thrombophilia when planning for a family will soon be standard practice."

Alan E. Beer, M.D.

Factor V Leiden (pronounced "factor five lie-dun") accounts for half of all cases of inherited thrombophilia. Identified in 1994, this gene mutation is the most common genetic defect associated with disease in the world, as well as the most prevalent cause of venous blood clots.

In white Europeans and North Americans, this mutation is present in approximately 4 to 7% of the general population. The highest rates are found in Europe, with a prevalence of 10 to 15% in southern Sweden.

In women with recurrent miscarriage, a rate of 20 to 27% has been reported.

The condition is characterized by a mutation in the gene for a clotting factor called factor V. Normally factor V is prevented from causing clots by a substance in the blood called protein C. The Leiden mutation makes the factor V molecule resistant to being broken down by protein C leading to increased stickiness of the blood. Thus, biochemically, factor V Leiden causes "activated protein C resistance."

A copy of the factor V gene comes from both parents. If one of these genes has the Leiden mutation, the risk of venous thrombosis is eight to ten times higher than normal. If both genes are affected the clotting risk during pregnancy is 34 times greater and without ongoing therapy and the chance of a thrombotic event over a lifetime is virtually 100%.

Studies have also shown that women with a history of recurrent miscarriage only have a livebirth rate of less than 40% (compared with 70% in the unaffected population) when this clotting disorder is left untreated.

Protein C and Protein S Deficiencies

"I have treated over 600 pregnant women with hereditary protein C or S deficiencies. These are potentially serious conditions and require treatment on day 6 of the cycle of conception, throughout the pregnancy and six weeks beyond."

Alan E. Beer, M.D.

Protein C functions as an anticoagulant by deactivating the coagulant molecules factor Va and factor VIIIa ("a" stands for "activated"). To do this, it combines with protein S on the surface of the blood platelets. If there is a lack of protein C or it is unable to interact properly with other molecules the risk of deep vein thrombosis is greatly increased. The incidence of protein C deficiency in women with two or more consecutive pregnancy losses ranges from 20% to 40%.

Prothrombin 20210 Mutation

Discovered in 1996, this is the second most common blood clotting abnormality, accounting for 18% of all cases of inherited thrombophilia. Between 1 and 4% of different populations are affected. For example, those in Southern Europe are twice as likely to carry the gene as Northern Europeans (in Spain, a rate of 6% has been reported).

This gene mutation leads to an increased amount of thrombin circulating in the blood, which can activate the clotting process and cause pregnancy loss. (The gene has a mutation at position 20210, hence its name.) It is a relatively mild risk factor for clots, but together with other factors such as oral contraceptives, stress, high blood pressure, obesity, smoking, or other blood clotting disorders, the incidence of thrombosis is five times greater than in unaffected people.

MTHFR Mutation
(Leading to Hyperhomocysteinemia)

"This is the most common abnormality in women with thrombophilia."

Alan E. Beer, M.D.

"Three months before I gave birth and several months afterwards I was in severe pain and vomiting. I was hospitalized for weeks at a time and lost a lot of weight. The doctors opened me up thinking it was an appendix problem and found large blood clot in my right ovarian vein. I got tested for MTHFR and was positive for two copies of C677T. I will be on blood thinners and folic acid forever but it sure beats lying in bed screaming in pain. I wish I had been tested earlier. Maybe they could have found the clot or might even have prevented it."

J. Arnold (Mother aged 33)

MTHFR stands for **M**etylene-**T**etra-**H**ydro-**F**olate-**R**eductase. Many people have a variant of this enzyme that is caused by a mutation of the MTHFR gene which is known as MTHFR C677T. It is a commonly inherited condition and most people with it may appear to be outwardly quite healthy. But for some women this is yet another microbiological feature of the non baby friendly body.

MTHFR is an enzyme in the cells that metabolizes and eliminates homocysteine, a toxic amino acid that damages the endothelial cell walls. Levels of homocysteine can increase if there is a deficiency of folate, B6 and/or B12. Those with the defective MTHFR gene are unable to process folate properly, so homocysteine concentrations build up, increasing their risk of arterial and venous thrombosis. Up to 20% of people with heart disease have abnormally elevated amounts of homocysteine in their blood. High concentrations are also found in approximately 30% of women with recurrent pregnancy loss.

Low levels of folic acid and vitamin B12 are also associated with this genetic mutation, which increases the risk of neural tube defects in the baby (e.g., spina bifida, where the bones around the spinal cord fail to close, encephalocele, where the skull is not fully formed and anencephaly, where both the brain and skull do not develop properly).

If the result for this test is "heterozygous," the defective gene has been inherited from only one parent. The incidence of this genetic condition in women with reproductive failure is approximately 25 to 30%. For pregnant women, the risk of complications is compounded if this genetic mutation coexists with other immune issues.

Some doctors are of the opinion that if a woman has tested heterozygous positive for this genetic variant and her homocysteine levels are normal before she gets pregnant there isn't a problem. However, testing levels at this stage is not necessarily relevant. During pregnancy, psychological stress and alterations in diet and metabolism can increase homocysteine levels. Therefore, a normal pre-pregnancy homocysteine result can be misleading.

If the MTHFR gene is found to be "homozygous," a mutated gene has been inherited from both parents, which can present a more serious prospect than inheriting a single gene. The homozygous MTHFR condition is estimated to affect 5% of Caucasians and is found in approximately 19% of patients with arterial disease, 11% with venous thrombosis and 14% of women with recurrent miscarriage.

Who Gets Inherited Thrombophilia?

"I suffered a brainstem stroke that left me unable to control my body from my neck down. It happened without warning; one moment I was supervising a student, the next I was face down, paralyzed and unable to speak. I felt completely calm. I knew what had happened as both my mother and her mother had suffered strokes."

M. Wilkinson (Teacher aged 49)

If one of your parents has an inherited form of thrombophilia the chance that you carry the defective gene is about 50%. If both your parents have the condition the odds rise to 75% or more.

Most people do not realize they have a blood clotting problem, yet they may have experienced related symptoms (e.g., poor circulation, migraines, cuts and blood draws that hardly bleed and memory problems). It is important to ask your parents and other close relatives if they have experienced such symptoms.

Anyone who subsequently tests positive for this condition should alert their immediate relatives and inform them of the risks. It is an absolute fact that one or both parents will carry a defective gene.

The medical profession is still largely unaware of many of the dozen or so forms of genetically inherited forms of thrombophilia that have been identified. Disappointingly, information about the risks, tests and treatment for these conditions is still limited. Added to this, there is no single test for all the different clotting disorders.

For a complete diagnosis, blood from both partners should be tested separately for each of the blood clotting problems mentioned in this chapter. This precaution should be taken not only to ensure the health of the baby, but also to safeguard the mother's own health until the birth of her baby and beyond.

7

Immunity to Pregnancy

"Women with this problem make antibodies to DNA or DNA breakdown products in the embryo or in the pregnancy. These antibodies form first in the blood as IgM. As the problem worsens they appear as IgG and live in the lymphatic system and lymph nodes. With more losses they form IgA antibodies which have their home and action in the organs, including the uterus. These same antibodies appear positive in women with lupus, rheumatoid arthritis, Crohn's disease and other autoimmune illnesses."

Alan E. Beer, M.D.

Antibodies that are formed against structures within the nucleus of the cell are known as antinuclear antibodies (ANAs). They specifically target the cell's DNA or components within it. If the nucleus of the cell is destroyed it will die. If enough cells are killed, organ tissue may be affected so badly that the organ can fail completely.

These antibodies are usually found in women whose immune system is targeting their own body tissue. ANAs can therefore indicate the presence of autoimmunity or autoimmune disease. They are also found in approximately 30% of women with recurrent miscarriage and in 20% of those who are infertile.

A single positive test for one autoantibody does not automatically indicate an elevated risk of infertility or recurrent miscarriage. However, for those who are already experiencing reproductive failure, the existence of one autoantibody is likely to indicate the presence of other antibodies that are detrimental to pregnancy. This is known as the "Reproductive Autoimmune Failure Syndrome." For example, those who test positive for ANAs are more likely to have elevated levels of natural killer cells and/or Th1 cytokines. This is why a positive ANA test is considered to be a marker for other categories of immune problem.

A Cell Destroying Experience

ANAs are often associated with hyperactivated NK cells which can cause an immediate inflammatory response against the embryo, thereby increasing the likelihood of implantation failure or early loss. Alternatively, the damage may occur later in the pregnancy when immune activity against the placenta destroys its ability to function. The inflammation is similar to that which is caused when the immune system deals with a splinter and the tissue becomes red and swollen.

If the fetus dies, more antibodies are produced, making the chance of conception even more unlikely next time round. These antibodies form first in the blood, then as the problem gets worse they start congregating in the lymphatic system and lymph nodes. With more losses, they may even start inhabiting the uterus where they will lie in wait, ready to sabotage future pregnancies. Effectively, the woman becomes immunized against having a baby.

Along with reproductive failure, ANAs can set the scene for autoimmune disease. For instance, virtually all women with systemic lupus erythematosus (SLE) test positive for antinuclear antibodies. SLE is not a rare disorder and worldwide it may be more common than rheumatoid arthritis.

This chronic, potentially fatal condition tends to flare up and then go into remission and because it involves uncontrolled autoimmune activity, the miscarriage rate for women with SLE is much higher than that of the general population.

The inflammation and cellular destruction caused by SLE can affect many systems of the body. Indeed, when ANA damage is seen in the placenta, the pathology report will often describe the tissue as being inflamed and weakened.

Some medications can also cause "drug induced lupus." Here, antibodies are made to histones (which are constituent parts of the chromosome) and a positive test result for these antibodies does not mean that any disease is actually present. Drugs that can provoke this reaction include hydralazine, Dilantin, procainamide and isoniazid.

Several other autoimmune diseases are characterized by the presence of ANAs. For example, they affect approximately 80% of patients with Sjögren's (pronounced "show-grens") syndrome. In this disease, the immune system creates antibodies to a virus that also target the exocrine glands, making sufferers unable to secrete saliva, sebum and tears. Joint or muscle inflammation and sleep disorders are other symptoms of this disease.

In addition, up to 95% of patients with scleroderma have ANAs. In this disease the connective tissues are attacked and the scarring that results makes the skin harden. Approximately 50% of those with alopecia areata (where the hair follicles are destroyed by auto-antibodies) are ANA positive. Those who have Raynaud's syndrome (featured in Chapter 10), juvenile chronic arthritis or the antiphospholipid antibody syndrome can also have these antibodies. In general, the presence of ANAs is associated with gastrointestinal, hormonal, blood, skin and rheumatic diseases.

The tendency to produce ANAs appears to be genetically determined in part, by a person's HLA tissue type. Their development can also be accelerated by viral or bacterial infection and environmental factors. For example, in a 2005 study, ANAs were detected in women with high blood levels of a chemical called bisphenol A (BPA), a substance found in common household items like food can linings and plastic containers, so the primary source of exposure for most people is via the consumption of BPA exposed food and drinks.

Research has additionally discovered that the mercury and silver in dental amalgam can induce an adverse immunological response. A higher than average incidence of ANAs has been detected in mercury sensitive individuals.

Having evaluated many patients with this category of immune problem, Dr Beer makes a further observation: "It is clear now that a positive ANA test also predicts an over activated immune response in general. I am coming to the conclusion that most patients with immune based infertility, pregnancy losses or IVF failures would benefit from immunotherapy until 12 weeks of pregnancy or longer."

IS YOUR BODY BABY FRIENDLY?

8

Antibodies to Sperm

"Antisperm antibodies occur in men and in women. For example, a woman whose partner has antisperm antibodies following a vasectomy often makes antisperm antibodies of her own. If she has failed two ICSI attempts it is 60% likely that she has immune problems that are causing these implantation failures."

Alan E. Beer, M.D.

Approximately 7% of women who are unable to conceive normally have produced antibodies to sperm. When this happens, a couple may also fail with assisted reproductive technologies such as intrauterine insemination, and experience multiple failed IVF attempts.

Antisperm antibodies can exist in either or both partners, in the blood, cervical mucus and ejaculate. Over 50% of men with low sperm motility and 66% of men with no live sperm have been found to carry these antibodies. There is an even higher incidence in those who have undergone a vasectomy or vasectomy reversal, where more than 70% of men can be affected.

These antibodies can be produced in response to obstructions in the vas deferens (the tubes that store and transport the sperm from the testes) or as a result of a congenital condition called obstructive azoospermia. Indeed, anything that causes a break in the normal blood/testes barrier can also trigger the formation of antisperm antibodies, including, for example, torsion (twisting of the testes), testicular cancer, infection or testicular biopsy. Sperm have unique surface antigens that elicit an immune response if they are detected by the immune cells in the man's blood.

The antibodies that are formed against sperm are designed to immobilize and destroy them. Studies have shown that antibodies that attach to the head of the sperm stop it from binding to the egg, while those that attach to the tail affect motility. In routine semen analysis, antisperm antibodies can be detected if the sperm clumps together when mixed with anti-IgG antibodies in a test solution.

Very occasionally (the risk is 1 in 1,500) this antibody coated sperm can produce a partial molar pregnancy (a complete mole has no fetal tissue present while partial moles have some fetal and some normal placental tissue).

Dr Beer described another aspect of this problem saying, "When two sperm fertilize the egg, two sperm pro-nuclei fuse with the egg pro-nuclei instead of one. Therefore, the genetic material is in triplicate. This results in a pregnancy with an abnormal growth pattern and a defective placenta. I have found this phenomenon is more common in men who have antisperm antibodies which 'glue' the sperm together, so two sperm may end up traveling and entering the egg jointly."

The woman can also develop reproductive problems by being exposed to antibody coated sperm and generating her own antibodies to it. These antibodies will then prevent the sperm from penetrating the cervical mucus. Instead, the sperm become stuck to it as if trapped on flypaper.

There is speculation that the rising incidence of antisperm antibodies in women may be due to delaying pregnancy until later in life, by which time they will probably have had several sexual relationships. This increases the risk of developing an immune sensitization. When antisperm antibodies develop, they will immobilize the sperm from her partner or any sperm donor. In other words, they are not partner specific.

This was demonstrated in a 1991 study in which the antisperm antibody levels of 109 prostitutes were measured and compared with those of 40 age matched women. Blood tests revealed that more than 40% of prostitutes had antisperm antibodies compared with just 5% among the control group and 61% of them eventually became infertile within nine years.

Despite the latest methods in the field of sperm retrieval, including intracytoplasmic sperm injection (when an embryo is created by injecting the sperm directly into the egg), some couples with this problem may still fail multiple IVF cycles. This is because women with antisperm antibodies are likely to have other cellular immunities that cause yolk sac damage to the embryo, implantation failure or miscarriage.

Tissue analysis of women with pregnancy loss who have been diagnosed as having antisperm antibodies often reveal changes in the placenta that are characteristic of other immune issues.

For example, Dr Beer observed that antisperm antibodies can be associated with antibodies to phospholipids. They are also a strong indication that the woman will have anti-DNA antibodies and elevated levels of circulating natural killer cells and CD19+/5+ B cells (that produce the antisperm antibodies). Such problems can manifest themselves as repeated IVF failure where the embryo implants but later miscarries early. Immunotherapy is an effective way of preventing these problems.

IS YOUR BODY BABY FRIENDLY?

9

High Natural Killer Cell Levels

"All of us are born with natural killer cells that defend us against cancer. When these natural killer cells see cancer cells they spit out a chemical called tumor necrosis factor alpha which shuts off the blood supply to the tumor and stops the cancer cells from growing and dividing.

Certain individuals have the ability to make 'natural killer like' CD57 cells that no longer play by the same rules. These cells are exactly the same kind that we find in the joints of patients with rheumatoid arthritis, in the organs of patients with lupus and in the bowels of patients with Crohn's disease. However, we also find them in the uterus and in the blood of perfectly healthy women who have been very unsuccessful in their reproduction."

Alan E. Beer, M.D.

Approximately 5 to 10% of the white blood cells in the peripheral blood are the "classic" CD56 natural killer (NK) cells. For many years, scientists considered these NK cells to be the "blunt instrument" of the body's immune system, providing a first line of defense against cells carrying cancerous mutations or infected with viruses, bacteria or fungi. Since then it has become clear that NK cells are not just restricted to immune surveillance but are involved in a variety of biologic processes ranging from reproduction to aging.

Natural killer cells are so called because, unlike T lymphocytes, they can spontaneously kill other cells without being sensitized to them first. NK cells identify their targets using a more general recognition system. They have two groups of proteins on their surfaces that interact with specific receptors on target cells. The first group activates the NK cell (switches it on) and the second can deactivate it (turn it off). In the presence of normal "self cells" they will therefore remain passive, but if they encounter what they consider abnormal "non self cells," they will become hyperactivated killing machines.

Reduced NK cell activity is associated with susceptibility to viral infections and tumors. So measuring the quantity and activity levels of these cells in a cancer patient will give an accurate idea of that person's ability to fight off the disease.

Conversely, an abundance of overactive NK cells and/or high concentrations of Th1 cytokines is associated with autoimmune disorders, reproductive failure and pregnancy complications. (Dr Beer referred to NK cells as "the Th1 autoimmune bad guys.") It also suggests the body may be under stress from infection or disease, situations which are consistent with a picture of poor immune function.

The body does need a certain level of NK cells to remain healthy. In pregnancy too, it is all about finding the right balance.

NK Cells in Pregnancy

"In normal, non-autoimmune pregnant women, levels of CD56+ NK cells are significantly suppressed at the time of their positive pregnancy test compared with their non-pregnant NK cell level. Pregnant women with a history of recurrent pregnancy loss have significantly higher circulating NK cell levels compared with those of normal pregnant women. The same problem is often seen in women with multiple failed IVF cycles."

Alan E. Beer, M.D.

Every month, NK cells travel from the spleen, lymph nodes and bone marrow to the uterine lining. Indeed, after ovulation and during early pregnancy, uterine NK cells (uNKs) make up the majority of the white blood cell population in the uterus and decidua (the special lining of the uterus that occurs during pregnancy). This NK cell population is functionally quite different to that of the NK cells in blood.

Uterine NK cells are defined as CD56+/CD16- cells as they generally lack the CD16 marker, which is associated with cytotoxicity (the toxic effect on cells), so they are not as prone to extreme killing tendencies.

The NK cells in the bloodstream, however, possess the CD16 marker, and are continually engaged in a search and destroy mission to wipe out foreign invaders. Those that are normally found in the uterus promote the growth of the embryo and protect it from harm.

These "beneficial" uterine NK cells locate themselves close to the outermost cells of the developing early embryo that go on to develop into the placenta. Here they secrete growth molecules that encourage placental development and promote implantation. Located primarily around the blood vessels, uNKs make structural changes that increase the capacity of the blood supply channels leading to the placenta/fetus.

Furthermore, uNKs release a spectrum of cytokines that enable them to influence the implantation process. Some are directed at restricting any T and B cell immune responses that may be aggressively targeted at the developing embryo, while others regulate the invasion of the embryo's "root system," so it does not burrow its way uncontrollably into the uterus like a cancerous tumor. Any disruption to these functions is likely to result in an unsuccessful pregnancy.

Although they have considerable destructive potential, uNKs deliver just 15% of the killing power of the NK cells that circulate in the blood. Yet this modest Th1 type immunity is all that is needed for the processes involved in the first 12 days of pregnancy. After this, they undergo a slow form of cell death and by week 20 have virtually disappeared.

In a normal pregnancy, around the time of implantation, peripheral NK cells show a decrease in both number and activity. In women with reproductive failure, the cytotoxic CD56+/CD16+ NK cells that are usually situated in the bloodstream are associated with higher rates of recurrent pregnancy loss, IVF failure and pregnancy complications such as preeclampsia and low birth weight

Blood circulating NK cells can release toxic Th1 cytokines, such as interferon-gamma and the potent variety, tumor necrosis factor alpha (TNF- alpha), tipping the immune balance to a cytotoxic one. Culture studies have shown that TNF-alpha disrupts cellular mitosis. This disruption stops cells from dividing and prevents implantation. Studies have also demonstrated that high concentrations of these cytokines in the endometrium are associated with delayed embryonic development and implantation failure. Evidence of such destructive activity is seen in chemical pregnancies, where a lab test indicates implantation has occurred long enough to raise the circulating blood level of HCG slightly before it drops back to zero.

High TNF-alpha concentrations can even activate the coagulation system and damage the lining of the uterus, the glands and the stroma (the tissue that nourishes the glands and placenta). In some instances, this can result in hemorrhages and blood cysts, accompanied by severe cramping and bleeding.

Later on in pregnancy, these effects can be disastrous, as Dr Beer explains, "Blood clots that form between the placenta and the uterus can lead to the separation of the placenta and a perfectly normal baby dies. Subchorionic hematomas can be associated with autoimmune activity that kills the cells of adjacent tissue. Women with autoantibodies and elevated levels of aggressive NK cells are more susceptible to these problems."

As the "warning siren" of the immune system, TNF-alpha alerts other cells of the immunological army that an unwelcome invader has arrived. CD3, CD4 and CD8 T cells, among others, then migrate to the uterus to join the battle. TNF-alpha also prompts the neutrophils and monocytes to secrete interleukins 1 and 6 and even more TNF-alpha. Up against this onslaught, a fledgling pregnancy stands little chance. Dr Beer always considered implantation to be the biggest hurdle for women with highly charged immune systems.

Unfortunately, the stimulation protocol in IVF can make the situation even worse, as high estrogen levels prompt the bone marrow to pour out more NK cells. As Dr Beer once said, "I am concerned with the very high levels of hormones that often inflame the autoimmune system at a time when I try to suppress it the most."

For women with a history of infertility who are undergoing IVF, there may be problems with egg quality and embryonic cell division. Smaller than normal or irregularly shaped gestational sacs, abnormally large gestational sacs and blighted ova are further evidence of Th1 cytokine mediated immune activity.

Some women with high NK cell/cytokine peripheral blood concentrations even notice other flu-like symptoms around the time of a failed implantation or miscarriage, including aching limbs, cramping, fever, fatigue and/or itchiness.

Because high numbers of cytotoxic NK cells can encourage the production of Th1 cytokines, NK numbers can serve as a useful marker for Th1-type immunity. Indeed, when peripheral blood concentrations of NK cells exceed 18%, there is a strong likelihood that the pregnancy will not succeed. If the baby does develop but is later rejected these circulating NK cells may then misinterpret any future fetal cells as the onset of cancer. The highest levels are found in women with:

- One or more liveborn child(ren) followed by secondary infertility or recurrent pregnancy losses. Dr Beer referred to these women as "the coaches of the Olympic team" as they often have some of the highest values
- Three or more implantation failures following IVF
- Three or more pregnancy losses
- DQ alpha genetic compatibility with their partner
- A pelvic disease in addition to an abnormal APA test result
- Antibodies to the thyroid gland

When appropriate treatment is provided, up to 85% of these women are able to deliver a healthy baby within three natural or IVF cycles.

Conditions Associated with an Inflammatory Immune Response

Thyroid disease

"Many women with antithyroid antibodies have activated NK cells that have caused the thyroid damage, as well as implantation failures, miscarriages or infertility. Even if the thyroid is treated, the NK cells remain active and need their own therapy. I do not just worry about thyroid antibody levels, I worry about the NK cell activity and levels that have caused the thyroid problems. All women with antithyroid antibodies have activated NK cells in my opinion, until proven otherwise."

Alan E. Beer, M.D.

The thyroid gland is situated in the neck and produces hormones that regulate metabolism and stimulate almost every type of tissue. Thyroid disease is an immunologically triggered condition where antibodies to the thyroid gland are produced. Those responsible are known as anti-thyroid peroxidase and anti-thyroglobulin antibodies.

Approximately 30% of women experiencing repeated spontaneous abortions test positive for one or both antibodies and are at more than twice the risk of miscarriage compared with women without them. They are also associated with reproductive failure in general.

Women with antithyroid antibodies (ATAs) may also have elevated levels of CD56+ NK cells, CD19+/5+ cells and activated T cells in their blood. Dr Beer observed that NK cells that damage the rapidly dividing cells of the thyroid ultimately cause miscarriages, implantation failure and infertility. That is why these antibodies are often considered markers for at risk pregnancies.

In addition to acting as a marker for reproductive problems, thyroid antibodies are linked to a predisposition to other autoimmune diseases. Women who are most likely to carry them include those with a personal or family history of thyroid problems or other autoimmune disorders, such as type 1 diabetes, or rheumatoid arthritis.

ATAs can be elevated in those with systemic lupus erythematosus and some studies have found a higher prevalence of thyroid antibodies in women suffering from clinical depression.

If this autoimmunity is allowed to develop over many years, thyroiditis can occur. This can take the form of an overactive thyroid, referred to as hyperthyroidism, or an underactive thyroid, which is called hypothyroidism. Both conditions have associations with high levels of NK cells in addition to blood clotting problems.

Because of all these associated health and reproductive risks, Dr Beer recommended that women with overly activate NK cells or ATAs have an annual thyroid evaluation to ensure these diseases were not developing. He also stated that antithyroid antibody testing should be routine in women with a history of two or more pregnancy losses and for those with thyroid irregularities. Some doctors have also suggested that ATA testing should be performed before any infertile woman starts their IVF cycle, as it may indicate that immunotherapy, not just thyroid hormone replacement is required.

As many doctors are still not aware of all the implications of a positive antithyroid antibody test , it is often up to the patient to ask the questions, do the research and push for the testing because of its wider implications.

Hyperthyroidism

When the body's immune system makes antibodies against thyroid tissue, too much thyroid hormone can be released into the bloodstream. A common form of hyperthyroidism is Graves' disease, which accounts for more than 85% of hyperthyroid cases.

Symptoms can include depression, fatigue, nervousness, sweating, an increased heart rate, raised blood pressure, weight loss, shaking, irritability, feeling hot, shorter or lighter menstrual periods and vision problems. Genetic factors are thought to determine the kind of symptoms a person experiences.

In the majority of cases, Graves' disease is stimulated by a particular virus that can activate the disease process. Antibodies to this virus have also been found in a high percentage of people with SLE and other autoimmune conditions. As the disease progresses, the problems associated with thyroid hormone over-production can swiftly move to the opposite end of the spectrum. When the damaged thyroid is exhausted, it shrinks and not enough thyroid hormone is produced, creating a condition known as hypothyroidism.

Hypothyroidism

As a result of increased NK cell activity, women with thyroid damage often display a Th1-dominant autoimmune profile. When the gland becomes inflamed, the damaged organ eventually stops generating enough thyroid hormone. The most common form of hypothyroidism is Hashimoto's thyroiditis. The onset of this disease is slow and it can be months or even years before the condition is detected.

An underactive thyroid can cause depression, fatigue, constipation, weight gain, dry skin, forgetfulness, a hoarse voice, mood swings, heavy menstrual periods and intolerance to cold. In many cases though, there are no physical signs of hypothyroidism and only a blood test will reveal its presence.

Treatment for hypothyroidism consists of thyroid hormone replacement drugs to prevent the symptoms and bodily changes associated with this condition. Pregnant women with hypothyroidism also need to increase their intake of thyroid hormone replacement drugs to protect their baby. Even a mild form of thyroid disease can potentially lead to serious complications including miscarriage, preeclampsia, gestational hypertension and premature birth. In addition, the baby's neural growth may be affected because the fetus depends entirely on its mother for thyroid hormones that are needed for healthy brain development.

However, treating the thyroid condition alone does not address the underlying autoimmunity that is directed against the thyroid gland. Hormone treated women can still suffer poor stimulation cycles, infertility, implantation failures, donor egg failures and miscarriages. In many women with immunologically related thyroid disease, successful pregnancy will not occur without immunotherapy.

Endometriosis

"I have found in 100 infertile women with minimal endometriosis that 60% had autoimmune abnormalities that were predictive of subsequent IVF failure. This was not found in 100 infertile women without the condition. The literature speaks clearly about the association between endometriosis and implantation failure. I therefore feel strongly that women with endometriosis and infertility need an immune work up prior to embarking on IVF."

Alan E. Beer, M.D.

Endometriosis is a leading cause of reproductive failure in many cases of "unexplained" infertility. Because its symptoms can easily be confused with common gastrointestinal distress symptoms and menstrual cycle pains, endometriosis is usually not diagnosed until a woman is over 30 years old. In the US, it takes an average 11 years for a woman to be correctly diagnosed To add to the difficulty of diagnosis, many patients with endometriosis don't present with any symptoms at all.

Estimates of the number of women of childbearing age with this disease range from 10 to 15% and of these 40% will be infertile. Even if only 10% are affected, this makes endometriosis one of the most common diseases in the world. According to the studies, this condition is often associated with high levels of autoantibodies and dysfunctional immune activity.

During a normal menstrual period, cells from the uterus are expelled through the vagina. If they enter other parts of the body they are destroyed by immune cells such as the macrophages or NK cells. In endometriosis, an abnormal decrease in NK cell cytotoxicity means the uterine tissue is not destroyed and continues to grow elsewhere. For example, it can enter the abdominal cavity and attach itself to organs such as the ovaries and fallopian tubes. Other sites for these endometrial growths (also known as implants) can include the bladder, bowel, vagina, cervix and vulva.

This migrant tissue responds to the menstrual cycle the same way as that of the uterine lining. Each month it thickens and sheds, causing pain and bleeding around the endometrial implants. As the blood has no place to go, it collects in pools, causing inflammation. This results in scar tissue formation or "powder burn" lesions that can block the fallopian tubes or interfere with ovulation.

These adhesions can even distort the surrounding organs and "weld" the fallopian tubes, ovaries and uterus into awkward positions. In many women, the uterine cavity can still look completely normal, while in others, adhesions can form on the walls of the uterus and create a less hospitable surface for implantation.

The immune cells that deal with the endometriosis release inflammatory TNF-alpha cytokines that attack the embryonic cells that will become the placenta. In fact, circulating levels of TNF-alpha in women with endometriosis are often much higher than they should be. This abnormal level of TNF-alpha acts to sustain the endometriosis by creating a favorable environment for the further implantation of endometrial cells and the progression of the disease. Its cytotoxic activity can also compromise egg development, fertilization and implantation.

Despite the fact that their TNF-alpha levels are high, women with endometriosis usually have normal or even low levels of circulating NK cells in their bloodstream. Dr Beer described this seeming contradiction: "Both the NK cells and macrophages located in the endometrium, uterus and peritoneum produce TNF-alpha. When these NK cells and activated macrophages are functioning in the tissue, we see a decrease in both numbers and cytotoxicity of the NK cells in the blood, but high TNF-alpha levels being produced in the affected organ."

Women with a family history of autoimmune disease are at greater risk of developing both endometriosis and immune mediated infertility. A study of over 3,500 women found that those with endometriosis were far more likely to suffer from additional autoimmunities; 20% had more than one other autoimmune disease, with over 30% of these suffering from fibromyalgia (at twice the rate of the general female population) or chronic fatigue syndrome (at 100 times the rate).

Many women with endometriosis also manufacture antiphospholipid antibodies and anti-organ antibodies (e.g., antithyroid antibodies). These can be detrimental to egg and embryo quality, and can affect the lining of the uterus, making it less likely for embryos to implant and increasing the risk of miscarriage for those that do.

Traditional surgical treatments and the use of hormones do not tackle the cause of endometriosis, just the symptoms. That is why the condition often reappears after treatment and even after a hysterectomy. As Dr Beer once affirmed, "Many of the patients I see have been treated by their doctors and had the endometriosis cleared out. The doctors pronounce them cured but when they try to become pregnant, they have an exceedingly high incidence of implantation failures and pregnancy loss. Removing the adhesions does not reduce the immune activity. We have to rely on other measures to do this. I will no longer treat endometriosis patients who also have other categories of immune problem without using anti TNF-alpha medication preconception."

Dr Beer's anti TNF-alpha treatment for patients with endometriosis has shown remarkable results with a 73% ongoing pregnancy success rate. Without this additional therapy the rate is just 45%.

Pelvic Inflammatory Disease and Tubal Blockages

"If a tubal blockage is due to infection or inflammation then I recommend immunological testing for women who are infertile. There is a 70% association with these conditions and the presence of autoimmune problems that are probably causing infertility."

Alan E. Beer, M.D.

In an ectopic pregnancy the normal passage of the egg to the uterus is blocked and the embryo implants itself into the wall of the fallopian tube. Such blockages can be caused by inflammation and scarring from tubal ligation (female sterilization in which the fallopian tubes are surgically tied) abdominal or pelvic surgery or infection.

The incidence of ectopic pregnancy is continuing to rise, mainly due to the increase in sexually transmitted infections that cause pelvic inflammatory disease (PID).

PID accounts for one in five of all gynecological admissions. It occurs when bacterial organisms travel from the urethra and cervix to the upper genital tract. Two of the most frequent sources of infection are chlamydia and gonorrhea. However, in some cases, bacteria that are normally present in the vagina and cervix can also be responsible.

The main symptoms of PID are lower abdominal pain and abnormal vaginal discharge. Other symptoms can include fever, painful intercourse and irregular menstrual bleeding. If chlamydia is the cause, there may be no obvious signs of infection (in either partner) even though damage to the reproductive organs may be taking place. Each episode of reinfection increases the risk of infertility and tubal pregnancy.

Sexually transmitted infections of the genital tract of pregnant mothers can double the risk of miscarriage in the first three months and are responsible for many premature and low weight births.

One of the most common forms of pelvic inflammatory disease is bacterial vaginosis or BV. This is a collective term to describe vaginal infection or inflammation caused by bacteria aggravated by yeast, viruses or chemicals. In severe cases, the infection can develop into inflammation of the uterus. Here, pro-inflammatory cytokines are secreted by leukocytes, including NK cells, which damage the lining of the uterus and create a hostile environment for the developing embryo.

Many common autoimmune disorders (e.g., Sjögren's syndrome, inflammatory bowel, Hashimoto's, Graves', Reiter's and Crohn's diseases) have been linked to chronic bacterial infections such as mycoplasma and chlamydia. The incidence of uterine resident NK cells is also higher in women with a known autoimmune disorder in addition to a pelvic infection.

Chlamydia

"Chlamydia is a cause of infertility and is an inducer of autoimmune responses that cause the body to attack the baby very early."

Alan E. Beer, M.D.

As the most common sexually transmitted infection in the U.S. and Europe, chlamydia now infects an estimated 10% of the sexually active population. Statistics show that chlamydia remains the most common type of sexually transmitted bacterial infection in England and it is the most common notifiable disease in the U.S.

Although repeated incidences are more likely to cause problems, a single infection can activate the NK cells, which then produce high levels of TNF-alpha and INF-gamma. The resulting chronic inflammation can lead to infertility, failed IVF attempts, ectopic pregnancy, miscarriages and pregnancy complications. As this infection often has no symptoms, women unwittingly are at risk of all of these issues if it is left untreated. This is why doctors test for chlamydia early on in the diagnostic process. Treatment with antibiotics alone may not overcome the reproductive problems associated with the inflammatory immune response this condition can generate.

Gonorrhea

The second most widespread sexually transferred bacterial infection is gonorrhea, which can infect the cervix, uterus and fallopian tubes and cause an increase in NK cell activity and TNF-alpha cytokine production. Inflammation in the fallopian tubes is associated with infertility and ectopic pregnancy. This disease can also affect the urethra, mouth, throat and rectum in both men and women. Again, there may be very mild or no symptoms of infection. However, if it remains untreated, gonorrhea can spread to the blood or joints.

Candida

"Candida is an immune activated condition. Women can react severely even to mild candida and have symptoms most of the time. This intense reaction inflames other categories of immune problem that can be detrimental to implantation and cause miscarriage."

Alan E. Beer, M.D.

Candida is a harmless form of yeast that lives in almost everyone's body. Problems can begin when the naturally "good" bacteria are killed off with antibiotics or overwhelmed by other factors that open the door for candida to overgrow, such as diabetes, pregnancy, poor nutrition, alcoholism, birth control pills, artificial hormones and antiseptic or perfumed bath additives.

When candida infects the vagina there is a thick white discharge along with inflammation and irritation. The accompanying symptoms of itching and burning are signs of a pro-inflammatory immune response within the cells of the vagina, caused by the candida IgA antibodies.

Also, if the body's immune defenses are severely breached, this normally harmless candida organism turns nasty. Instead of remaining hidden away in the bowel where it survives on dead tissue, it becomes a pathogenic fungus thriving on living tissue and growing out of control.

The fungal form of candida can produce root-like structures that bore into the intestinal walls, enabling toxins and partially digested proteins to escape into the bloodstream. When this happens, the immune response is fierce. IL-1, IL-6, TNF-alpha and more IgA antibodies are rapidly fired out, the macrophages are mobilized and battalions of NK cells are deployed. This immunological onslaught can soon exceed the actual degree of threat. If the battle is prolonged, all kinds of allergic and autoimmune reactions may eventually take place, including food sensitivities, arthritis, asthma, hives, acne, eczema, hay fever and bronchitis.

An intestine that is over-run with candida is also more vulnerable to colonization by aggressive bacteria, which may increase the risk of miscarriage and preterm birth.

Herpes

"Women with herpes often have elevated and cytotoxic NK cells in their blood and in their tissues."

Alan E. Beer, M.D.

Herpes comes in two strains: herpes simplex virus-1 (HSV-1) and herpes simplex virus-2 (HSV-2). Herpes simplex virus-1 can cause cold sores on the lips and can occasionally cause infection in the genital area. Herpes simplex virus-2 causes genital disease.

Genital herpes is a highly contagious infection that is usually spread via intercourse with a person who has infected sores. Approximately

12% of the US population tests positive for herpes virus HSV-2, making it one of the world's most common sexually transmitted diseases.

The first outbreak of herpes can last for several weeks, after which the virus retreats to the nervous system where it remains dormant until a trigger such as stress or illness reactivates it. In a 2004 study of infertile women, the herpes virus was detected in 64% of the 42 women who were examined. Their peripheral NK cell and TNF-alpha levels were also found to be elevated.

Dysplasia (Genital warts)

"The virus that causes dysplasia, in my experience, increases the chances of NK cells populating the reproductive tract. These produce TNF-alpha, which causes infertility and implantation failure."

Alan E. Beer, M.D.

Cervical dysplasia is defined by the presence of abnormal or pre-cancerous cells on the cervix. Mild dysplasia is the most common form and is a tissue response to the human papilloma virus (HPV). Many strains of HPV have been identified. Some cause genital warts and others may not, but they can still alter the cells of the vagina or cervix.

Severe forms of dysplasia have a higher probability of becoming cancerous and therefore require treatment. However, even after the surface of the cervix has been burned or frozen off, the virus can remain. In fact, it is possible for the HPV virus to lay dormant on the cervix for up to 20 years before warts develop or cell changes take place. HPV infection can create immunologic dysfunction that has been linked to miscarriage and infertility.

Allergies

"High eosinophil levels indicate an allergic problem and perhaps an immune etiology for pregnancy loss."

Alan E. Beer, M.D.

An allergy is a reaction against a substance that is normally tolerated by most people. When a virus or bacterium enters the body, antibodies are produced to destroy the invader. In the case of common allergies, or hypersensitivities something similar happens, except this time antibodies are directed at a threat, or "allergen," that is eaten, inhaled or touched (e.g., grass, pollen, animal hair, food or dust mites).

Allergies or hypersensitivities affect approximately 30% of the U.S. population. Genetic markers have been identified that show some people are more prone to these kinds of immune reactions than others.

Most allergies are of the "classic" Th2 dominant variety, where IgE antibodies are produced in response to an allergen. Such allergic reactions include hay fever, skin inflammation (e.g., hives and eczema), asthma and anaphylaxis. In this kind of allergy, when an irritating substance enters the body, IgE antibodies are produced in response to IL-4 cytokines. Antibodies then attach themselves to mast cells that line the surfaces of the skin, mouth, nose, sinuses, lungs and intestines, a process known as "allergic sensitization." So the next time the allergen arrives, an immune reaction is primed, ready and waiting.

The IgE antibodies cause the mast cells' membranes to rupture and release histamine and a hormone-like substance called prostaglandin D_2, which interacts with receptors on Th2 cells. This process stimulates an inflammatory response, which causes the blood vessels to dilate and smooth muscles to spasm. In asthma for example, the muscles of the bronchi contract, narrowing the air passage.

In extreme allergic reactions, so much histamine is released that not only do the bronchi contract, but the blood pressure also drops dramatically. This is called anaphylactic shock and can be fatal in rare cases. Anaphylaxis is most often triggered by allergens in foods, drugs and insect venom.

A sudden influx of inflammatory cytokines mobilizes a division of leukocytes called eosinophils. Operating within the frontline innate response, the normal role of eosinophils is to defend against parasites and infection. To do this they have an arsenal of chemical weaponry that makes them a potent fighting force, as well as a potential liability.

Eosinophils possess granules containing destructive enzymes and chemicals that promote inflammation and release yet more cytokines of their own. Although they are good at killing invaders like parasitic worms, peripheral tissue is often caught in the crossfire. For example, eosinophils are responsible for the damage that is caused to the lining of the lungs in asthma. When allergens are hormones, this can lead to infertility, premature menopause and multiple IVF failures.

The onset of hives is a symptom that Dr Beer has observed in women with hypersensitivity to hormones, particularly progesterone. As he relates, "I have learned that women with chronic hives have the strongest allergies that make pregnancy very difficult."

Irritable Bowel Syndrome and Crohn's Disease

"Crohn's disease is also strongly associated with Th1 cytokine production and can lead to recurrent miscarriage, especially if the disease is chronically active or relapses after surgery."

Alan E. Beer, M.D.

Irritable bowel syndrome (IBS) affects approximately 7% of people in the U.S. However, because many cases are likely to have gone undiagnosed, the prevalence may be as high as one in five – with the majority of sufferers being women. It is speculated that this syndrome arises when ordinary bacteria that is normally confined to the large intestine migrates to the small intestine, causing bloating after meals, as well as diarrhea, constipation and abdominal pain.

When bacteria within the small intestine cross the lining of the gut and enter the body, the immune system responds by increasing the levels of inflammatory TNF-alpha cytokines in the surrounding tissue. The response is often so intense that it can produce a flu-like illness, headaches, muscle and joint pains and chronic fatigue.

In some autoimmune women, these symptoms occur only during miscarriage or an immune threatened pregnancy, where they are a sign that the pregnancy is in danger. Despite its debilitating symptoms, IBS is considered a relatively mild disorder that does not permanently harm the intestines, unlike inflammatory bowel disease.

Cytokines secreted by Th2 cells normally prevent an aggressive immune response to the antigens in food and bacteria that come into contact with the lining of the intestines. In Crohn's disease, which is a type of inflammatory bowel disease (IBD), there is a shift towards a Th1-mediated response and the NK cells secrete TNF-alpha, which leads to chronic hyperstimulation and inflammation of the bowel. Whole sections of intestinal smooth muscle cells can become encased in a dense overgrowth of fibrous collagen, resulting in narrowing and obstruction. In severe cases, large parts of bowel have to be removed.

It is caused by excessive TNF-alpha output that encourages the release of other inflammatory cytokines by activating immune cells like the macrophages and neutrophils.

Stress and depression, as well as certain kinds of foods, are known to aggravate the condition. Symptoms may include fever, abdominal pain, diarrhea and fatigue. Many people with IBS or IBD have found that excluding certain foods from their diet and relaxation therapy can help control its symptoms.

It is known that a hypercoagulable state often exists in those with IBD. Dr Beer has found that women with IBD, who have an inherited or acquired blood clotting disorder combined with excessive TNF-alpha output are at greater risk of experiencing implantation failure and miscarriage. He has also noticed that the incidence of uterine resident CD57 cells in women with bowel disorders is higher than in women who do not have these conditions.

If IBD is active and untreated during pregnancy, the risks of spontaneous abortion, premature delivery and stillbirth are significantly increased.

Stress

"I have studied women who gave up trying to conceive and adopted or sought a surrogate. I tested them a year after their child arrived and their NK cells were normal. A successful pregnancy, or a significant reduction in stress can decrease NK cell levels."

Alan E. Beer, M.D.

The theory that doctors should provide their patients with tender loving care (TLC) is often cited as a "medical" solution for women who have successively failed with IVF or experienced recurrent pregnancy losses. A limited number of poorly designed trials that involve self or pre-selected groups and small sample sizes prompted this idea (see Chapter 15). While it may be true that psychological support can help calm immune hyperactivity to some degree (Dr Beer encourages his patients to undergo relaxation and other holistic therapies) these approaches are not "cure-alls" for immune-based infertility and recurrent pregnancy loss. More potent immune treatments are usually needed to ensure a successful cycle and a safe pregnancy.

A key issue that is often overlooked by infertility doctors and psychologists alike is that some women react more acutely to stress because of their immunological make up. Autoimmune women tend to have higher levels of CD8+ T cells, higher levels of toxic TNF-alpha, higher autoimmune inducing Th1:Th2 ratios and lower serotonin levels – the same markers that are seen in women with stress triggered miscarriages.

In other words, women who are at high risk of miscarriage already have greater susceptibility for stress "built in" to their physical constitution before they ever experience a loss. This is why patients with illnesses characterized by a hyperactive immune system often suffer from stress and depression.

Chronic stress can in turn, reduce the immune system's ability to respond to anti-inflammatory signals, escalating the problem even further. Indeed, researchers at Rice University interviewed 99 people who had lost a spouse in the last two weeks and took blood samples.

Those who were suffering prolonged grief had 53.4% more inflammation in their bodies than those who were not.

The fact that psychological stress seems to have an adverse affect on the pregnancies of some women, but not others, is also evidence of a specific immune profile that involves genes for stress activated and inflammatory responses. This is demonstrated by the results of animal experiments, which show that only certain breeds of mice lose their pregnancies when subjected to environmental and psychological stressors. Such abortions can largely be prevented with immunotherapy.

A common human genetic variant that over regulates the availability of serotonin is another key factor in explaining the body's hyper-reactivity to stress and excessive Th1 cytokine production. Antibodies to serotonin can also create similar problems.

In view of all these considerations, "stress" (with all its physio-logical and psychological symptoms of depression, migraines, increased TNF-alpha levels and blood clotting risk) could be considered to be evidence of genetically determined inflammatory immune activity that could lead to a myriad of health issues from stroke to miscarriage. Yet, chronic stress (including social isolation stress) can have the opposite effect in some women, temporarily depressing the immune system and leaving the body more vulnerable to opportunistic infection and ironically, pregnancy.

These opposing actions may explain the conflicting conclusions of various studies concerning stress, IVF outcome and miscarriage. Some have found a strong association when the markers for inflammatory response are measured, while others have found no association when psychological parameters are used.

An association between stress and a negative pregnancy outcome all depends on how "stress" is defined, reported and assessed and if genetic and immunological factors are taken into consideration. When stress appears to influence the course of a pregnancy, it is possible the symptoms that are being evaluated are simply those of subclinical autoimmunity.

In view of these variables, the theory that psychological stress alone causes miscarriage and infertility becomes quite questionable. Anxiety, depression, obsessive thinking, hypertension and sleep problems can all be symptoms of fundamental immune dysfunction, examples of which are featured in more detail in the following chapter.

10

Antibodies to Hormones and Neurotransmitters

"Central nervous system and endocrinal disorders can indicate immune activity that is associated with infertility and pregnancy loss. Infertile women and women experiencing recurrent miscarriage, often have significantly higher levels of NK cells and CD19+/5+ B cells."

Alan E. Beer, M.D.

CD19+/5+ B lymphocytes are responsible for a large amount of autoantibody production and their presence is strongly associated with autoimmunity. For example, elevated numbers of circulating CD19+/5+ cells correlate with high levels of antiphospholipid antibodies in some APS patients, and are involved in altering the immune profile of women who experience recurrent miscarriage.

In addition to producing the antiphospholipid and antinuclear antibodies of previous categories, these cells can also generate antibodies against hormones and neurotransmitters.

Antibodies to Hormones

The monthly reproductive cycle has four stages: the follicular phase, ovulation, the luteal phase and menstruation. During the follicular phase, follicle-stimulating hormone (FSH) is released from the pituitary gland. This tells the ovary to mature an egg and produce estradiol and progesterone to stimulate the growth of the uterine lining. Hormones from the ovaries then signal the brain to decrease the output of FSH.

Around the day of ovulation estradiol levels reach a peak. This prompts the pituitary gland to secrete luteinizing hormone (LH), which triggers the ovary to release an egg (ovulation). During the luteal phase, the body prepares itself for pregnancy. If the egg is not fertilized, or the embryo fails to implant, menstruation will follow. The glandular layer of the endometrium, called the decidua, sheds itself with each menstrual flow.

In addition to generating antibodies against phospholipids, DNA, sperm and histones (featured in the previous categories), CD19+/5+ cells can generate antibodies to the hormones that are essential for pregnancy. These include estradiol, progesterone and human chorionic gonadotropin (HCG). A reduction of these hormones can lead to luteal phase defects, which essentially means there are too few days between ovulation and menstruation. When this happens, the lining of the uterus may not reach the right stage of development at the right time so when an embryo arrives it is not thick enough, or there is not enough blood flow to its deeper layers. Implantation is then unlikely to succeed and if it does, an early miscarriage will probably follow.

Antibodies to hormones can affect all the stages of the monthly cycle and make the ovaries resistant to stimulation. High FSH and estradiol levels three days after the first day of menstruation are signs that antibodies to hormones could be at work. For example, in one study of women undergoing IVF, 92% of low responders had antibodies to follicle-stimulating hormones, 65% had antibodies to luteinizing hormones and 70% had ovarian antibodies.

In such cases, heavy doses of fertility drugs are often needed to generate a response during ovarian stimulation. Even so, fewer eggs are likely to be retrieved at the time of egg recovery. They are also likely to be slow to divide after fertilization and to be fragmented and fragile after being frozen and thawed.

Should the embryo attempt to implant, these antibodies may target the hormones that enable the uterine muscle to grow and keep the tissue of the decidua firmly in place. In this event, the likely outcome is partial implantation and a very low HCG reading, factors that often suggest an immune etiology for the pregnancy failure.

Antibodies to Estrogen

Estrogen is a group of hormones produced in the ovaries, comprising estrone (E1), estradiol (E2) and estriol (E3). Estrogen regulates the menstrual cycle and promotes cell division and the growth of the endometrial lining. It is also initiates the development of the female sexual organs and retains a strong influence over the health of the breasts, ovaries, cervix, fallopian tubes and vagina.

During the first part of the menstrual cycle, estrogen encourages the development of blood-rich tissue in the uterus. It then stimulates the maturation of the follicle in the ovary, softens the cervix and triggers the production of vaginal secretions that provide lubrication during intercourse and allow the sperm to swim.

Too little estradiol can restrict the development of the uterine lining so that it rarely gets above 7 mm (healthy levels are 10 to 14 mm), disrupt the muscle function within the uterus, and prevent blood flow to all these areas at the time of implantation.

Further evidence that estrogen is in short supply includes non ovulatory cycles, irregular periods, vaginal dryness and hot flashes. The problems associated with a severe deficiency (e.g., after the menopause) can be more serious, and include urinary problems, fluid retention, weight gain and loss of bone density.

Because estrogen receptors are found on the surfaces of all the cells in the body, this hormone can influence the onset of a host of disorders including endometriosis, polycystic ovaries and uterine fibroid tumors, and can exacerbate autoimmune disease. Estrogen can also act as the "on switch" for receptor sites on some hormone dependent cancer cells.

Once again, it is all about finding the right balance. Being a hormone that is essentially "pro growth," estrogen needs to be regulated. That is why another factor comes into play to offset and moderate its effects: a hormone called progesterone.

Antibodies to Progesterone

Progesterone is produced by the corpus luteum (the tissue left in the ovary after ovulation). It acts on the uterus to stimulate and maintain uterine functions that encourage embryonic growth, implantation and the formation of the placenta. It then continues to contribute towards fetal and placental development throughout the duration of the pregnancy. It also counteracts the negative effects of estrogen, offering protection against ovarian, endometrial and breast cancer, in addition to autoimmune disease.

Progesterone is often referred to as "the hormone of pregnancy" as it plays a pivotal role in achieving and maintaining the right conditions in which the baby can thrive. As its name implies, progesterone is "pro-gestation." As well as preparing the endometrium for a possible pregnancy, progesterone inhibits T cell activity by working as an immuno-suppressant. Consequently, low levels of this hormone during the first eight weeks of pregnancy indicate a strong likelihood of miscarriage.

A small number of women were also experiencing skin reactions such as hives and eczema just before their menstrual cycle: a condition known as autoimmune progesterone dermatitis. Other common symptoms associated with this allergy included asthma and migraines.

A relative absence of progesterone can create a state of estrogen-dominance that can add yet more fuel to the inflammatory process. For example, levels of pro-inflammatory estrogens, particularly estradiol, are often significantly elevated in those with rheumatoid arthritis or SLE. Estrogen stimulates the production of nitric oxide, which makes the blood vessels dilate, thereby putting pressure on the surrounding tissues and causing pain and inflammation.

Progesterone therapy can help offset this imbalance, modulate the immune response, restore a healthy ovulatory pattern and altogether make the body more baby-friendly. Dr Beer usually prescribed daily progesterone suppositories after the embryo transfer in an IVF cycle, and/or during the first 16 weeks of pregnancy.

Antibodies to HCG

"Women with a positive skin test for HCG often have a very high incidence of CD57 cells in the uterus and may suffer implantation failures or early miscarriages."

Alan E. Beer, M.D.

Human chorionic gonadotropin (HCG) is made soon after conception and plays a critical role in implantation. It is produced by the embryo in conjunction with the placenta to stimulate the production of estrogen and progesterone. It also acts to inhibit the secretion of LH and FSH.

The cause of the immune attack against HCG is thought to arise from its close resemblance to LH suppressor molecules. A reaction to LH suppressors could therefore potentially stimulate an antibody reaction to HCG. Under these circumstances, the NK cells release cytokines that activate the macrophages. The macrophages then alert the T-helper cells, which prompt the CD19+/5+ B cells to produce antibodies to HCG.

Antibodies to HCG are found in the blood of some women with infertility. So effective is their action that these antibodies have even been developed for use as a contraceptive vaccine.

Premature Ovarian Failure

"Women with ovarian antibodies have overly active NK cells. It is the secretion of TNF-alpha by these NK cells, or by antibodies to hormones and neurotransmitters that causes ovarian resistance or ovarian failure."

Alan E. Beer, M.D.

Approximately one in a hundred women is affected by premature ovarian failure and up to 20% of this group have a family history of the condition. A few cases are due to Turner syndrome, where a chromosomal defect is responsible for a complete lack of ovarian development, but in the majority cases, the cause is never diagnosed.

It is now believed that many cases of premature ovarian failure are caused by an autoimmune disease that depletes the ovarian follicles and attacks the eggs, inflicting DNA damage.

Antiovarian antibodies can impair the function of proteins on the ovarian cell surface and disrupt normal ovarian processes. Therefore, their presence is often a marker for premature ovarian failure. This is defined as being the end of normal ovulation and menstruation before the age of 40 (menopause normally occurs around the age of 50).

Studies have shown that in many cases of premature ovarian failure the woman will have an additional autoimmune disorder, the most common being hypothyroidism. Others include asthma, chronic active hepatitis, systemic lupus erythematosus (SLE), Crohn's disease, diabetes, Sjögren's syndrome, Myasthenia Gravis, rheumatoid arthritis, vitiligo, alopecia and Addison's disease.

Women with elevated antiovarian antibody levels are often poor responders to ovulation induction when undergoing IVF and have lower pregnancy success rates. In one study, 58% of women with failed IVF cycles had antiovarian antibodies, compared with 25% of those who were successful. Cycle day 3 FSH levels may be elevated because the ovaries are not producing enough estrogen and LH levels can often be high, even if the follicles do grow successfully.

Another indication that antibodies against the ovaries and hyperactivated NK cells are present is irregular periods. Half of all women with this kind of autoimmunity also experience symptoms similar to those of menopause, including hot flashes, night sweats, lack of libido and dryness of the vagina that can potentially lead to vaginitis or cystitis. Abnormal hormone secretion is associated with an increased risk of depression, osteoporosis and cardiovascular disease. It should therefore be treated whether or not conception is the goal.

During the early stages of ovarian failure, some healthy follicles may continue to develop and normal concentrations of reproductive hormones might be maintained. Eventually though, cellular destruction by antiovarian antibodies will speed the decline of the already dwindling reserves of healthy follicles, menstruation will cease and the ovaries will begin to shut down. As long as the condition does not reach the stage of premature menopause, the damage may not be permanent and can sometimes be treated. In Dr Beer's experience, three months of immunotherapy is usually needed to make pregnancy possible for this patient group. Indeed, he found that around 30% of his immunologically treated patients conceived naturally while waiting for their next IVF cycle.

How Autoimmunity, Obesity and Infertility Can Interrelate

More than 60% of American women are now obese or overweight. As we are all aware, being overweight is an increasing problem for men, women and even children (30% are now overweight or obese, up from 19% in 1980). This is an extremely serious threat to health, as the percentages of instances where obesity is linked to disease show:

- Colon cancer – 42%
- Cardiovascular disease   70%
- Breast cancer – 50%
- Gall bladder disease – 30%
- High blood pressure – 26%

For severely overweight women, the risk of death from an obesity-related condition is 50% higher than for those who are a healthy weight, and the risk of osteoarthritis is four times higher. Obese women are twice as likely to get breast cancer, four times more susceptible to endometrial cancer, (the risk is even greater for those with diabetes) and over a third more likely to suffer from rheumatoid arthritis. The chances of dying from cervical, ovarian or gallbladder cancer are also increased. This is because obesity creates changes at a cellular level that present a risk to health and to pregnancy.

As fatty tissue expands, it creates inflammation, producing elevated serum levels of C-reactive protein, IL-6 and TNF-alpha, the markers for autoimmune and cardiovascular disease. Due to this increased inflammatory activity, obesity also carries more risks for women who are pregnant, with a greater incidence of miscarriage, preeclampsia, hyperinsulinemia (high blood sugar) and gestational diabetes. Add to this estrogen dominance, and many other biochemical changes that are associated with obesity and things can become very difficult for overweight women hoping to become pregnant naturally or with IVF.

It is estimated that 30% of all cases of infertility worldwide and the poor results that are seen in IVF are related to conditions that involve obesity. Specialists have predicted that the industrialized nations' already low fertility rates are set to plummet further due to an "obesity crisis."

However, it should not be automatically concluded that weight problems are self inflicted and infertility is some kind of punishment for a lack of self control. Obesity can have an autoimmune connection. Some of the autoimmune diseases associated with extreme weight gain include hypothyroidism, polycystic ovary syndrome, type 2 diabetes and depression. Furthermore, the obesity that these conditions promote can lead to a vicious circle of hormonal imbalance and further weight gain that can make pregnancy a virtual impossibility for some women.

The ovary makes estrogen in variable amounts within the normal menstrual cycle. When extra estrogen is generated elsewhere this can be problematic. Fat cells convert the steroid hormone androstenedione into estrogen-like hormones. This extra stream of estrogen can upset the normal ebb and flow of the hormonal pattern and interfere with ovulation. Symptoms of this non baby friendly hormonal state include irregular, heavy and prolonged menstrual cycles (due to the extra estrone and estriol produced by the fat cells).

Side effects that are more serious include failure to ovulate or hormonal disturbances that prevent a pregnancy from continuing. Too much estrogen can also create pre-cancerous changes in the uterus, making the uterine lining thicker, but not in a way that is conducive to implantation. These potential health risks can usually be reversed by treating the autoimmunities that are causing the weight issue and the hormonal imbalances associated with it. This involves more than simply going on a diet and exercising more as Dr Beer explains, "It's not so much the weight, but the hormonal imbalance induced by autoimmunity that is the problem."

There are two autoimmune conditions in particular where the body's failure to use insulin properly results in a vicious circle of ever-increasing weight and hormonal imbalances: type 2 diabetes and poly-cystic ovary syndrome. Both share the same kinds of symptoms and health problems and both are treated the same way. Their many similarities have led to speculation that they could be variations of the same disease.

Type 2 Diabetes:
Both the Result and Possible Cause of Obesity

"15% of the women I see have developed type 2 diabetes. These individuals need to be treated with a glucophage called metformin to bring their free insulin levels down. Free insulin doesn't control the blood sugar it does only one thing, it makes new fat cells and it puts them on the thighs, the butt and the hips.

Women can jog and women can eat 500 calories a day. They will lose weight in their face, their neck, their breasts and their arms, but the fat on their legs, butt, thighs and hips will stay there. Many couples come to me and the husband says 'My wife has kind of given up. She is putting on weight. She can't be exercising enough. She must really be cheating on her diet,' and all the time it's due to a chemical imbalance."

Alan E. Beer, M.D.

According to the U.S. Center for Disease Control, as of 2015 almost one in 10 US adults has diabetes and more than a third has prediabetes.

Type 2 diabeties is the most common type of this disease and despite its description as "adult onset diabetes" it is increasingly being seen in children and teenagers. As the condition mirrors the increasing weight problem within the American population, obesity and diabetes are often referred to as twin epidemics and some doctors refer to the medical problem they create as "diabesity." However, the relationship between obesity and diabetes is not quite so simple.

Insulin is a hormone that is needed to convert sugar and starches into energy. If the body does not produce or use insulin properly, it can lead to diabetes. Around 95% of people with diabetes have the type 2 variety. This disease is a combination of insulin resistance, (when the body does not use insulin properly) coupled with hyperinsulemia (which means having too much "free insulin" in the bloodstream). In type 2 diabetes, the body gradually loses its ability to metabolize glucose (or sugar) when its cells' insulin recognition systems partially shut down because of immune activity directed against the insulin receptors.

The function of insulin is to activate other cells to absorb glucose. When this fails, blood levels of glucose build up and the pancreas tries to produce more insulin to deal with the situation. This excess of "free insulin" acts as a toxin within the body. It speeds up cell production on the artery walls, creating conditions for abdominal obesity, hypertension and ultimately, heart disease.

Increased body fat adds a further level of insulin resistance and creates a syndrome in which a person's weight can spiral out of control. This is because insulin blocks fat burning and promotes fat storage. Therefore, type 2 diabetes can be both the result and the cause of obesity, and free insulin levels must be controlled before the weight problem is resolved.

The diabetic state also creates conditions that can aggravate the immune system. Increased levels of Th1 cytokines and activated CD4+ and CD8+ white blood cells are commonly found in those with type 2 diabetes. All this pro-inflammatory activity is associated with the possible development of antibodies to phospholipids, yet another obstacle to a successful pregnancy.

Furthermore, a high level of free insulin suppresses the production of "insulin growth factor" which binds to receptors on the placenta to stimulate the output of glycodelin (a placental protein, also known as "placental protein 14" or PP14). Glycodelin suppresses NK cell activity in the uterus, so when glycodelin levels are low, NK cell activity increases. This is one of several reasons why reproductive failure is more prevalent among diabetics.

There are many other ways that an insulin imbalance can compromise both fertility and health in general, some of which are described in this summary of the following related condition.

Polycystic Ovary Syndrome: Another Disorder Weighted by Insulin Resistance

"Women with polycystic ovarian disease and ovarian cysts have a higher incidence of autoimmunity of the type that leads to insulin resistance (high fasting free insulin levels), autoimmune thyroiditis and recurrent pregnancy losses.

Alan E. Beer, M.D.

Polycystic ovarian syndrome (PCOS) is a pre-diabetic condition that is often associated with weight gain. The syndrome affects up to 10% of women of reproductive age and is usually inherited, although it can have an autoimmune component. It is the most common form of female infertility in the United States and around 40% of the sisters and 35% of the mothers of affected women have the syndrome to varying degrees.

Male relatives also show a greater incidence of type 2 diabetes, obesity, premature baldness and high blood pressure. With so many so potential risk factors, PCOS is not just a reproductive problem, it is an important health concern.

In this disorder, the ovaries become up to three times larger than normal and contain multiple small cyst-like structures about 4 to 9 mm in diameter, hence the term "polycystic" meaning "many cysts." Approximately 25% of women with the syndrome have polycystic ovaries that can be seen by ultrasound, but other than this, most remain asymptomatic.

Once again, insulin resistance is the main "active ingredient" in this condition. In fact, the discovery that insulin resistance plays a pivotal role in polycystic ovary syndrome is one of the most important advances in the quest to control this disorder. Elevated levels of insulin prompt the ovaries to produce testosterone and other male hormones (androgens) and not enough progesterone. This can lead to poor endometrial development, which can prevent the embryo from implanting.

Other fertility problems can manifest themselves as failure to ovulate, irregular periods and poor egg/embryo quality in IVF. Symptoms that are commonly seen are the growth of excessive body hair, weight gain and acne.

Up to 75% of women with PCOS also have insulin resistance and up to half will become obese due to the stimulation of fat cells by the high levels of free insulin. Approximately 10% will also go on to develop type 2 diabetes by the age of 40.

Additional problems can include high blood pressure, hardening of the arteries and high blood fat levels. In a 2004 study, 36.8% of women with PCOS also had elevated levels of C-reactive protein, a marker for cardiovascular problems. In fact, women with PCOS are at seven times greater risk of a stroke or heart attack, independent of obesity.

Furthermore, an excess of insulin can interfere with the normal blood clotting balance, leading to restricted uterine blood flow. It also reduces glycodelin output, the protein that inhibits NK and T cell activity. Therefore, low levels of this key protein can increase the chance of miscarriage.

For women with untreated PCOS, these immune problems combined with abnormally activated or high NK cell numbers can increase the risk of miscarriage by between 30% and 50% during the first trimester. The risk is even greater for those with a history of recurrent loss.

Although the hormonal aspects of PCOS are well understood by reproductive endocrinologists, the immune changes that can lead to pregnancy failure (even after the woman has received hormone treatment) are not well known, as this information is relatively new. For example, Dr Beer has observed several PCOS related cellular dysfunctions are associated with autoimmunity, including higher circulating levels of inflammatory mediators such as TNF-alpha.

The most effective treatment for PCOS is metformin hydrochloride (Glucophage is a brand name), the same drug that is used to treat type 2 diabetes. Metformin increases the body's sensitivity to insulin and allows it to be used more efficiently. It also reduces the amount of glucose produced by the liver, and the amount of glucose absorbed from food through the stomach. By controlling levels of insulin, metformin helps to elevate levels of glycodelin, which regulates the NK cells, thereby lessening the risk of immune mediated infertility and miscarriage.

In Dr Beer's experience, women treated with this safe oral medication achieved lower free testosterone levels, normal FSH and LH ratios, weight loss, a reduction in male pattern body hair, lower blood pressure and reduced levels of "bad" blood fats, e.g., LDL cholesterol. Metformin can even correct blood clotting problems to a degree. In some women, these changes alone are sufficient to restore fertility.

Antibodies to Neurotransmitters

Neurotransmitters are chemical substances that regulate brain, muscle, nerve and organ functions by acting as messengers between neurons: the impulse transmitting cells in the central nervous system. There are approximately 10 billion neurons in the human brain and health problems can be caused by anything that affects the flow of information between them.

Neurological disorders, also known as central nervous system disorders, are very common. Among the most recognized of these are Alzheimer's, Parkinson's disease and multiple sclerosis. What is not so well known however, is the range of other problems, including infertility that can arise when antibodies to neurotransmitters take effect.

Several different neurotransmitters play a role in female fertility, namely serotonin, endorphins and enkaphlins. Serotonin is probably the most significant in terms of the scope of functions that depend upon it as it provides the cells of the brain with hundreds of thousands of informational connections that influence everything from movement to mood.

In the uterus, serotonin regulates blood vessel elasticity and acts as a vasodilator causing vessels to expand. In other parts of the body, serotonin acts as a vasoconstrictor, narrowing the vessels and regulating the function of platelets (the blood cells that help blood to coagulate and close a wound). It also causes smooth muscles to contract, such as the abdominal muscles that push food along the gastrointestinal tract.

CD19+/5+ B cells make many autoantibodies, including antibodies to neurotransmitters and hormones. Normal numbers of these cells range from between 2% to 10% of the lymphocyte population. Women who have difficulty conceiving or suffer early pregnancy losses can have levels well above 10%. This can lead to problems of restricted blood flow through the vessels and capillaries of the uterus, which can disrupt the early stages of pregnancy.

Abnormally low serotonin levels can also accompany the myriad of health problems that women often experience alongside reproductive failure. These include migraines, depression, hypertension, anxiety, obesity, fibromyalgia, chronic fatigue syndrome, achiness in the small joints and muscles (usually in the morning), sleep disorders, night sweats and worsening premenstrual syndrome (PMS) or menopausal symptoms. In fact, there are many similarities between the immune profiles associated with these neurotransmitter disorders which is demonstrated in the following examples.

When Autoimmunity Gets Depressing

"Symptoms in women who have antibodies to serotonin and neurotransmitters include increasing depression that has no apparent reason. 15% of the patients I see with activated NK cells will stop making enough serotonin. Levels of this neurotransmitter should be in the 100 to 200 range, but in these individuals, I may find that it is less than 5. Serotonin in adequate levels is necessary to build a strong, thick uterine lining for implantation and placentation."

Alan E. Beer, M.D.

Research has revealed yet another spin off from the disordered immune system. Feelings of anxiety and depression could be more than psychological in origin; they could be the result of another immune ambush in the body, this time against the neurotransmitter serotonin.

Studies have also shown that women deplete their serotonin more rapidly than men do (and don't replace it as quickly) and that a significant reduction of this neurotransmitter can make them vulnerable to worry, depression and obesity.

Serotonin (or 5HT) is a "messenger molecule" that passes a signal from one neuron to another by binding to molecules called receptors, after which, serotonin is released. These receptors have distinct roles in regulating pain, sleep, digestion, cardiovascular function and temperature and influence many body systems, including blood clotting and blood vessel behavior.

Best known for its role as a mood controller, serotonin keeps us happy and controls feelings of anxiety. Its also has a lesser known influence on female reproduction.

Around the middle of a normal 28-day cycle, endorphins and enkaphlins (natural opiates and pain relievers) help prepare the uterine lining so blood can enter to nourish the embryo. Serotonin relaxes the vessels in the uterus, increasing the blood circulation so the embryo can implant successfully. Serotonin may also play a role in egg maturation and the early cellular development phase of the embryo.

In addition, serotonin is an important regulator of TNF-alpha production. If serotonin levels are too low, these inflammatory cytokines can multiply out of control. This is one reason why depressive disorders are often associated with inflammatory conditions (e.g., heart and autoimmune diseases) and why antidepressant medication has been shown to regulate the inflammatory immune response.

As a side effect of inflammatory immune activity, depression, especially in pregnancy, is very significant. First, a lack of serotonin means that the blood vessels in the uterus may not be relaxed enough for nutrients to pass properly through the placenta to the baby. Second, TNF-alpha levels may not be adequately controlled. Indeed, several studies have described a link between depression and bleeding in pregnancy, preeclampsia, retarded fetal growth, early labor, low birthweight and other birth complications.

Another health problem that often goes hand in hand with depression is obesity. In experiments, increased serotonin availability or activity tends to curb the desire to eat. Conversely, if levels of serotonin are reduced, there is a compulsion to eat more. Low levels of serotonin are also associated with increased sensitivity to stress, a negative emotion that is commonly linked to weight gain. This is one reason why conditions like anxiety and obesity are often successfully treated with antidepressants.

Drugs to treat low serotonin levels include "serotonin reuptake inhibitors," also referred to as SSRIs. Normally, serotonin is used once and then pumped back into the nerve cell that released it. These drugs interrupt that process so that more serotonin is able to reach the target receptors, thus increasing the availability of serotonin in the brain and bringing it up to a more comfortable working level.

To achieve a baby friendly body, the problem of the cytokine producing NK cells that underlies the serotonin deficit needs to be addressed. The most crucial factor is taming the natural killer cells and CD19+/5+ cells that are so high they are inhibiting the serotonin producing nerve cells from functioning properly.

Autoimmunity Can Be a Real Headache

"Neurotransmitters are important molecules that model the uterus the correct way for implantation. Antibodies to these neurotransmitters decrease serotonin levels, which often results in recurring migraines."

Alan E. Beer, M.D.

Migraine headaches are the most common type of vascular headache in women. Not only are they more prevalent in those suffering from depression, but in Dr Beer's experience, they were mainly seen in women with a history of endometriosis, mitral valve prolapse, infertility, IVF failure and recurrent miscarriage.

Thanks to advanced scanning techniques, it is now clearly apparent that migraines are caused by an interference of the blood flow patterns. The size of the cerebral arteries and blood vessels is partly regulated by serotonin, which has the ability to constrict the blood vessels in the brain. Serotonin is released into the blood following a trigger mechanism such as exposure to stress, chemicals or certain foods. This makes the blood vessels in the brain contract or spasm.

The kidneys then process the serotonin, which causes its level to drop significantly. The vessels of the brain then dilate and rapidly fill with blood which puts pressure on the surrounding nerves, causing pain and inflammation and a headache that can last for hours or even days. This kind of migraine is more common in women between the ages of 25 and 45 and can be severe enough to cause loss of appetite, nausea and even vomiting.

The body needs a comfortable working level of serotonin to cope with any fluctuations (above 100 nanograms per milliliter). If levels are consistently reduced, any sudden demand can tip the balance into a deficit until more serotonin becomes available. Those with antibodies to serotonin are susceptible to migraine attacks because their working levels of serotonin become too low.

With such a low threshold, any fluctuation downwards can lead to vascular problems because there is not enough of this neurotransmitter to keep the blood vessels evenly controlled. Furthermore, because serotonin can influence the output of TNF-alpha, if its availability is limited, levels of inflammatory cytokines can spiral upwards. High concentrations of TNF-alpha and the cells that produce it are often present in those with migraines and during a migraine attack, cytokine levels can escalate dramatically.

Because inflammatory cytokines and antibodies to neurotransmitters are the hallmarks of other classic manifestations of autoimmunity, those with the antiphospholipid syndrome, SLE, thyroid disease and immune-mediated reproductive failure, often suffer from migraine headaches.

Drugs that are directed at eliminating the pain, such as aspirin and non steroidal anti-inflammatory drugs like ergot alkaloids, only address the symptoms and not the serotonin deficiency that is ultimately responsible. Serotonin reuptake inhibitors (antidepressants) can help restore serotonin availability to healthier working levels where normal fluctuations can be comfortably tolerated. However, the NK cells will need to be controlled or the cycle of autoimmunity, low serotonin and infertility is likely to continue.

Migraines can also be aggravated by restricted blood flow as a result of thrombophilia. Blood thinning medication can help prevent migraine attacks and create more favorable conditions in which pregnancy can occur.

Raynaud's Syndrome

"Women with Raynaud's disease have antibodies to hormones and neurotransmitters and often need immune treatment. Many women with Raynaud's also have inherited thrombophilia and require anticoagulant therapy. Vascular problems of endometrial blood flow often accompany this disorder and lead to implantation failure."

Alan E. Beer, M.D.

Vascular dysregulation associated with reduced levels of serotonin is an underlying factor in migraine headaches. It is also a feature of another circulatory problem: Raynaud's syndrome. Women with inherited thrombophilia are particularly prone to this condition, which is characterized by a lack of blood flow to the extremities of the body, such as the fingers and toes.

In this syndrome, an over reaction to cold, or occasionally to stress, triggers the release of serotonin from the nerve endings and blood platelets where it is stored. This causes the small blood vessels to constrict dramatically. Deprived of oxygenated blood, the fingers, nose, ears and toes will turn white then blue. Finally, they start throbbing and tingling and turn red when the area warms up and the blood rushes back in.

In most cases, these symptoms are mild but in 30% of individuals, the condition is more severe. The entire hand may become affected (instead of just the tips of the fingers) and responds with painful spasms when exposed to cold. This often occurs when there is a preexisting autoimmune disease. For example, Raynaud's syndrome is experienced by up to 95% of people with scleroderma (which itself is strongly associated with the over expression of autoantibody producing CD19 B cells).

Microvascular circulatory restriction can have a negative impact on early pregnancy. Not only does poor blood circulation in the uterus make implantation less likely, but if a pregnancy should happen, it will have difficulty progressing. Any process that adversely affects blood flow can damage the placental and uterine blood vessels, meaning the fetus may not be able to grow properly or even stay alive.

Immunotherapy with anti-inflammatory and antidepressant medications can help to moderate the immune response and restore serotonin to normal levels, while anticoagulation therapy can help improve blood flow, all of which increases the chances of a healthy pregnancy.

The Wreckage That Is Left After a "B Cell Blitz": Fibromyalgia and Chronic Fatigue Syndrome

"Women suffering from chronic fatigue syndrome, in my experience, have activated NK cells and antibodies to hormones and neurotransmitters, which increase dramatically after an IVF transfer and incur even more pronounced symptoms. We see this particularly in women whose estradiol levels exceed 2,000 pg/ml. Antibodies to hormones and neurotransmitters also underpin the symptoms of fibromyalgia. I have not found one woman with this condition who did not have abnormal immune activity that was contributing to her implantation failures or losses."

Alan E. Beer, M.D.

Chronic fatigue syndrome (CFS), which is also known as ME (Myalgic Encephalomyelitis) and fibromyalgia are medical conditions that have only recently been taken seriously by doctors. CFS, in particular, has sometimes been viewed with skepticism. Sufferers have often been told that their feelings of severe exhaustion, muscle pain, anxiety, migraine headaches, depression, poor circulation and sleep problems are just a figment of their imagination or an excuse to take time off work.

Since the late 1980s, there has been an enormous amount of progress in the understanding of these diseases, mainly due to the research associated with AIDS. These disorders are now acknowledged as real, physical, immunological illnesses. Indeed, it has been suggested that CFS should be reclassified as "chronic fatigue immune dysfunction syndrome" because 60 to 80% of T cells are activated, compared with those in a healthy person where 80% are resting.

Women between the ages of 20 and 50 are primarily affected by fibromyalgia (myalgia means "muscle pain"). This disease is characterized by "hot spots" of pain at various locations around the body, which typically include the lower back, hips, shoulders, neck and arms. Apart from this, many of the symptoms and clinical characteristics of fibromyalgia closely match those of CFS. In both conditions, there are elevated levels of antibodies to serotonin. As a result, circulating blood levels of serotonin are significantly lower than average, with up to two-thirds of sufferers experiencing prior or concurrent major depression.

As well as its effect on blood vessels (as detailed in its role in migraines and Raynaud's syndrome), serotonin is a regulator of the production of TNF-alpha. If serotonin levels fall, these inflammatory cytokines are left to multiply out of control. High cytokine levels are typically associated with CFS and fibromyalgia. Besides inflammation, excessive cytokine activity can induce flu-like symptoms including fever, achiness and fatigue.

The result of all this volatile immune activity is the disruption of the central nervous system by an "antibody factory" that is constantly being fueled by hyperactive T cells and excessive amounts of TNF-alpha. It has been speculated that triggers for all this immunological mayhem can include exposure to a viral or bacterial infection, or a reaction to environmental toxins such as pesticides or other industrial chemicals, which are mentioned in the Addendum.

Another marker for fibromyalgia is the presence of elevated levels of antinuclear antibodies. In addition, antibodies to phospholipids have been detected in 90% of those with the disease and are equally prevalent among CFS sufferers. Indeed, the results of a retrospective study of over 400 chronically ill patients revealed that 83% had one or more coagulation protein defects. Women with these conditions who are prescribed low dose heparin (an anticoagulant that is also mildly immunosuppressive) often notice an improvement in their condition.

A Summary of Conditions and Symptoms Associated with Antibodies to Hormones and Neurotransmitters

"In many women, the following situations and complaints are discounted or minimized by reproductive endocrinologists or Ob/-Gyn doctors. These symptoms are not figments of the imagination. They are real and demand attention and work up."

Alan E. Beer, M.D.

Dr Beer discovered a common link between many seemingly unrelated diseases states often associated with antibodies to hormones and neurotransmitters.

Specific medical conditions include:

- Fibromyalgia or achiness in the small joints and muscles, usually in the morning
- Raynaud's syndrome
- Thyroid disorders (even those controlled by medication)
- Premature ovarian failure
- Migraines
- Depression
- Chronic fatigue syndrome
- Adult onset diabetes

Other symptoms and problems often associated with autoimmunity and low serotonin levels:

- Anxiety and panic attacks
- Sleep disorders (including night sweats)
- Irritability
- Severe PMS

- Sweating at night especially over the chest area
- Irregular cycles
- Anovulatory cycles

Problems encountered during IVF:

- Poor ovarian stimulation and reduced egg quality and numbers
- Slowly dividing embryos
- Fragmented embryos that often do not survive the freeze/thaw process
- Two or more implantation failures

Test results that often indicate autoimmunity associated with low serotonin levels:

- A uterine lining of less than 8 mm when tested on day 13 or 14
- The three layers of the uterine lining fail to develop, or blood circulation fails to reach zone three
- Hormone levels fall significantly in the middle of the cycle
- High estradiol levels and follicle-stimulating hormone levels on cycle day 3
- Low progesterone levels
- High prolactin levels

11

Hope for Older Mothers To Be

"I have treated many women aged 40 and above, the oldest being 48. In the 40 to 42-year-old age group, around half of women who return to IVF after previously failing three IVF cycles deliver a baby within two cycles of treatment. If we use donor eggs in older individuals the success rate is even higher. So I can no longer have long discussions with women who are worried about their age, because to me, as long as they are menstruating and producing eggs there is a possibility of a child in their home."

Alan E. Beer, M.D.

A growing number of women are delaying childbearing until their late 30s and early 40s. It is well known that the incidence of chromosomally abnormal embryos increases as a woman ages. What is not so well known is that the loss rate of chromosomally normal fetuses also increases.

When a woman ages, immunological abnormalities become more common as her immune system starts shifting from a baby friendly Th2 response to a less baby friendly Th1 pattern. In other words, it moves away from the reproductive mode to the pathogen defense mode of an older woman.

In many such cases, immunotherapy can temporarily reset the immune balance so the body is more receptive to pregnancy. Immuno-therapy has been shown to reduce the rate of miscarriage in older women and to improve the success rates of those receiving donor eggs.

In IVF, the ovarian response to fertility treatment can predict the likely outcome in women with both a normal and abnormal ovarian reserve. Therefore, age is not the absolute determining factor in predict-ing a woman's chances of success. Important indicators of potential cycle outcome are follicle-stimulating hormone (FSH) and estradiol concentrations on cycle day 3. If the FSH level is below 12 and the estradiol level is 35 or below, a fertile cycle will probably follow. If either one or both of these levels are higher, the cycle is unlikely to be successful.

When half of all cycles have high FSH and estradiol numbers and periods start to be missed, menopause is approaching and the ovaries are starting to close down. At the age of 47 (about four years before the average age of menopause) some cycles will still be ovulatory ones, but most of these will not produce good quality eggs.

The actual age at which menopause begins depends to a large degree on heritability and the variation between women is probably genetically controlled. In a study of women aged 45 and over, who had conceived spontaneously and experienced successful pregnancies it was discovered that they possessed a distinctive genetic profile. So to assess how much longer a woman will remain fertile she should look to her own mother as a guide.

A Case of Bad Eggs? The Age Old Question

"I believe that some eggs in older women perform less well and are more prone to genetic abnormalities, but everything I know about older women has told me that they can become mothers safely up to the age of 45.

The older half of my patient population is close to 40 years of age and has failed IVF more than three times. These women are not simply those who have tried to conceive for over a year without success. They are the toughest cases to crack, having been trying for many years before finally turning to me as a last resort."

Alan E. Beer, M.D.

Many women who fail repeatedly with fertility treatments are told their problems are due to age and poor egg quality. As one patient puts it, "The IVF world believes that women nearing 40 are over and beyond the hill. It's like a done deal: you are downhill from now on and your eggs are no good so your only options are donor eggs or embryos, surrogacy or adoption."

According to the 2013 "ART Fertility Clinic Success Rates Report," women trying to conceive via IVF at age 40 using their own eggs have less than a 30% chance of becoming pregnant and less than a 20% of giving birth to a live baby. For those aged 42 and older, the rate drops to about 6%. At this stage, the vast majority who fail will probably give up. Yet there may still be hope for these women, thanks to new discoveries in immunotherapy and more aggressive protocols to prevent hyperactive immune cells damaging the eggs.

Based on the analysis of ovarian tissue samples carried out during the 1950s, the female fetus has up to seven million egg cells. By the time she is born she has only one or two million left. This number dwindles until only 400,000 or so remain at puberty and virtually none by age 50. Consequently the ovary is considered to be one of the fastest aging organs in a woman's body.

Challenging the notion that women are born with all the eggs (also called oocytes) they will ever have, evidence from animal studies now suggests that there may be a continual death and renewal of eggs and not a finite number as is commonly believed.

Researchers at Harvard Medical School discovered, by observing mice, that the ovaries harbor a previously undiscovered type of stem cell that can form new eggs throughout adulthood, much like the sperm that is constantly being reproduced in the male testes.

In this 2004 study, whose finding have since been confirmed by other research teams, the scientists saw that a third of the ovarian follicles in young adult mice were dying, yet their egg supply did not run out. This meant that new eggs were being made to replace the ones that had been lost. To prove that the stem cells were responsible for this regeneration, the researchers treated the ovaries with a drug that paralyzed the stem cells. There was a 95% reduction in the number of immature eggs because they were no longer being replenished.

Associate Professor Ray Rodgers, former President of the Endocrine Society of Australia, supports the discovery, stating, "The ovary can be regarded as a tissue in which endocrine organs, follicles and corpora lutea continually develop and regress. This makes the ovary unique, since other than the placenta, all the other endocrine organs in adults have completed development in fetal life or at puberty."

According to this theory, reduced fertility with advancing age occurs because the stem cells die off and fewer, poorer quality eggs are produced. As the remaining stem cells are older, they are more likely to contain chromosomal aberrations and DNA abnormalities.

Although stem cell technology to rejuvenate human eggs is in the early research stages and scientists still cannot grow new human eggs, the possibility that new eggs are generated at all, means steps can be taken to promote their healthy development.

The first attempts to analyze the chromosomal content of human female eggs were made in the 1970s but resulted in limited data owing to the inadequacy of the testing procedures. Since the 1990s, using advanced methods it has been possible to produce results that are more consistent. It is now thought that for women aged 40 to 45, chromosomal defects could affect between 70 and 80% of their eggs, compared with just 17% in women aged 20 to 25 and 35% of those in women aged 26 to 35.

Chromosomes contain a single coiled molecule of DNA, the blueprint of a human being's make up. The coding order of the DNA determines the characteristics of the genes. Twenty-three chromosomes or "genetic packages" are found inside the nucleus of each human cell. DNA damage has been shown to be involved in a variety of genetically inherited disorders and later in life, aging and cancer occur because of chromosomal anomalies caused by DNA damage and faulty DNA repair mechanisms.

Chromosomal aberrations due to defective DNA are either inherited ("germline" mutations) or the result of changes in body cells ("somatic" mutations). Aneuploidy, when there are irregularities in the number or composition of one or more chromosomes, is a common cause of problems such as Down's syndrome (trisomy 21) or Turner syndrome. The majority of aneuploidy associated birth defects result from errors in chromosome segregation (when the chromosome should separate into two identical parts), during egg and sperm production, or in the early cell divisions following fertilization.

It is hypothesized that DNA damaging agents, such as radiation, environmental toxins and free radicals, are behind the inability of some chromosomes to segregate successfully. These same harmful influences are also responsible for DNA fragmentation, a factor that is now considered more frequently associated with age related infertility than aneuploidy.

By administering treatments to encourage DNA repair mechanisms and advising reduced exposure to toxic environmental agents, Dr Beer observed an improvement in the egg quality and fertility levels in older women. He noticed that in many cases, the problem with egg quality originated from the fluid in the follicle surrounding it and an abnormally high level of TNF-alpha cytokines in this fluid had a damaging effect on the egg.

These observations have been supported by subsequent studies involving the analysis of the follicular fluid of infertile women. The consensus being that exposure to excess TNF-alpha is associated with deterioration in egg quality and poor fertilization.

Dr Beer used to say that TNF-alpha "stains the egg as wine does a rug." The egg then becomes dark and brittle and is less capable of being fertilized. The embryos that result are often fragmented, have a tough, mottled "shell," are slow to divide and fragile when frozen and thawed. Dr Beer noted all these phenomena when carrying out biopsies at his clinic.

When the woman's TNF-alpha IL-10 cytokine ratios are above 40 her eggs will often display signs of DNA damage. In these circumstances, patients are advised to have treatment that allows time for these damaged eggs to be ovulated out. Eggs deeper within the ovaries that are protected from TNF-alpha exposure can then mature and rise to the surface. The woman can start trying to conceive when she is in a "safe window of opportunity."

For women worried that their eggs are more likely to be chromosomally defective, Dr Beer has found that if there is DNA damage in their embryo or egg, the pregnancy will fail in a matter of two or three days, or at the most, a week. He has also noticed, "The incidence of Down's syndrome and genetic abnormalities in the fetuses of older, immune treated women is two times less than the life tables predict for women in their age group. So what we are doing is not making it more likely for them to have an abnormal child."

In women with TNF elevation and prior infertility, Anti-TNF-alpha therapy significantly reduces TNF-a / IL-10 ratios and increases their pregnancy rates. It has beens shown that the highest IVF success rates are achieved when the last anti-TNF injection is given 61–120 days before the day of IVF transfer. This suggests that much of Humira's benefical effect is related to improvement of egg quality (a preconception effect) rather than an effect at implantation.

Dr Beer also found that when couples had failed IVF three times and then got pregnant on their own, the peak time for these women to get pregnant was 17.4 weeks after the start of anti-TNF therapy, (switching to IVIG at implantation). Again, this suggests that the benefit effect of anti-TNF therapy occurs preconception.

For women who continue to undergo IVF treatment, assisted hatching may be necessary, since immune toxins can harden or thicken the zona pellucida, making it difficult for the egg to "hatch" independently. (Women with endometriosis are particularly prone to this problem, which can lead to a higher incidence of immune damaged eggs and lower implantation rates.)

Since the discovery of the 17.4-week preconception treatment period, even Dr Beer admitted that he had to rethink his definition of a "hopeless case," commenting, "This figure really surprised me; I was not expecting it. It tells me that when the reproductive system has been labeled broken and irreparable, we may have over called the diagnosis because for these women, there is now a real chance of success."

12

Immune Problems and Pregnancy

By Alan E. Beer, M.D.

A positive pregnancy test can mark the end of one long and stressful journey for most women, and the beginning of another. Every blood test and scan is both welcomed and dreaded and the ultrasound screen is scrutinized with concern. Only when a healthy baby is safely wrapped up and placed in their arms can these women finally celebrate and stop imagining the worst. This is what it feels like to have a new pregnancy after years of suffering failure and loss.

I wish there was a magic time when I could say to my patients, "You and your baby are out of the woods," but this science is too new for complacency. I treat every hard won pregnancy with more than a degree of caution, watching closely for indications of potential dangers and taking steps to avoid them.

If problems are not detected early and treated promptly, the baby could suffer intrauterine growth retardation, miscarriage or premature birth. I never want to be in a position where I have solved one problem for the couple, only to see another one passed on to their innocent child because of a lack of proper follow up care. I always worry for the next thing to go wrong in pregnant women with autoimmunities, especially those with prior losses and IVF failures.

Throughout the nine months, I recommend a series of ultrasounds and blood tests to monitor the health of both the mother and her baby. Some doctors might not be as concerned about so much extensive testing and say it is a waste of money because they cannot or will not provide treatment unless something is overtly wrong. Unfortunately, I have found that subclinical problems in pregnancy that might be considered "common" and "nothing to worry about" can present quite a different prospect for those with immune disorders.

For example, migraines, skin rashes or aching joints tell me that there is inflammatory activity going on and that sounds alarm bells to me. Low amniotic fluid volume, subchorionic hemorrhages or cervical incompetence are more examples of unregulated immune activation. In such cases, I will recommend my patients are given IVIG – an option most Ob/Gyns are not familiar with.

Of course, I would rather not see these situations at all. That is why my immune treatment protocol starts early; often well before the first missed period. My patients must start home pregnancy testing on cycle days 23, 25, 27 and 29 (cycle day 1 being the first day of the last menstrual period). The test should be observed for one hour and if a faint positive is seen, a blood beta HCG reading will confirm the result. Waiting to test after a missed menstrual period is usually too late to start therapy in many immune activated women.

In my patients, the NK cell cytokine assays are also done at the time of a positive pregnancy test to determine if IVIG or other treatments are needed to help the pregnancy continue. Antiphospholipid antibody and anti-DNA/histone antibody tests are then scheduled every two weeks during the first trimester and then monthly.

Patients taking anticoagulant medications require a monthly baseline CBC (complete blood count) and APTT (Activated Partial Thrombo-plastin Time) test, which measures the time it takes blood to clot. These tests are carried out twice at two weeks apart and then once monthly. Progesterone levels are also recorded at the time of a positive pregnancy test, and then weekly for 16 weeks. All these assessments should be done at the referring physician's office and the results forwarded to our center.

This testing and treatment protocol may seem extensive to those unfamiliar with my program. However, I have found that these protocols, developed as a result of 25 years' clinical experience, are the best way to give the pregnancy a safe start in high risk immune patients.

To check the development of the fetus, ultrasounds are scheduled every two weeks from around 5 to 6 weeks of gestation. In my experience, an elevation of the NK cells in the mother retards the growth of new placental cells throughout the pregnancy. The baby does not know this is happening unless the problem is untreated for four weeks. An ultrasound allows me to determine if the placenta is undergoing this type of immune attack.

After the first trimester, scans can be performed on a monthly basis to assess the condition of the placenta, amniotic fluid levels, cervical length and the presence of subchorionic hemorrhages. The baby's heart rate, growth, internal organs and spine are also checked to ensure these are normal.

A quadruple screen (consisting of four blood tests) should be performed at approximately 16 weeks' gestation to identify the possibility of open neural tube defects or other chromosomal problems. A detailed level 2 ultrasound also looks for physical markers associated with chromosomal anomalies.

If both the quadruple screen and level 2 ultrasound are normal, I do not recommend an early amniocentesis unless absolutely necessary. Unfortunately, this procedure has resulted in the loss of more healthy babies from rupture of the membranes in my high risk patients than the diagnosis of a severe defect. However, an amniocentesis test in the third trimester of pregnancy is relatively safe, and must be carried out when required.

During the last month of pregnancy (and in some cases as early as 29 weeks), my patients undergo a twice weekly non stress test. A monitor is placed around the mother's abdomen to measure the baby's heart rate accelerations in response to fetal movement. The biophysical profile is an even more comprehensive evaluation that combines both the non stress test and a detailed ultrasound evaluation.

A few weeks before the end of the 40-week term, the placenta will be reaching its maximum lifespan or may even have started to exceed it. Over the years, I have seen many placentas that are small for their age, with infarction (tissue death) and signs of calcification. There is a persisting pathology in almost all the placentas of women with autoimmunity that can give rise to fetal distress during labor.

Calcification, or "grittiness," is a sign of placental aging and inflammatory immune activity. The more calcification there is, the less placental tissue will remain to deliver nutrients and oxygen to the baby. Problems arising from placental calcification can include reduced amniotic fluid level, intrauterine growth retardation, and placental abruption. The good news is that with proper monitoring and diagnosis, these complications can often be reduced or prevented with aggressive immune therapy.

Even though immunotherapy can provide something of a safety net, I am convinced there comes a point when it is much safer for the baby to be outside the uterus rather than in it. I have known infants to die in utero at 38 weeks, and babies to become terribly injured by breathing in meconium when mothers have been allowed to labor late. (Meconium is a mixture of the baby's feces and amniotic fluid that can block and irritate the airways.) Babies that are left too long in the womb with a poorly functioning placenta can be starved of oxygen and may face the serious possibility of brain damage or stillbirth.

Because spontaneous labor and fetal distress is most likely to occur in the final two weeks, controlled delivery where labor is scheduled and induced around 38 weeks, is often the safest course of action in many of my patients. At this stage of gestation, the baby is virtually fully grown and able to enter the world healthy and strong.

My own data has shown that for 220 births, the average age at delivery was 37.8 weeks. 50% were delivered by C-section and the average birthweight was 7 lbs 1 oz. For this group, the average age of the mother at conception was 34.4 years. I believe their immune conflicts induced many of these early deliveries.

Despite these potential hazards, some women still believe the best way to bring a baby into the world is in a "natural," low tech environment, without medication and with minimal intervention such as anesthetic or surgery. However, for immune patients, this choice is risky to the point of reckless. I am extremely concerned when I hear a woman say that she wants to stay at home and rely on a midwife for the delivery, or insists on a vaginal birth no matter what. This may be an option for low risk groups – but not for immune patients, who must consider themselves to be in the high risk category.

I will only agree to a natural labor provided my patient is in a hospital environment where specialist nurses and anesthesiologists are available around the clock and emergency procedures can be carried out immediately. A vaginal birth after a previous C-section is also too dangerous for my patients and I urge them not to consider it. Most doctors will argue, but I cannot tolerate dead or damaged babies caused by stress, when I know the medical set up is there to ensure their safe arrival.

The Inherent Risks (and Benefits) of Autoimmunity

Pregnancy loss, infertility and implantation failure can indicate that there are problems in the mother that could be passed on to her child. Because many maternal autoimmune conditions often go undiagnosed, most women would not associate developmental or health problems in their son or daughter with an autoimmune condition that might have been inherited from themselves.

Sadly, today mental health problems affect approximately 10% of U.S. preschool children and according to research, 5% of children aged 6 to 12 are given Ritalin (methylphenidate) to control their hyper-activity. This and other anxiety problems like obsessive compulsive disorder, depression and autism are thought to be autoimmune in origin, as several studies have shown. So, for the sake of children yet to be born, it's really important that you know if your body is baby friendly, and whether there are any immunities that are affecting your own system that could be passed on to your child.

Having studied the progress of many thousands of pregnancies, I have learned that, if the mother has untreated autoimmune problems before she conceives, there is an eight-fold greater likelihood that her child will suffer from hyperactivity, autism or attention deficit disorder. Such immune imbalances in the mother can be successfully treated, with "good antibodies" in the form of IVIG prior to conception and during pregnancy. This precaution greatly reduces the risk of trans-ferring harmful antibodies to the unborn baby.

There is no doubt that the susceptibility to develop an autoimmune disease can be inherited, and affects more women than men. Yet only a few women with this genetic tendency will actually develop a classic autoimmune disorder. If they do, many are still able to become mothers and can even experience a remission of the symptoms during their pregnancy, as in rheumatoid arthritis for example.

Women who do not have an overt autoimmune disease, just an immune system that overreacts when they try to become pregnant, can also benefit from preventative therapy and become mothers of healthy babies. They may have antibodies and hyperactive lymphocytes of the kind seen in autoimmune disease patients, but without any symptoms of illness. However, when these women are observed 26 years after childbearing is finished, I have found that although they may not suffer from classic autoimmune conditions, approximately 15% of them go on to develop a malfunctioning thyroid, 15% develop low serotonin levels and 15% develop gestational or adult onset diabetes; the autoimmune risks are still there.

In the past, I have worried that, through immunotherapy, we may increase the gene pool for autoimmunity. I have monitored mothers long after they have finished their families, with the oldest children in my program now having reached their mid-20s. An analysis of outcomes of several thousand cases did not reveal a higher incidence of serious autoimmune disease or cancer in the mother or her child. In fact, the incidence of cancer was higher in the father of the baby, who was not treated in any way.

It could even be considered that, in some ways, genes for autoimmunity may actually do more good than harm. An aggressive immune system can be a survival mechanism, increasing disease resistance and fighting off cancer. Just as thrombophilia presents certain health risks to the mother and her baby, dying of hemorrhage during childbirth is certainly less likely for a mother with an aggressive clotting system. Moreover, low serotonin and antibodies to hormones and neurotransmitters that induce obsessive thinking, aggressiveness and increased drive may actually be beneficial to many of us struggling in the real world.

These "benefit" cases of autoimmune disease never make it to the doctor's office, so it is possible that we see a negatively skewed overall picture of autoimmune genetics. As I mentioned earlier, many who are genetically prone to autoimmunity may never suffer from it. It is possible that during their lifetime, they find a partner who is completely genetically dissimilar to themselves, or they may never be exposed to any disease trigger, such as a particularly stubborn infection.

Because autoimmunity has survived in the gene pool for thousands of years, there has to be a reason for this and there may be more advantages to autoimmune genetics than we know. That said, one of my objectives has always been to find ways of identifying those whose pregnancies need special vigilance because the mother may carry antibodies that might cause harm. I know for certain, there are at least five categories of immune problem that can afflict couples and their babies. There may be even a sixth or seventh that has yet to be discovered.

I have now collected a huge volume of data on many hundreds of my patients and their infants and compared their wellbeing to those who have not been exposed to immunotherapy. From monitoring the health of the babies born in my program, I can confirm that there have been no new diseases, disorders, growth or developmental problems in the children of immune treated couples compared with those of untreated couples. Other than the fact those who had been under my care took their babies to the pediatrician four times more frequently during the first year than the control group, there were no indications of any major health problems. Scientifically it was almost a bit disappointing that increased parental vigilance was the only significant data to emerge from the analysis.

So this chapter is not a warning about the hazards of having children for those with autoimmunities. It is a reminder of the dangers that can lie in store when their conditions are not recognized, and a positive reassurance that with the right tests and treatment, the health of both the mother and her baby can be ensured.

IS YOUR BODY BABY FRIENDLY?

13

Comprehensive Immune Testing

Several diagnostic procedures should be carried out to determine whether immunological factors are preventing successful pregnancy. Blood tests can detect the presence of antibodies in one or both partners. To identify the cause of a previous miscarriage or stillbirth, the placental tissue sample that was obtained at the time, can also be re-evaluated by an experienced immunopathologist to determine whether immune destruction took place at the pregnancy site itself.

As most of Dr Beer's patients are also under the care of a reproductive endocrinologist, Ob/Gyn or other primary healthcare provider, the patient receives a combination of expertise in regular fertility treatment or gynecological management plus the added benefits of immune evaluation. Such partnered care is possible for all patients, wherever in the world they may live. (Blood samples are regularly shipped to laboratories in the U.S. for testing.)

By studying the patient's health records and analyzing the larger pattern found in blood work, history and tissue, it is possible to accurately deduce which of the five categories of immune problem are present, if any, and formulate the optimum treatment program.

The first step for couples seeking treatment for unexplained infertility or repeated losses is to contact a fertility center that specializes in reproductive immunology. This allows immune problems, if they exist, to be identified first so repeated heartache and expense can be prevented. In some cases, these couples may only require immune therapy to become pregnant naturally and successfully carry their baby to term without having to pay thousands for an IVF cycle.

There are now hundreds of such clinics around the world (most are listed in the Reference Section of this book). Many of these clinics are either run by, or employ doctors with specific training in reproductive immunology. These "top rated" immune educated specialists are the driving forces behind fertility centers with the highest success rates

Leading figures in this field include John Couvaras M.D. at *IVF Phoenix*, Carolyn Coulam, M.D. at *The Reproductive Medicine Institute* in Illinois, Geoffrey Sher at *The Sher Institute for Reproductive Medicine*, Joanne Kwak-Kim M.D. at *Reproductive Medicine and Immunology* in Illionois and Jeffrey Braverman M.D. at *Braverman IVF and Reproductive Immunology* in New York.

In the UK, Dr Mohamed Taranissi, Dr Hassan Shehata and Dr George Ndukwe have been offering their patients immune therapy for years and continue to deliver some of the highest success rates in the UK. And in Canada, Dr Michael Virro at *The Markham Fertility Centre* is demonstrating similarly high success rates.

Despite their more challenging patient caseloads, these centers are maintaining increasingly higher success rates than those where reproductive immunology is not provided, for subjective or commercial reasons; a failed IVF cycle means repeat business.

Despite decades of research and many thousands of supporting studies, there is still a minority of "Luddite" fertility doctors who claim they are not familiar with the science, or worse, refute the whole idea of treating immune issues that have been unequivocally proven to cause pregnancy failure. These seemingly oblivious practitioners continue to subject couples with immune related infertility and loss to years of wasted time, but more unforgivably, successive miscarriages and numerous failed IVF cycles.

According to a 2008 survey of doctors at 217 fertility clinics, show that 93% think the understanding and use of principles of reproductive immunology is important for human reproduction. Yet in around half of fertility clinics worldwide, the solutions that have now been proven for decades are still not being put into practice.

When a miscarriage after IVF is chromosomally normal, 39% of physicians will simply repeat the same IVF protocol and 45% will not modify their approach even after three failed embryo transfers. In the words of Albert Einstein, "The definition of insanity is doing the same thing and expecting different results."

There is also a category of fertility specialist who is "pro" reproductive immunology and will refer couples for blood and/or tissue tests at an earlier stage: after two failed IVF cycles or the loss of one chromosomally normal baby. Patients with autoimmune disorders are also likely to be fast tracked for tests to identify blood clotting disorders and to identify the scale and type of abnormal immune activity. A list of these doctors can be found on the immunology support group's Yahoo website in the Resources section and at the end of this book.

Access to immunotherapy is available to all couples anywhere in the world, providing their Ob/Gyn, fertility doctor or physician is willing to collaborate with a reproductive immunologist at one of the centers listed in this book. Blood can then be shipped to specialist laboratories in the U.S. in thermal packaging which keeps the samples fresh.

To identify the cause of a previous miscarriage or stillbirth, a placental tissue sample from the time the loss occurred can also be re-evaluated by an experienced immunopathologist to determine whether the immune destruction took place at the pregnancy site itself.

By identifying the larger pattern that is revealed through blood work, health records and tissue samples, it is possible to accurately determine any categories of immune problems that may be present and formulate the optimal therapeutic program going forward.

Blood Tests

In an initial immune work up, a series of blood tests are ordered. Blood is drawn into test tubes which have different colored tops to designate the type of test that will be performed. They are then labeled and shipped to specialized testing facilities in the US (although some basic tests are available locally). Most results are available within a week and are sent to the reproductive immunologist's office for assessment. A standard set of immune blood tests includes the following:

Leukocyte Antibody Detection (LAD)*

The Leukocyte Antibody Detection (LAD) test measures the level of antibodies in a woman's blood that react with foreign white blood cells. These antibodies are also called blocking antibodies because they block the woman's immune system from attacking the fetus during normal pregnancy. If the results of this test reveal an inadequate response, the woman will be unable to produce these antibodies, which protect the fetus from rejection and stimulate growth of the placenta.

In this test, the man's white blood cells (leukocytes) are mixed with serum from the woman, and serum antibodies that attach to the leukocytes are marked with a dye. The solution is then placed in a device called a flow cytometer, which channels the cells down a narrow stream of fluid. As they pass in front of the eye of a laser, cells marked with dye are registered by computer. It takes about 10 seconds to collect data on 10,000 cells to see if they have blocking antibodies attached.

The Reproductive Immunophenotype

This is a unique panel of tests originally devised by Dr Beer to determine the concentrations of white blood cells whose percentages, when elevated, are predictors of future pregnancy loss. This applies to infertility patients preparing for IVF or ART (assisted reproductive technologies), women who conceive naturally and suffer repeated miscarriages, or those who are unable to become pregnant. This test is gradually being adopted by other laboratories and includes an analysis of the following:

CD3 (Pan T cells)
Normal Range: 63 – 86%
These cells are among the most important in our immune system. Their percentage is low when the immune system is weak and normal when the immune system is healthy. Infertile patients and patients with recurrent pregnancy losses often have values in the high normal range. Elevated CD3 cell levels are associated with autoimmune diseases such as thyroiditis, SLE and rheumatoid arthritis.

CD4 (T-helper Cells)
Normal Range: 31 – 53%
CD4 T-helper cells plan and direct the various missions of the other lymphocytes. In women with infertility or miscarriage, these cells are in the high normal range. If they are low in number, the patient needs a further immunological evaluation to study the cause of this deficiency, as it could be an indication of a serious health problem (for example, CD4 cells are killed off in those who have AIDS).

CD8 (T-Cytotoxic Suppressors)
Normal Range: 17 – 35%
These cells help to moderate the activity of Th-1 lymphocytes. In women with miscarriage and/or infertility, their percentage is often low.

CD19 (B Cells)
Normal Range: 3 – 8%
Percentages of these cells are usually high normal or very elevated in women with immune mediated infertility or recurrent pregnancy loss, reflecting production of pathological (autoimmune) antibodies.

CD56+/CD16+ Natural Killer Cells
Normal Range: 3 – 12%
Natural killer (NK) cells of this type produce TNF-alpha that kills the rapidly dividing cells of the embryo and placenta, leading to IVF failure, a blighted ovum or a chemical pregnancy. Levels are often elevated in women with infertility and recurrent miscarriage.

CD56+ Natural Killer Cells
Normal Range: 3 – 12%
These NK cells can be activated by a pregnancy that fails or a fertilized embryo that degenerates. Percentages of 12% or greater usually predict a poor reproductive outcome.

CD3/IL-2R+ Cells
Normal Range: 0 – 5%
These cells are usually elevated in patients who reject a kidney or a bone marrow graft. Women who have, or may be developing an autoimmune disease, also have above average levels of these cells.

CD19+/5+ (B-1 Cells)
Normal Range: 2 – 10% of B Cells
CD19+/5+ cells produce, among others, antibodies to hormones and neurotransmitters. Hormones that can be affected by the activity of these antibodies include serotonin, estrogen, progesterone and growth and thyroid hormones.

Patients whose CD19+/CD5+ antibody levels exceed the normal range often stimulate poorly with gonadotropins (e.g., Metrodin-HP, Gonal-F and Follistim). In addition, they may have immunological symptoms such as joint pains, finger stiffness, headache, lethargy, malaise, fever, depression and occasional bouts of hives.

These cells are often elevated in women with autoimmune disorders and in those who reject a bone marrow transplant from a compatible donor. They are also associated with embryonic damage or loss.

Natural Killer Cell Assay
In this assay, NK cells from the woman's blood are separated and cultured at different dilutions with target cells they can kill. For example, when the killing ratio is stated as being 50:1 this means there are 50 times more NK cells than target cells. The target cells used are from an embryonic cancer cell line and have many similarities to placentas and embryos. They are tagged with a dye so that the flow cytometer can detect them.

After two to four hours of culturing the NK cells with the embryo-like targets, the dye will have been taken up only by the DNA of the cells that have been killed. The cell suspensions are then put into the flow cytometer, which precisely counts the percentage of dead to live cells at the different dilutions.

Examples of normal percentages of cells killed would be: 50:1 – 10%, 25:1 – 5% and 12:1 – 2.5%. Examples of abnormal ratios would be: 50:1 – 40%, 25:1 – 20% and 12:1 – 10%. Any killing percentage above 15% will damage the embryo. The aim is to reduce the killing power of the natural killer cells to below 15% before the cycle of conception.

Antinuclear Antibody Test (ANA)

If a patient tests positive or borderline positive for antinuclear antibody (ANA), it is possible that she is suffering from an immune imbalance associated with an undiagnosed autoimmune disease. (This test is often weakly positive in women experiencing infertility or recurrent pregnancy losses.)

An ANA result is considered "positive" when the titer is 1:40 or higher. A "titer" is the measurement of the concentration of an antibody in a solution. The number given shows how many times the fluid has to be diluted before the ANA is no longer detected. A titer of 1:40 shows that it took 40 dilutions of the plasma before the ANA disappeared.

In another experiment, the antibodies in the blood sample are marked with a dye that allows their reaction to various proteins within the nucleus to become apparent under the microscope. Evidence of antibody activity appears as a recognizable constellation or pattern, which is then described as "homogeneous," "nucleolar" or "speckled." Various patterns are associated with autoimmune disorders and/or miscarriage.

Anti-DNA/Histone Antibodies

Strands of DNA wrap themselves around proteins called histones. If antibodies are directed at the histones, they form a speckled pattern. This pattern is associated with autoimmune disorders and/or miscarriage.

Antiphospholipid Antibodies (APA)*

The presence of APA is detected using a test called an "ELISA" (enzyme linked immunosorbent assay). A patient blood sample being tested for antiphospholipid antibody is added to tubes containing specific phospholipids and a dye. If the blood contains a specific antiphospholipid antibody, the antibody will bind to only this one type, changing the color of the test solution.

Specialist laboratories usually test for three classes of antibody (IgG, IgM, and IgA) in relation to six types of phospholipids: cardiolipin, serine, ethanolamine, phosphatidic acid, inositol and glycerol (18 tests total). This far exceeds the level of testing provided by non-specialist laboratories that often only perform the cardiolipin and lupus anticoagulant (LAC) screening tests, missing many important APA diagnoses.

The importance of carrying out the complete 18-test panel cannot be over-emphasized. Any positive APA result means other immune problems may be present, and there is a 50% likelihood of elevated NK cells or Th1:Th2 cytokine ratios (see below).

Lupus Anticoagulant Antibodies (LAC)*

The "lupus anticoagulant" test, an older screening test to evaluate whether the patient has antiphospholipid antibody, can also be performed. These antibodies are commonly found in patients with lupus. However, women who do not have lupus can also produce a positive test result, especially if they are experiencing recurrent pregnancy losses.

The LAC interferes with blood clotting in a test tube by binding to phospholipid. Coagulation tests are used to assess the length of time it takes for blood to clot, such as the "Russell Viper Venom Test". These tests are less sensitive than the APA testing described above.

Antisperm Antibodies

Antibodies to sperm should be suspected if sperm are dead or not moving in the cervical mucus. There are several methods to determine the presence of antisperm antibodies.

If women are experiencing recurrent miscarriage, antisperm antibodies are unlikely to be present because they would block fertilization. Even in women who fail to conceive, antisperm antibodies are less likely to be the cause compared to other abnormalities described in this chapter.

Antiovarian Antibodies

Antibodies that react with ovarian tissue may also cause recurrent pregnancy loss and pregnancy failure. These antibodies can sometimes be associated with structural egg defects that are not detected by chromosomal analysis. In addition , antiovarian antibodies can be associated with elevated TNF-alpha, CD19+/5+ levels and NK cells that can contribute to implantation failure, independent of the poor egg quality. In any case, the presence these antibodies indicates that immune therapy may offer hope for successful pregnancy. Even in cases where donor eggs are needed (and they may be needed only in the more severe cases), women with antiovarian antibodies likely require immunotherapy if successful pregnancy to occur. Donor eggs will fail just as their own if underlying immune imbalances are not corrected also.

Methylene-Tetra-Hydro-Folate-Reductase (MTHFR)

MTHFR metabolizes and eliminates homocysteine. Patients with a defective MTHFR gene cannot process folate properly. If homocysteine levels build up, the risk of arterial and venous thrombosis is increased. When the result for this test is "heterozygous," the defective gene has been inherited from one parent and will be found in just one strand of DNA. If the gene is found to be "homozygous," a mutated gene has been inherited from both parents and will be found in both DNA strands.

The MTHFR defect is detected using the standard polymerase chain reaction (PCR) test. Developed in the early 1990s, the PCR is the most sensitive test there is for analyzing DNA and is a commonly used in the field of forensic science. Enzymes known as polymerases (which are present in all living things) are able to copy genetic material from blood, hair or tissue. Any variations in the DNA copies can then be analyzed for genetic mutations.

Th1:Th2 Cytokine Assay

This assay simply counts the quantities of each type of cell. The result is given as two ratios: The ratio of tumor necrosis factor-alpha (TNF) secreting cells to interleukin 10 (IL-10) secreting cells and the ratio of interferon-gamma (IFN) secreting cells to IL-10 secreting cells.

Depending on the reference laboratory used, the TNF:IL-10 ratio is generally be below 30 and the IFN:IL-10 ratio is generally below 20 before patients are advised to try to conceive.

Other Tests

In addition to the specialized tests detailed above, several others are required to create a full immunological profile. These include tests for serotonin, fasting free insulin, immunoglobulin levels, antithyroid antibodies and thrombophilia (including factor V Leiden and prothrombin gene mutations).

Tests marked* are only provided by specialist reproductive immunology laboratories such as ReproSource Fertility Diagnostics and Rosalind Franklin University Clinical Immunology Laboratory. These tests are often omitted in a standard work up for immunological problems.

Placental Tissue Analysis

"The placental tissue provides a roadmap of the problems that were experienced from the beginning. It also helps us to find out if immune abnormalities existed even before the pregnancy was initiated. It is important that a proper diagnosis is made and that patients are treated appropriately; otherwise, there is a high likelihood they will lose another pregnancy. This evaluation enables us to help our patients end their long journey of disappointment."

Alan E. Beer, M.D.

Unfortunately, most miscarriages do not occur in convenient places like a hospital. Nonetheless, when a miscarriage takes place at home or in a non medical setting, it is still possible to analyze the tissue providing it has been correctly stored. The tissue should be put in a sterile, sealed container in the fridge (not the freezer) and then taken in a cool bag to the doctor's office as soon as possible. It can then be preserved in formalin (formaldehyde) and sent to the laboratory for testing. If a miscarriage is imminent, there may be time to ask for a small jar of the formalin to be provided for home use.

Another option when a pregnancy fails is to have a dilation and curettage (D&C) to remove the pregnancy tissue. In some cases, this is required if the products of conception are not completely expelled during a natural miscarriage, or if there is a significant delay after the diagnosis of a failed pregnancy.

In either case, (natural miscarriage or D&C), the placental tissue can be saved and sent to a pathologist who embeds it into a paraffin block, which is then cut into slices around 5 microns thick (a micron is one thousandth of a millimeter). These sections are stained and examined under a microscope and a basic pathology report is sent to both the patient and her doctor. After the pathology evaluation, the paraffin blocks and slides are saved indefinitely as part of the patient's long term medical record.

Each category of immune problem corresponds with two or three abnormal tissue features that are apparent in the pathology specimen. A great deal of what is determined relies upon the skill and judgment of the immunopathologist, who assesses each specimen drawing upon their experience in interpreting these biopsies.

When a Couple's Tissue Types are Too Similar

Women who have a close genetic match with their partner are more likely to experience problems during the first weeks of pregnancy including:

a) Inadequate invasion of the trophoblast
The early trophoblast is the cell of the embryo that begins to invade or "root" into the uterine lining. This process is very aggressive in a normal pregnancy. The trophoblast grows through the three zones of the endometrium, into the decidua and into the muscle of the uterus. When this process is weak and the placenta attaches incompletely, implantation failure or pregnancy loss will follow. This deficiency can be detected in some pathology specimens.

b) Inadequate blood vessel conversion by the trophoblast

A few days into the pregnancy, the trophoblast is directed to the arteries that have grown into zone three of the endometrium (the layer closest to the endometrial cavity). A maternal blood supply to the fetus is established, at which time some women may experience slight spotting or "implantation bleeding."

The trophoblast grows inside the blood vessels and replaces their linings. It then grows into the muscle of the artery, which prevents it from constricting and shutting off the blood supply to the baby. This process is easily observed in the pathology specimen. If it has not occurred at the proper time and on the proper day, the blood vessel conversion is deemed "inadequate." If it has occurred promptly and is well established, it is judged "adequate."

c) Improper formation of the syncytium

As well as establishing the growth of the placenta, the trophoblast cells adapt to enable food to be transferred to the baby. They fuse together to create a "dialysis" membrane that acts as a filter through which food is passed to the baby and waste is transferred back to the mother. This process is called "syncytium formation" and is simple to detect.

d) Lack of an implantation site

The "intermediate" trophoblast is a collection of cells that "glue" the embryo to the uterus and invade its walls to anchor the placenta. To locate the implantation site, antibodies against the intermediate trophoblast are applied to the tissue. If the implantation site is not found the pathology report may state, "The sample cannot be evaluated because the implantation site is not present." This does not mean the embryo did not implant, it means the implantation site was not seen in the tissue. It may have passed spontaneously, or was not part of the pathology specimen.

Blood Clotting Disorders

Women who have a genetically inherited or acquired blood clotting tendency are more susceptible to implantation failure, miscarriage, preeclampsia and unexplained fetal death. Evidence of inflammation that is associated with thrombophilia can also be detected during placental pathology.

a) Vasculitis of decidual vessels
Vasculitis (in this case, inflammation of the blood vessels that feed the placenta) is caused by the presence of antiphospholipid antibodies.

b) Thrombosis of decidual vessels
Inflammation in the placental blood vessels caused by antiphospholipid antibodies increases the risk of the formation of clots (thrombi). The pathology report will grade this as "extensive," "moderate" or "mild." Any level of thrombosis is too great. Antibodies to the baby and components of placental DNA can cause inflammation in the placenta which is graded "severe," "moderate" or "mild."

Other Signs of Abnormal Immune Activity

When examining a tissue sample that has been preserved following the loss of a pregnancy the pathologist looks for evidence of the following:

a) Decidual necrosis
Necrosis refers to cell or tissue death. This is graded this as "severe," "moderate" or "mild." Decidual necrosis means that the tissue attached to the developing placenta disintegrated.

b) Villitis
Villitis is inflammation in the tissue of the root system of the placenta known as the villus. The inside of the villus contains the blood vessels of the placenta that will eventually join with the larger vessels and the

umbilical cord. Antibodies to DNA can cause inflammation of the entire villus.

c) Intervillositis
When the inflammation is severe it spreads from one villus root to another and there is inflammation between them.

d) Decidual inflammation
This type of tissue and placental injury is similar to that which is seen in patients with antinuclear antibodies. However, the cells that cause the inflammation are not antibodies, they are the monocytes, lymphocytes, plasma cells and granulocytes. The damage they inflict is categorized as "severe," "moderate" or "mild."

e) Fibrin deposition and fibrinoid formation
This analysis can indicate when the injury to the placenta took place. After decidual necrosis, the placenta tries to heal itself by forming scar tissue where the injury has occurred. Fibrin is deposited in the placenta and when it has aged, it forms fibrinoid. This is easily seen in the decidua and placenta and is reported as being "severe," "moderate," "mild" or "absent."

f) Trophoblast morphology
The placenta has many different structures that enable it to attach to the uterine wall (similar to the way a plant puts down roots). Seven or eight different cell types and "root" structures are involved. Their overall form (morphology) is easy to see under the microscope and is described as "normal" or "abnormal." Abnormal morphology can be caused by the immune attack and/or a genetic abnormality that is incompatible with life. If a chromosomal problem is suspected, a high resolution process known as the FISH procedure is likely to confirm its presence.

14

Immunotherapies

The following treatments work across a range of problems can be combined as to address the various abnormalitites associated with autoimmune mediated reproductive failure. Not all these therapies will be required, as each patient's treatment plan or "protocol" is designed according to their blood test results, uterine tissue analysis and history. In some cases several months of therapy may be needed before a patient is cleared for conception. However, many women may only require immunotherapy – with or without IVF – during the month in they are trying to conceive.

The treatments described here are not necessarily all provided at the Alan E. Beer Center. They have been included to ensure that this book provides a comprehensive a resource in a field that is highly complex and rapidly evolving. Therefore, the effective and safe practice of clinical reproductive immunology should only be carried out by clinicians who are constantly absorbing the latest research advances in immunology, reviewing the literature, attending meetings and engaging with other immunologists.

Intravenous Immunoglobulin G (IVIG)

"IVIG is a powerful and safe tool to modulate abnormal responses of the immune system. It is used for patients who need immune rejuvenation and has the wonderful property of lessening rejection reactions in patients with transplants. It also calms autoimmune damaging responses in patients with diseases like rheumatoid arthritis by decreasing the natural killer function by 50%, although this is short lived and subsequent infusions are usually required."

Alan E. Beer, M.D.

Immunoglobulins are antibodies that are made by the B cells. Immunoglobulin G is found in most tissues and plasma. It is the most abundant of all the immunoglobulins, being the antibody for viruses and bacteria.

Since 1981, intravenous immunoglobulin G (IVIG) has been given to patients with viral infections, immune deficiencies and autoimmune disorders to modulate their immune response and bring their immunoglobulin levels within normal range. It is also routinely used to help prevent the rejection of transplanted organs and bone marrow.

IVIG is made from the blood of up to 50,000 healthy donors. After being washed and processed to remove the red blood cells, the remaining clear serum, composed primarily of IgG antibodies, is screened for a range of infections including hepatitis and HIV. It is then drip fed through a catheter inserted into a vein in the top of the hand or lower arm, via a process called infusion.

IVIG floods the body with "good" antibodies that combat the effects of those that are harmful, thereby helping to protect the embryo or fetus from rejection. It also assists in controlling activated T cells, which are major producers of Th1 cytokines. As a potent suppressor of NK cells, it shifts the Th1:Th2 balance to the more baby friendly Th2 state. Furthermore, IVIG helps to deactivate the B cells that produce the autoantibodies associated with poor reproductive performance.

It is prescribed for patients when:

- The NK cell assay cytotoxicity 50:1 is over 15%
- The CD56 NK cell assay numbers are over 12%
- Th1:Th2 and TNFa:IL-10 ratios are over 30 (or in some cases over 20)
- CD19+/5+ cell levels are over 10% of total B cells
- There are low levels of blocking antibodies (determined by the LAD test)
- There is a high titer ANA result
- There is a positive test for antithyroid antibodies
- Intrauterine growth retardation is associated with an immune etiology
- Low amniotic fluid is linked to an immune etiology
- The patient experiences a subchorionic hemorrhage or hematoma
- The patient has an active autoimmune disease

- APAs have not responded to treatment with heparin, corticosteroids and low dose aspirin
- The patient has antibodies to ethanolamine or serine
- A replacement for steroid treatment is needed
- Implantation failure continues despite corticosteroid treatment

At present, the most consistently effective treatment for reducing NK cell numbers and activity for both IVF and recurrent miscarriage patients is IVIG. The key active ingredient of protective antibodies in IVIG varies between bags from the same manufacturer. It occurs in much higher concentrations when the serum is collected from women who have had normal pregnancies. (Interestingly, the rejection rate in kidney transplant patients is lower when IVIG from pregnant women is used.)

In addition, there are differences between various IVIG products. For example, eight times more of Bayer's Gamimune infusion is needed to achieve the same immune suppression as Baxter's Gammagard. Furthermore, studies have also shown that if IGM antibodies are collected they are a much stronger active ingredient than the IGG rich antibody product that is commercially available today. Dr Braverman at *Braverman IVF and Reproductive Immunology* in New York is working on these issues to improve the efficacy and quality of IVIG. With an IGM product higher success rates should be possible using lesser quantities which equates to a lower cost.

Administration

IVIG is usually prescribed at 400 mg/kg body weight with dosing frequency determined by NK cell number and activity, antibody levels and other determining factors. A qualified nurse gives the infusion, which takes around three hours. During the first stage of the infusion, an antihistamine product such as Benadryl is normally given intravenously to minimize the chances of an allergic response.

One or more treatments may be required during a cycle of conception, depending on the severity of a patient's immune problems. Because the effects of IVIG are transient, the procedure may need to be repeated every 21-28 days during pregnancy.

The NK cell assay is carried out 7 to 10 days after each infusion. When there are two normal results three to four weeks apart, the therapy can be stopped, although testing is still continued monthly. This is because around 15% of women can develop activated NK cells after 24 weeks and may require further infusions.

It is important to note that not all IVIG infusions are the same. For example, eight times more Gamimune is needed to achieve the suppression of Gammagard.

Side effects

Before the first treatment, a patient's IgA levels must be tested. In the rare event that IgA levels are low, IVIG is not administered as it may cause kidney damage or anaphylactic shock.

IVIG is usually well tolerated, although a few patients may experience headaches, chills or flu-like symptoms. These side effects are usually short lived and often relate to the rate of infusion. When the rate is slowed down, the symptoms tend to subside. Subsequent infusions are normally better tolerated.

IVIG can be safely administered during pregnancy; as Dr Beer testifies: "IVIG is totally safe for the baby and protects its life. It is also given to newborns with weak immune systems." Indeed, there is much written on the beneficial "immune re-booting" effects of IVIG as those who receive it will have fewer, milder, more controllable infections than they had before starting the therapy. These protective antibodies will remain in the circulation for 3-4 weeks.

Over two million IVIG administrations have been carried out in the U.S. for a range of conditions without a single transmission of HIV. The Beer Center prescribes more than a thousand infusions a year and reports that serious complications are extremely rare.

Intralipid

Intralipid is an emulsion containing essential fatty acids Omega 3 and Omega 6 that helps remove the danger signals that over activate the immune system that contributes to IVF and implantation failure. Made from a mixture of 10% soybean oil, 1.2% egg yolk phospholipids, 2.25% glycerin and water, intralipid is approximately 10 times less expensive than IVIG. Its other appeal is that it's not a blood product and therefore comes without the perceived, albeit negligible, risk of disease transfer.

Fertility centers who have adopted this therapy are seeing very impressive results. For example, at The Sher Institute for Reproductive Medicine over 60% of the patients achieved viable ongoing pregnancies, prompting the center to virtually abandon its use of IVIG in favor of intralipid claiming that it performs as well and if not better than its more costly counterpart for increasing IVF success rates. However, data from the Beer Center suggests that it is not as effective at preventing later pregnancy complications such as recurrent miscarriage, preterm birth and preeclampsia, as its more expensive counterpart IVIG.

Nonetheless, some fertility centers report great success using a combination of intralipid plus Neupogen® injections to reduce inflammatory cytokines, enhance the uterine lining and improve egg quality.

Administration

An intralipid infusion via a drip in the arm to is given 7 to 10 days before embryo transfer to reduce NK cell activity associated with auto-immune issues such as antiphospholipid antibodies and/or antithyroid antibodies. Another infusion is given after a positive pregnancy test. In cases where a couples' genetic material is too similar these infusions are repeated at 2 to 4 weekly intervals until the 24th week of pregnancy. The procedure takes around 3 to 4 hours and is usually administered in the patient's home by a trained nurse.

N.B: Patients who are allergic to eggs or soybean oil should never be given intralipid for obvious reasons.

Side Effects

Side effects include fever, shivering and chills (rare) and nausea or vomiting (affecting less than 1% of patients). In such cases, the infusion should be discontinued. Adverse effects occurring in less than 1 in a million infusions include anaphylaxis, skin rash and urticaria, rapid breathing, circulatory effects (high or low blood pressure), abdominal pain, headache and tiredness. Overall, intralipid is considered to be extremely safe.

Neupogen®
(filgrastim, G-CSF or C-GSF)

Neupogen® is a man-made form of granulocyte colony-stimulating factor (G-CSF), a substance naturally produced by the body. It stimulates the growth of neutrophils, a type of white blood cell important in the body's fight against infection. It is usually used for cancer patients to help increase white blood cells that are depleted by chemotherapy.

Neupogen® has been shown to increase the number of good quality eggs during an IVF cycle. Recent studies have shown that the best quality eggs come from the follicles with the highest level of G-CSF. Patients treated with Neupogen® have higher pregnancy rates and higher average pregnancy hormone levels, most likely due to a a more robust initiation of placental development.

Neupogen® also also prevents the maturation of the dendritic cells in the uterine lining. When dendritic cells are mature they take information about the embryo to the lymph nodes and present it in a way that causes the mother's immune system to mount a response against the embryo.

It has also been shown to increase the thickness of uterine lining in women who have previously failed to achieve a minimum thickness of 8mm prior to an embryo transfer.

Administration

In cancer patients a whole vial (300 mcg or 480 mcg) is usually administered daily. The off-label use of Neupogen® as a treatment for infertility and miscarriage involves a much smaller dose based on the patient's weight. Protocols are still being developed, but here are a few examples:

1. A subcutaneous dose of 100 mg/day started at 6th day after ovulation. The patient is assessed by ultrasound and treatment is continued until the 35th day after ovulation for a total of about 30 consecutive days.

2. 10 to 13 injections starting at the beginning of a natural conception cycle or the day after transfer of an IVF cycle.

3. 100 mg/day starting from 3 days before ovulation.

Side Effects

This drug has been used at low doses to treat women with immune related pregnancy failure since the 1990s. To date studies have shown no significant risk to mother or baby exposed to this drug.

Lymphocyte Immunization Therapy (LIT)

"LIT does one thing: it induces antibodies to paternal T and B cells, the same immunity that occurs naturally in women who have delivered a full term liveborn child. It does not cripple you or cause you to be at risk for other problems."

Alan E. Beer, M.D.

LIT is an immunization procedure using white blood cells extracted from the blood of the male partner or a donor's blood. Prior to the procedure, blood from the patient and her partner is screened for HIV1, HIV2, hepatitis A, hepatitis B, hepatitis C, cytomegalovirus and others. The "vaccine" is then prepared at a specialist facility where the blood is washed three times with sterile saline and the CD3 T cells and CD19 B cells are isolated by centrifugion. The final volume of less than 0.6 cc of prepared cells in suspension is then injected under the surface of the woman's skin.

This treatment will usually result in the formation of blocking antibodies in the recipient, a reduction in NK cell killing power and a shift from a Th1 to a Th2 cytokine immune response. This combined effect lessens the impact of all five categories of immune problem and is used to treat:

• Low blocking antibody levels (LAD test IgG T cells or IgG B cells are below   50%)
• Elevated number of CD56 NK cells (above 12%)
• Elevated NK cytotoxicity (NK cell 50:1 activity above 15%)

Administration

The cell preparation is injected just under the skin. Four injections are usually given – two on each forearm. About five or six days later, the injected areas will itch slightly, like a positive allergy test. The reaction will "peak" at around 10 to 12 days.

A month later, the process is repeated and is typically followed by a milder response. The leukocyte antibody detection (LAD) assay is then performed. This two part test will determine if the woman has made blocking antibodies to her partner's T and B cells. If a positive result is not achieved after the first immunizations, booster paternal immunizations are recommended. Alternatively, donor lymphocytes (which are also screened for transferable viruses) may be mixed with the male partner's lymphocytes to produce a stronger immune response.

The effects of LIT will last for six months, after which "booster" immunizations can be given to extend its benefits for a further six months. If pregnancy is achieved, treatment may be administered every five to seven weeks to control NK activity and boost blocking antibody levels to keep the baby immunologically protected.

LIT is currently not approved by the USA Food and Drug Administration, however it is available in many countries outside of the U.S. such as the UK, Canada and is standard treatment in Europe and Asia.

Side effects

Commonly reported side effects include a raised itchy red rash at the injection site that may last for around two weeks. In very rare cases, cellulitis may develop (a spreading skin infection, which can be accompanied by chills and sweats). However, a survey of over 4,500 women who had used LIT from 1996 to 2003 found no incidence of serious side effects, and there were no reported cases of anaphylaxis, autoimmune disease or graft versus host disease following LIT.

Corticosteroids
(Prednisone & Dexamethasone)

Steroids are naturally occurring fat soluble hormones that are made in the adrenal gland. Synthetic versions of these chemicals are produced from a man-made form of cortisone, which gives these drugs their generic name of "corticosteroids." The therapeutic dose is much larger than the amount of cortisone that is normally present in the body. As a result, the minor functions of the hormone become exaggerated in order to decrease the release of cytokines by the white blood cells. (These drugs are not the same as anabolic steroids, which can be misused for the purpose of weight gain and muscle building.)

Corticosteroids have been used for over 50 years to treat inflammatory and autoimmune disorders. They are also commonly used to promote fetal lung maturity in premature babies and to prevent graft rejection. As a conventional treatment for autoimmunity, corticosteroids can relieve the symptoms of severe allergies, arthritis, lupus and other types of rheumatic diseases. They also help inhibit NK cell activity and provide an effective "first base" treatment for women with elevated levels of antinuclear antibodies.

Their beneficial effect is associated with a reduction of inflammation as well as some moderate suppression of the immune response. When NK cell activity is aggressive, additional IVIG and/or anti-TNF-alpha therapy is normally required.

Prednisone and Prednisolone
(Methylprednisolone)

The body naturally produces the equivalent of 8 mg per day of prednisone which suppresses the inflammatory process. Some reproductive immunologists will prescribe prednisone or prednisolone, which although not quite identical drugs, are used in the same way. Prednisone does not pass through the placenta easily and the small quantity that does get through is broken down by enzymes, so the fetus is only exposed to trace amounts.

Dexamethasone

"I use dexamethasone in the NK assay to prevent the NK cells from undergoing cell division and increasing in number. "

Alan E. Beer, M.D.

Although prednisone therapy is a moderately effective means of depressing NK cell activity, dexamethasone is better at restricting NK cell division and it is generally better tolerated than prednisone. Dexamethasone can have a positive impact on ovarian response and follicular development by reducing the production of androgens (male sex hormones) by the adrenal glands.

Administration

Corticosteroids are normally taken a few weeks before the time of conception. In general, the lowest possible effective dose is prescribed. For example, with prednisone, the dosage is described as "low dose" at less than 10 mg a day, medium at 10 to 20 mg a day and high at more than 20 mg a day. The medication is taken in the morning (with or after breakfast to avoid irritating the stomach) to follow the body's own natural rhythm of cortisone production.

Early successes for the treatment of immune induced reproductive failure were reported with high dose corticosteroids (40 mg prednisone daily) and low dose aspirin. However, long term exposure to high doses of steroids can have adverse side effects. As treatment lasting more than three months is regarded as long term, and these drugs can be taken for up to 24 weeks of pregnancy, more moderate doses of prednisone (10-20 mg/day) or dexamethasone (1 mg/day) are usually prescribed. (One mg of dexamethasone is equivalent to approximately 7 mg of prednisone.)

Side Effects

All corticosteroids cross the placenta, some more than others, which is why physicians are very careful when prescribing them during pregnancy. Corticosteroid exposure in animal experiments has shown an increased incidence of cleft palate and other pregnancy complications, such as intrauterine growth restriction and shortening of the head and the lower jaw. However, as human doses are lower than those used in experiments, most studies of women who have taken corticosteroids during pregnancy do not show a large risk.

In a survey of literature on corticosteroid use and birth defects from 1952 to 1994, the frequency of malformations in the offspring of 475 patients was 3.5%, which included two cases of cleft palate. The incidence of cleft palate and/or cleft lip is about 1 or 2 per 1,000 for steroid users, compared to 1 per 2,500 in the general population.

Steroids can also increase the appetite and cause extra fat to be deposited around the abdomen. Patients are therefore advised to be careful about their calorie intake and exercise regularly when taking these drugs. In rare cases, corticosteroids can induce gestational diabetes and a monthly fasting blood sugar testing is sometimes needed while on this medication.

Dexamethasone can also increase the blood pressure in sensitive individuals and may occasionally induce an insulin reaction if blood glucose levels fall excessively, although this is only likely when taken in addition to drugs that stimulate insulin production.

With long term use, corticosteroids can have a bone thinning effect, which is why it is important to take them with a calcium supplement of 500 mg twice a day. A good quality multivitamin containing vitamin D will help the body to absorb the calcium.

Another important point to remember is that the body can become temporarily reliant on these drugs if they are taken for more than two weeks. Abrupt withdrawal may result in corticosteroid insufficiency symptoms such as fatigue, weakness, nausea, vomiting, and hypertension. Therefore, the dose should be tapered down before it is discontinued completely.

Regular Molecular Weight Heparin
(Multiparin)

Regular molecular weight or "unfractionated" heparin is a natural, water soluble anticoagulant. Developed in the 1940s, it was the first generation of heparin compounds, and even today it is sometimes used for anticoagulation therapy when surgical procedures are required. However, its use has largely been replaced by therapy with low molecular weight heparin (see below).

Administration

This drug is usually injected subcutaneously (although in other medical situations it can be given intravenously). 5,000 units are normally administered once or twice daily, starting on day 6 of the cycle of conception. An initial trial dose of 1,000 units is advised before the therapeutic dose to make sure there are no adverse reactions, although allergy to heparin is uncommon.

Side Effects

As regular heparin inhibits many factors in the coagulation cascade, it is associated with a slightly higher risk of bleeding problems than the more modern heparins. As with the low molecular weight varieties described earlier, bruising at the injection site is very common.

Long term use of unfractionated heparin has been associated with osteoporosis and spontaneous fractures in patients receiving more than 15,000 units a day for more than six months. However, at lower doses these risks are diminished, though calcium supplementation is still recommended. Regular heparin is a large molecule that does not cross the placenta and appears safe for the fetus. Furthermore, it cannot be transferred to the baby through breast milk.

Low Molecular Weight Heparin
(Lovenox, Clexane, Fragmin & Arixtra)

"Lovenox does not thin the blood and make you a bleeder; it just keeps your blood from clotting too quickly. Lovenox and a newer, synthetic variety called Arixtra are far superior to standard heparin and are associated with fewer pregnancy complications in the mother and the baby than when regular heparin is used."

Alan E. Beer M.D.

Low molecular weight heparins like Lovenox and Fragmin emerged in the late 1980s and are more purified forms of heparin. Their main advantage is their predictable anti-coagulant activity, reduced incidence of bleeding and increased safety in pregnancy. For those with inherited thrombophilia, regular heparin may be not be the best choice as it does not diffuse through the placenta as effectively as these newer varieties to reduce the risk of placental abruption during the second trimester.

Low molecular weight heparins, including a synthetic version called Arixtra, are prescribed for patients with acquired and/or inherited forms of thrombophilia. Arixtra (Fondaparinux sodium) is another manmade anticoagulant that works by inhibiting just a small part of the coagulation cascade and, like Lovenox and Fragmin it is highly effective in preventing deep vein thrombosis. However, unlike the other heparin formulas, Arixtra is not manufactured from animal products, so it is less likely to cause an allergic reaction.

Administration

A typical dose of Lovenox or Clexane would be 30 or 40 mg once or twice a day administered as a subcutaneous injection (just underneath the skin). For Arixtra, the dose is usually 2.5 mg daily or 5 mg in exceptional cases. Injections are started on day 6 of the cycle of conception. In IVF, they are stopped the night prior to the egg retrieval and are restarted immediately after the procedure.

Patients with inherited or acquired thrombophilia usually take these drugs through the first trimester of pregnancy or beyond, depending on their history and follow up test results. Some patients may continue to take these blood thinners throughout gestation to avoid fetal complications that may arise from placental blood clotting.

Side Effects
Almost all patients experience some bruising at the injection site, but in the doses that are prescribed, there is a low risk of uncontrolled bleeding. In some cases, however, heparin can cause an allergic reaction with symptoms that may include hives, chills, fever, dermatitis, asthma or, very rarely, anaphylactic shock. These potential side effects are significantly reduced with Arixtra, which is a synthetic formula.

Even though there is a very low risk of osteoporosis with the low molecular weight heparins and Arixtra, patients are still advised to take a daily calcium supplement to protect against this potential side effect. Routine monitoring to check, for example, blood platelet counts and antiphospholipid antibody levels is also recommended for the duration of this therapy. When used correctly, the administration of these anticoagulants in pregnancy is generally considered safe.

75 mg or 81 mg "Low dose" Aspirin

Aspirin is an inexpensive, widely used over-the-counter drug, yet it is still an important addition to most immune treatment protocols. Aspirin is a non-steroidal anti-inflammatory drug that works at a different level than heparin to stop platelets from clumping together and causing a clot. It also assists in widening the blood vessels by relaxing their walls. The result is improved blood flow and circulation around the body, including the uterus and ovaries. A randomized clinical trial carried out at the Harvard Medical School hospital in 2004 has also demonstrated that low dose aspirin triggers the body to generate its own anti-inflammatory compounds to fight inflammation and disease.

Aspirin therapy has been shown to produce better implantation and pregnancy rates in trials. Improved IVF cycle outcomes have also been seen when it is taken during the ovarian stimulation phase.

Aspirin therapy is usually started on cycle day 6 of the cycle of conception and taken throughout the entire pregnancy. Although aspirin is able to cross the placenta, the dose is so small that the fetus is unlikely to be affected. Indeed, there is currently no evidence to show that aspirin exposure causes fetal abnormalities. However, it has demonstrated a beneficial effect, by significantly reducing the incidence of stillbirth and preeclampsia.

Administration

To protect the stomach from excess acidity, soluble forms of low dose aspirin are dissolved in water before they are taken. Those labeled "enteric coated" can be swallowed whole as they have a special outer layer that acts as a buffer to protect the stomach and prevent the drug from being absorbed too quickly. Antacids (indigestion remedies) should not be taken at the same time as aspirin.

Side Effects

In approximately 2.5% of people who take this drug (compared to 1.4% who do not), aspirin therapy carries a risk of bleeding or ulceration of the stomach or intestines. It should therefore be avoided by anyone with stomach ulcers or a known bleeding tendency. The risk of side effects is slightly increased when it is taken in addition to corticosteroids. In rare incidences, aspirin may cause gastrointestinal problems.

Sildenafil Citrate
(Vaginal Viagra)

Viagra has been shown to increase blood flow to the uterus as well as thickening its lining. When there are problems in these areas, particularly in women with endometriosis, healthy embryos fail to implant, resulting in multiple failed IVF attempts and chronic infertility. Treatment with Sildenafil Citrate has been known to help women conceive naturally, thus avoiding IVF altogether.

Administration

20 - 25mg sildenafil vaginal suppositories are inserted high in the vagina four times a day for up to a week, starting soon after the end of a menstrual cycle. (A local pharmacy can prepare these suppositories using oral tablets.) When absorbed vaginally, Viagra immediately enters the uterine blood circulation in a high concentration to improve blood flow and estrogen delivery to the inner endometrial lining. In an IVF cycle, the embryos are transferred a week after treatment.

Side Effects

When administered orally, Viagra absorbs from the upper gastro-intestinal tract and enteres the systemic circulation. In women with coronary, neural or peripheral vascular disease, it can result in serious complications. The adverse effects of oral sildenafil citrate include headache, flushing, blurring of vision, nausea, and dyspepsia.

Administered as a suppository there are few if any side clinical effects except for very rare cases of vaginal irritation.

Anti-TNF Agents
(Enbrel, Humira and Simponi)

"Humira is an antibody that has a human sequence that is only directed against the TNF-alpha molecules that kill or cause disease. We simply do what pregnancy does naturally early on, so that the baby can live long enough to establish its own down regulation of the immune system through the placental production of Inter-leukin-10. Once a woman becomes pregnant, the placenta of the baby will produce IL-10 to moderate aggressive immune activity for the remainder of the pregnancy."

Alan E. Beer, M.D.

TNF blockers Enbrel® (etanercept), Humira® (adalimumab) and Simponi® (golimumab) were originally developed for the treatment of rheumatoid arthritis. By blocking the action of TNF-alpha, these drugs tip the immune balance from a Th1-dominated, to a more baby friendly Th2 state, which encourages successful implantation and reduces the risk of miscarriage. In patients with cytokine damaged eggs, anti-TNF-alpha medications are usually taken for several months until healthy eggs are produced.

TNF blockers are recommended when the patient has:
- Elevated Th1:Th2 ratio on the cytokine assay (TNF:IL-10 ratio over 30 and/or INF:IL-10 ratio over 13)
- Failed past cycles with LIT and IVIG

To ensure that the correct time is given to try to conceive naturally or embark on an IVF cycle, the patient's Th1:Th2 ratio is monitored at regular intervals. The highest IVF success rates are seen in patients when anti-TNF-alpha medications are taken preconception and IVIG is given before the embryo transfer.

Administration
Enbrel is self administered by subcutaneous injection once or twice a week. Humira is self administered by subcutaneous injection once every two weeks. Simponi is self administered by subcutaneous injection once a month. At the end of the prescribed course, a blood test is performed two weeks after the final injection to evaluate the Th1:Th2 cytokine ratio.

All TNF blockers must be stored in a refrigerator and kept cool during transportation (i.e., stored in an insulated bag with an ice pack). They should never be frozen or left in direct sunlight.

Side Effects
Because TNF blockers suppress the immune system, those with active infections should not start treatment until they have recovered. Due to an increased risk of infection, a negative test for tuberculosis (skin test or blood test) must be provided before these medications can be prescribed.

The most common side effects are injection site reactions, upper respiratory and sinus infections, rashes and headaches. Other side effects can include joint pain and/or flu-like symptoms and fatigue for the first 30 days, dizziness, queasiness and night sweats. In rare cases, these drugs may cause heart palpitations or high blood pressure. However, the majority of patients remain unaffected. Positive health effects include increased energy and decreased joint pain. Symptoms reported by fertility patients include longer cycles, delayed ovulation, mid-cycle spotting and heavier menstrual flow.

There have been rare cases of certain kinds of lymphomas in patients taking Humira, Enbrel and other TNF blockers. To date, however, there has been no evidence of lymphomas in more than 1,000 Beer Center patients treated with short-course TNF blockers.

The data suggest that these drugs do not affect the fetus in the first trimester, but as the pregnancy continues more of the medication is able to cross the placenta. To err on the side of caution, these drugs are usually prescribed pre-conception.

Metformin (Glucophage)

Metformin is used to regulate blood sugar levels. As well as reducing the amount of glucose produced by the liver, it reduces the amount of glucose that is absorbed from food and allows insulin to process it more effectively in the blood.

This drug is prescribed for the treatment of non insulin dependent diabetes mellitus or type 2 diabetes. It can decrease insulin resistance, reduce abdominal obesity in some cases, and contribute to weight control by suppressing the appetite. Metformin can also help to promote ovulation, restore fertility, improve uterine blood flow and lining thickness and decrease miscarriage rates in women with PCOS. One study has reported an ongoing pregnancy success rate for this patient group of 83% with metformin versus 34% without. Metformin is considered safe to take during pregnancy.

Side Effects

The dose that is usually prescribed is 500 mg twice a day. Up to 20% of women taking metformin experience abdominal discomfort, cramping, diarrhea and nausea, which is more likely to occur during the first few weeks. To help avoid these symptoms, tablets should be taken with a full glass of water at mealtime. As a decrease in vitamin B12 may also occur with metformin (associated with anemia), it is advisable to accompany this medication with vitamin B12 supplements.

FaBB
(Folic acid 2.2 mg)

This high dose vitamin supplement is prescribed for those with inherited thrombophilia and in particular the MTHFR genetic mutations (C677T and A1298C). Studies have shown that increasing folic acid intake can reduce homocysteine levels and help protect against thrombosis and high blood pressure. Folic acid supplementation can also reduce the risk of neural tube defects such as spina bifida, and improve the baby's health in general.

FaBB replaces Folgard RX, which has been discontinued. It contains three major vitamins: folic acid 2.2 mg, vitamin B6 25 mg and vitamin B12 500 mcg.

Administration
FaBB tablets should always be taken with a meal. The usual dose is one tablet daily for those who are heterozygous for the MTHFR genetic mutation (one inherited gene) and two a day for those who are homozygous (with two inherited genes).

Side Effects
In rare instances, FaBB may cause diarrhea or drowsiness. An allergic reaction is unlikely.

Vitamin D
(ergocalciferol-D2, cholecalciferol-D3, alfacalcidol)

Vitamin D is a fat soluble vitamin which belongs to the steroid hormone family. There are two main forms: vitamin D2, which you can get through your diet and vitamin D3 that you synthesize after sun exposure which represents 95% of your vitamin D production.

Women who do not get enough direct sun exposure or have dark skin are at risk for vitamin D deficiency. People with digestive problems like celiac disease, liver problems, or Crohn's disease are also more likely to require supplementation.

Research has shown that sufficient vitamin D levels reduce the risk of miscarriage in women who have suffered previous losses. A lack of this vitamin D also plays a significant role in autoimmune disease and other inflammatory disorders such as endometriosis and pre-eclampsia.

Calcitriol, the active form of vitamin D, influences over 900 genes including those that regulate cell growth, the immune response and cell death. Vitamin D and its receptors are present in the ovaries where they stimulate the production of estrogen and progesterone. The uterus also synthesizes the active form of vitamin D, so a major deficiency can adversely affect pregnancy outcome.

Administration

A 25(OH)D blood test to determine vitamin D concentrations must be carried out before supplementation.

Guidelines from the Institute of Medicine increased the recommended dietary allowance of vitamin D to 600 international units (IU) for everyone ages one to seventy and 800 IU for adults older than seventy to optimize bone health.

The safe upper limit is 4,000 IU but doctors may prescribe more than this to correct a vitamin D deficiency. Cholecalciferol is considered safe to use during pregnancy when used at therapeutic levels. Cholecalciferol supplements are usually taken once a day with food. Regular blood tests are required to check calcium levels when taking this medicine.

Side effects

Women should not self medicate with vitamin D supplements before or during pregnancy unless they are supervised by a qualified medical professional. It is possible to overdose on vitamin D which can lead to too much calcium building up in the body, which can weaken bones and damage the heart and kidneys. Excessive consumption of vitamin D has been associated with fetal abnormalities in animals at doses 4 to 15 times of those recommended for human use.

Other potential side effects associated with overdoseage include loss of appetite, nausea, vomiting, diarrhea and increased thirst, headache, fainting and lack of energy, increased sweating, itching, rash and hives, increased urination and excessive urinary calcium excretion.

IMPORTANT

Patients should always carry identification stating which drugs they are taking and the amount and frequency of administration. Doctors and dentists should also be informed of these treatments. Any concerning side effects should be reported to the patient's prescribing doctor immediately.

IS YOUR BODY BABY FRIENDLY?

"Innovators are rarely received with joy and established authorities launch into condemnation of newer truths; for at every crossroads to the future, are a thousand self appointed guardians of the past."

Betty MacQuitty
Victor over Pain: Morton's Discovery of Anaesthesia

"People with infertility and pregnancy losses have taught me so much and have provided the solid data that has pointed the way to successful treatment and parenthood for them. This data is sacred to me and makes it easy for me to smile at 'the self appointed guardians of the past' who have given my work mixed reviews on occasion."

Alan E. Beer, M.D.

IS YOUR BODY BABY FRIENDLY?

15

Immunotherapy:
Rejected by a Body of Opinion

New ideas in the fields of science and medicine go through a succession of stages before they are accepted. Ridicule is followed by violent opposition before the whole concept is finally accepted as evident. Since 2006, when this book was first published, reproductive immunology is closer to the final stage. According to data collected from 434 fertility doctors around the world, 93% think "the understanding and use of principles of reproductive immunotherapy is important for human reproduction."

However, the pace of change in day to day practice is still not fast enough. for. In their bid to take home a baby, those suffering from chronic infertility or recurrent miscarriage still have to enlist the help of reproductive immunologists via an online search, indicating that there is still a desperate need for immune testing and treatment that is not being met at a grass roots level.

In her book entitled *Miscarriage, What Every Woman Needs to Know*, Professor Lesley Regan describes how doctors have to look their patients in the eye after their "umpteenth" miscarriage and tell them the only advice they can offer is to "keep on trying because they have no idea why it happened."

Half of Dr Beer's patients were self referred at that time because their doctors refused to accept an association between pregnancy failure immune dysfunction. And unbelievably today, reproductive immunotherapy is still being dismissed as pseudo science by some so called "experts" with some even threatening legal action against its practitioners.

Dr Beer, during his lifetime, was quite bewildered by the hostility that was directed towards this field of medicine and him personally. He commented, "These doctors have dismissed immune reasons for infertility and miscarriage yet they believe in immune responses to everything else. I simply do not understand it."

One element that may contribute to the opposition to reproductive immunology is the fact that it threatens the booming multi billion dollar infertility treatment market. In many cases, women are able to bypass IVF, which can cost upwards of $20k per cycle, and sustain a successful pregnancy using immunotherapy alone for a fraction of the expense.

For women with immune disorders, IVF is unlikely to be successful without the additional treatment they require. In the worst case scenarios, the woman ends up with an emotionally devastating miscarriage or keeps repeating the same ineffective IVF protocol until she is financially and emotionally drained.

Professor Rob Norman who pioneered frozen egg technology says, "There's the phenomenon of the IVF treadmill. You just keep running on it and can't get off. My estimate is that probably 40 to 50% of people can get pregnant without IVF... by tracking their fertility cycle, losing weight... or getting assessed properly." According to Dr Beer's data, 30% of IVF patients are able to get pregnant on their own when treated immunologically."

Dr Geoffrey Sher, Medical Director of the Sher Institute for Reproductive Medicine (SIRM) describes the reproductive immunology controversy as a "political football." He has noted how the same critics that disputed immunological factors as being involved in recurrent miscarriage have now turned their attention to the IVF arena to discredit immunological testing and treatments. Unfortunately, it is ultimately the patient who suffers, as the following experiences demonstrate:

Experience no.1
After my third successive miscarriage we were interviewing potential Ob/Gyns to work with Dr Beer. One told met, "Immune issues are nothing to worry about because every time a miscarriage occurs it's due to genetic reasons." This was said while our normal genetic karyotyping report was sitting in front of her. She told me that Dr Beer was "a quack who would take my money and provide no help." My follow up question was, "Exactly how many patients have you helped with my condition and how much research have you had published on the subject of recurrent miscarriage?" Silence followed.

Experience no.2

We were working with Dr Beer and my lab reports were on the doctor's desk. They showed that the only thing that I had tested positive for were immune issues, nothing genetic, hormonal, or infectious. He told me, "Your problem is obviously genetic and you should consider IVF." I was 28 at the time and had conceived naturally four times in a year and miscarried every time. He said immune treatments were a waste of money and referred to them as 'voodoo medicine.' He agreed to monitor me if we got pregnant on our own but wanted nothing to do with immunotherapy. He strongly pushed us to do IVF but we got pregnant on the first try naturally with Dr Beer's protocol.

I went back to the same RE in the hope of him monitoring me with my second "Beer baby." He had the nerve to sit there and say in front of my husband and my son in his stroller, "You aren't going to do that voodoo medicine again are you?" Then he looked over my chart and said we should try IVF with preimplantation genetic diagnosis (another $10k added) because of genetic problems. I asked, 'What genetic problems are you referring to exactly?' He explained that most miscarriages are because of genetic reasons.

A genetic counsellor told us during our lab review that everything had been normal with the lost baby and with our karyotyping.

Experience no.3

After I lost my third baby my Ob/Gyn refused to draw blood to test for some of the common immune issues like APAs and ANAs and so forth. She told me that they were worthless since there was no treatment.

Experience no.4

I have seen and interviewed eleven doctors over the last five years. I have found three that were tolerant of Dr Beer's collaboration, four were bitterly opposed to me working with him and four said I could do what I wanted but they wouldn't help me with any of it.

Experience no.5

Our rheumatologist is livid about Dr Beer's protocol. She says it's criminal and has no idea what he's talking about. She kept asking where the research was and if he was published. I said, "Yes, he is published, I can send you articles.' She said, "I don't have time to read them or go any further." The she repeated, "Nothing is wrong with you. A positive ANA doesn't mean anything." She urged us to see another specialist at a 'top' university and made remarks about Dr Beer being out for the dollar saying he should be sued.

She told me she was going to send my protocol letter to some committee of Ob/Gyns and to her research friends (at 'top' universities) so they could take action, to which I said, "I don't want you circulating my information in this way." She said, "I feel an obligation to speak up about this and I can mention your case without identifying you or your specifics."

She left a phone message for us mentioning that my husband and I, being well educated people, might be the ones to take action. This really upset me. I don't want to take any action, particularly against the only person has seemed to care. I just want a healthy baby. Is that so crazy? So now, not only are my husband and I further beaten down by the system, I've potentially and completely unintentionally stirred up some firestorm for Dr Beer. I could just cry.

Experience no.6

I thought I would share a few quotes from my recent visit to an IVF clinic in Vancouver: "Immune treatments are ridiculous." "There are no studies supporting any success with immune treatments." "Reprouctive immunologists are just good sales people." They said, "Keep trying. You can't call it failure until after 15 embryos are transferred." "Have you considered donor eggs?" "Have you thought about adoption?"

Experience no.7

I found out I was pregnant, after many early losses. My doctor knew of my autoimmune problems so I asked him if I would need blood tests to check that baby aspirin was enough or if more aggressive treatment was needed. He told me he wasn't going to order any blood work, just weekly ultrasounds. I kept insisting that I should be checked as the baby's growth rate was slow.

My doctor assured me everything was normal and that I should stop taking the baby aspirin because it had already done its job. I again asked to be tested to see if my antibody panels were elevated. He told me that any testing while I was pregnant would be invalid and refused to do it. He told me to come back the following week for another ultrasound.

When I returned, they found no heartbeat. At some point over the weekend my baby had died. I confronted him with the fact that I should have been treated more aggressively and his only comment was that I was welcome to see another doctor.

As is evident from these experiences, these women were failed by doctors who believe that they alone should be in charge of their patient's welfare. Some physicians are barely able to conceal their resentment towards what they see as a defiant and misguided mob of self referred women armed with a little knowledge from the Internet and no idea of the potential dangers that they are about to unleash upon themselves. Others consider their business to be under threat if women decide to pursue immunological treatments instead of traditional IVF options or hormonal management.

Finding a doctor who agrees to work with a reproductive immunologist is quite an achievement in itself for many couples. Because regular obstetric care is still required throughout pregnancy, some patients even resort to withholding information about the drugs they are taking so as not to upset their RE or Ob/Gyn, which is an extremely dangerous thing to do. To enable women to receive the professional and informed care they need throughout their pregnancy, a list of collaborating doctors worldwide is included at the end of this book.

The media has published the opinions of opponents of reproductive immunology using headlines like, "Treatments exploit hope for baby" and "Infertile couples warned of 'useless' tests." Much of this adverse publicity emerged in the wake of the publication of a British review of reproductive immunology by the Royal College of Obstetricians and Gynaecologists in 2003.

Professor Lesley Regan, who coauthored the review, said in an interview at the time, "It is a major concern to clinicians in the U.K. that patients are turning up to appointments armed with information downloaded from the web and wanting these unvalidated immunological tests. It is clear that the advice given on many websites is strongly influenced by the personal prejudices of doctors practicing non evidence based medicine. Much of the data they provide has never been exposed to the rigorous scrutiny of peer review. These couples are emotionally vulnerable and there is currently no scientific evidence to justify the use of these tests and treatments."

Citing the disagreements that exist on the subject of thyroid antibodies, she comments, "For years and years people thought that this was a problem, particularly since women who have thyroid disease often can't get pregnant. Having thyroid antibodies doesn't actually affect the outcome of the pregnancy, hence screening for thyroid antibodies doesn't seem to be very sensible." Apart from the test for the antiphospholipid syndrome, even today, some sixteen years after the release of this review, Professor Regan believes other tests have not been researched sufficiently enough to be considered "evidence based" and in a 2010 interview for the Guardian newspaper she stated, "They (women who have lost two successive pregnancies or more) walk into the clinic wanting an abnormal test result. I have to work hard to convince them that finding nothing wrong is good news. These (losses) could be down to chromosomes or age. But it really is better not to find a problem... Some people are incredibly resistant to the truth and I do find myself feeling gloomy, perhaps when there are issues of age or weight, or if there is an underlying problem I just can't identify, but I have to be tough. For example, last week I saw five (women)... with very late uterine deaths or still-births and that does wipe you out... I never find myself inclined to say to the women, 'You should stop trying now' or 'It's never going to work', because most people reach that point themselves."

One critic, who asked to remain anonymous, stated that he objected to reproductive immunology because of "the absence or lack of support from peer reviewed clinical trial studies and the strength of the confounding placebo effect in women provided with good supportive care." He also added, "While the hypothesis of a relationship between immune disturbance and reproductive failure is undoubtedly attractive, with the exception of the antiphospholipid syndrome in recurrent miscarriage, it is unfortunate that there is still a paucity of good data to support this view."

Professor Peter Johnson, Head of the Reproductive Immunology Group at the University of Liverpool and Editor-in-Chief of the *Journal of Reproductive Immunology,* agrees that the immune system undoubtedly plays an important role in the way the body normally adapts to allow a pregnancy. However he also says, "Clinical investigations and treatments that are without a sound scientific basis mislead patients, often at high cost, exacerbating their emotional rollercoaster ride. In addition, these empirical approaches can create a smokescreen, masking real research advances to the detriment of future patients. The reason why (immunotherapy) has become very popular, particularly in private medicine and in the United States, is that it appears to offer hope to a lot of women who are putting pressure on their doctors and there is money to be made from it."

Dr Beer responded to these comments stating, "Any doctor that plays on the vulnerability of couples with losses to get their money and give them false hope should be in jail. Unfortunately, many doctors who deal with reproductive health still do not understand immune problems or believe that they even exist. These same doctors say that until double-blind studies are done they are not interested.

"Double-blind, randomized, controlled studies, meta-analyses and prospective controlled studies do exist. That is why the American Society for Reproductive Immunology has sanctioned and advocated immune testing and therapy. All of the tests I do have been certified. The laboratory I use is a reference laboratory with an international reputation and the data that I use is correct and not in dispute."

In a double-blind, randomized, placebo controlled trial, patients with similar characteristics are randomly divided into two groups. One group receives treatment while the other is given a placebo. Neither the researcher nor the participant knows who is receiving treatment until the end of the study. Professor Regan says that patients who have miscarried need evidence coupled with "the benefit of pooled knowledge" and encourages them to participate in such trials, assuring them they will not be guinea pigs or, if they are in a control group, receive no treatment. Her view is that the principle of these studies is to compare one type of treatment with another and even if the woman does not take home a baby her miscarriage will not have been in vain as it may help other women in the future.

These objectives sound admirable, but in reality, when women know the options that are available, they refuse to take part in such a lottery. As Dr Beer explained, "Would you enter a double-blind study? I have tried this and patients say, 'No way am I taking a placebo or having inferior treatment and risking my baby's life.' They want no part of a double-blind study. They know my success rates and they come to me because of this."

In fact, the pool of knowledge to which Professor Regan refers already exists. In 1994, the Ethics Committee of the American Society for Reproductive Immunology (ASRI) found that conducting a large, multi center, randomized, placebo controlled, double-blind trial of immunotherapy was impossible to execute because the number of recurrent miscarriage patients and physicians working with them was relatively small. Indeed, some women with recurrent pregnancy loss have diseases that are so uncommon there will never be a randomized controlled trial that relates specifically to their condition.

The ASRI therefore carried out a meta-analysis of hundreds of published and unpublished trials involving control groups. Particular attention was focused on the randomization and blinding of each study and two independent biostatistical teams then assessed the data. Both came to the conclusion that immunotherapy was of "significant benefit." Interestingly, the use of chemotherapy for the treatment of breast cancer was similarly fraught with controversy until a meta-analysis of over 20,000 women generated a convincing result.

Moreover, according to a subsequent 1996 ASRI meta-analysis concerning the treatment of recurrent spontaneous abortion, "When the role of recurrent chromosome anomalies was discovered and taken into account it could be seen that immunotherapy might be more than 90% effective in those who usually abort chromosomally normal embryos."

16

Critics of Reproductive Immunology

Much of the negativity that surrounds reproductive immunology has been generated by the publication of the 2003 guidelines: *"Immunological Testing and Interventions for Reproductive Failure"* and the 2011 guidelines: *"The Investigation and Treatment of Couples with Recurrent First-trimester and Second-trimester Miscarriage"* by Profes-sor Lesley Regan and her colleagues, on behalf of the Royal College of Obstetricians and Gynaecologists (RCOG).

A 2004 brochure from The Recurrent Miscarriage Clinic at St Mary's Hospital in London, (the largest miscarriage clinic in the world), which is run by Professor Regan, stated that this center had four purposes:

1. To identify women with an underlying cause for their pregnancy losses.

2. To conduct... studies to determine the optimal treatment for women with an identified cause for their pregnancy losses.

3. To practice evidence based medicine and "avoid subjecting those women with no identifiable cause for their miscarriages to treatments of no proven benefit."

4. To "identify those women whose miscarriages remain unexplained despite detailed investigation."

According to Professor Regan, this last group has a 75% chance of a successful pregnancy outcome with supportive care alone, which is still cited as a treatment approach in the 2011 guidelines.

As women with unexplained miscarriages account for some 60% of those with recurrent losses at St. Mary's, this success rate would only apply to 75% of this 60%, i.e., 45% of all patients attending the clinic, which calls into question the standard of diagnosis that is being provided. The brochure concluded that this 75% success rate with supportive care proves that the use of immunotherapy is unnecessary as do the 2011 RCOG Guidelines.

In a 2004 paper published in the British Medical Journal, Professor Regan, a self professed "debunker of immune theories," advised that, "New treatments aimed at natural killer cells in women with reproductive failure is unfortunately not backed up by the science." Despite an accumulation of over a dozen year's of evidence to prove the vailidity of immunological testing and treatments for recurrent miscarriage Professor Regan's opinion remains unchanged.

Her resistance to the discoveries within the now well established field of reproductive immunology and firm belief that only her own research is relevant along with studies from those who share her entrenched personal opinions was confirmed in a 2007 interview for The Daily Telegraph newspaper in which she said, "An observation made by a patient leads us to posing a question and then designing an experiment to try to answer it."

In 2018, the American Society for Reproductive Medicine (ASRM) also produced a report, "The Role of Immunotherapy in In Vitro Fertilization: A Guideline." Their paper similarly dismisses reproductive immunotherapy advising, "the use of immunological testing in the general ART population cannot be recommended." This verdict is entirely based on a 1999 paper by Dr Joseph Hill III, *"Immunologic tests and IVF: "Please, enough already"* (more about Dr Hill later) and a 2001 paper by Dr William Kutteh who was an ASRM Star Award Winner in 2017.

It is perhaps of note to mention here that the ASRM receives large donations from the companies that make the fertility drugs used in IVF (e.g. Gonal-f®, Ovidrel®, Endometrin etc.) as well as funding from major fertility center chains (e.g. Myovant and Prelude Fertility). The infertility treatment market will be worth $2.05 billion by 2022, mainly generated by fertility treatments costing around $20,000 per stimulated cycle. As Professor Gab Kovacs, former Medical Director of Monash IVF states, "This (invasive treatment) is the key to generating income for an IVF clinic. Reproductive immunotherapy threatens this market as it eliminates the need for such invasive treatment in many cases."

Two eminent professionals were asked for their opinions on the statements made in these recent RCOG and ASRM guidelines :

David A. Clark, M.D., PhD, DiplABIM, FRCP(C), FRCP Edin. – David Clark is Professor of the Departments of Medicine, Pathology,

CRITICS OF REPRODUCTIVE IMMUNOLOGY

Obstetrics and Gynecology and the Graduate Program in Medical Sciences at McMaster University in Hamilton, Ontario, and a Professor at the Institute of Medical Sciences at the University of Toronto.

Professor Clark has been the President of both the American Society for Reproductive Immunology and the International Society for Immunology of Reproduction, and is a Fellow of the Royal Society of Medicine in London and an MRC scientist. His published works include over 500 book chapters, articles and abstracts, the majority of which are featured in peer reviewed journals.

He is on the editorial boards of the *American Journal of Reproductive Immunology* and the *Journal of Assisted Reproduction and Genetics* and has spoken and lectured on the subject of reproductive medicine at over a hundred conferences, symposiums, society meetings and universities around the world.

Professor Clark says, "I prefer to base my opinion on all of the available facts, appropriately analyzed, using state of the art statistical methods. As Rory Collins (Oxford University) has stated, one has to consider the overall effect of all of the data. There may be some that merit discarding, but only after careful evaluation and I am always prepared to change my opinion if new information becomes available."

Carolyn B. Coulam, M.D. – Dr Carolyn Coulam is internationally recognized for her contributions to medical and scientific education and research. In 1986, she established the reproductive immunology and reproductive biology laboratories at the Center for Reproduction and Transplantation in Indiana. Ten years later, she was appointed National Director of Reproductive Immunology at the Center for Human Reproduction in Illinois. In 2000, Dr Coulam joined the Sher Institute of Reproductive Medicine as Medical Director and Director of Laboratory Research. She was Director of Recurrent Pregnancy Loss at the Rinchart Center for Reproductive Medicine in Chicago and Research Director at Millenova Immunology Laboratories. Dr. Coulam is now part of the fertility specialist team at The Reproductive Medicine Institute which has seven centers in Illinois.

In addition to her role as Managing Editor of the *American Journal of Reproductive Immunology* she has more than 200 articles in peer-reviewed journals to her credit. Dr Coulam also edited the major reference textbook *Immunologic Obstetrics* and her 1986 paper

"Incidence of Premature Ovarian Failure" set the standard by which the rate of this condition is determined.

> **"To diagnose antiphospholipid syndrome it is mandatory that the woman has two positive tests at least 12 weeks apart for either lupus anticoagulant or anticardiolipin antibodies..."**
>
> *RCOG 2011 Opinion Paper*

Dr Coulam: "These two tests alone cannot identify the presence of all the underlying immune problems that can lead to recurrent miscarriage. The frequency of autoantibodies is significantly greater in women with reproductive failure and a panel of tests for antibodies to six additional phospholipids is recommended to determine the presence of APAs. There are 21 markers for immunoglobulins and, if any are elevated, this can indicate the existence of an autoimmune process that can trigger pregnancy loss. If only the anticardiolipin antibody is measured, just 4% of the positive APAs are detected and 81% of women will have the diagnosis missed."

Professor Clark: "Currently, antibodies to serine are thought to be one of the most significant antibodies with respect to pregnancy loss. Several mechanisms have been postulated to explain how such antibodies might cause abortions in the first trimester. Antibodies such as these may also interfere with the anticoagulant surface properties of the trophoblast and inhibit the development and function of the placenta, leading to implantation failure for women undergoing IVF."

A sample of studies that show testing for antibodies other than lupus anticoagulant and anticardiolipin is of clinical significance:

Coulam, C. et al.: *Journal of Assisted Reproduction & Genetics*, Nov; 14(10):603-8, 1997
APAs were detected in 22% of 312 women with implantation failure compared with 5% of a control group of 100 women. Anticardiolipin antibodies were found in 4% of women with implantation failure, but

CRITICS OF REPRODUCTIVE IMMUNOLOGY

18% had positive values of other APAs. "A complete APA panel using seven isotypes is necessary for diagnosing implantation failure..."

Gleicher, N. et al.: *Mount Sinai Journal of Medicine*, Jan; 9(1):32-7, 1992

326 patients with reproductive failure were tested for the presence of lupus anticoagulant and 15 types of autoantibodies. The investigation concluded: "Patients suspected to suffer from reproductive failure due to abnormal autoimmunity have to be screened not only for lupus anticoagulant and/or selected antiphospholipid autoantibodies, but with a more comprehensive autoantibody profile."

Ulcova-Gallova, Z. et al.: *American Journal of Reproductive Immunology*, Aug; 54(2):112-7, 2005

Blood samples from 1073 women after one IVF failure, 853 women after two or more IVF failures, 627 women with three and more spontaneous miscarriages or missed abortions and 412 women who had undergone diagnostic laparoscopy were compared with 391 healthy fertile women. Patients with multiple IVF failures and those with repeated spontaneous miscarriages had significantly higher levels of phospholipid antibodies against inositol and L-serine. 25% were positive for three or more APAs. The authors concluded: "Determination of APA only against cardiolipin in reproductive failure is not sufficient for obstetric/gynecology diagnosis as the primary antiphospholipid syndrome."

Comment: In isolation, a positive APA test is not an absolute predictor of immune mediated reproductive failure. Each APA marker has its own clinical significance when put in the context of a patient's history. Rather than being interpreted in isolation, it is a useful tool when viewing the overall reproductive picture.

Further supporting studies can be viewed in the Notes section.

> **"A single prospective study has shown that the presence of thyroid antibodies in euthyroid women with a history of recurrent miscarriage does not affect future pregnancy outcome."**
>
> *RCOG 2011 Opinion Paper*

Professor Clark: "There are several reports of an increased incidence of antibodies against the thyroid in women with pregnancy failure. Dr Sher published a randomized controlled trial of patients with antithyroid antibodies and compared their success rate with IVIG plus heparin to that of heparin alone. The success rate was significantly higher in the group that received IVIG. This would suggest the statement in the RCOG report is incorrect. If there are antithyroid antibodies, appropriate treatment may improve the success rate."

Comment: This statement is based on a 2000 study by Professor Regan. This study included 870 women with a history of three or more pregnancy losses. A livebirth rate of 58% for women with or without antithyroid antibodies is not particularly high. This low success rates indicates there were other problems in both groups that remained undiagnosed and untreated. Health problems encountered during pregnancy concerning these women or their babies were not revealed.

Studies that show the thyroid antibodies do affect pregnancy outcome and that screening for them is useful:

Bussen, S. et al.: *Human Reproduction & Embryology*, 15 (3):545, 2000
In a study of 24 women with three consecutive IVF failures, the incidence of thyroid antibodies was "significantly increased." The report concludes: "Since these autoantibodies seem to be distinct and independent markers for reproductive failure their identification provides the opportunity to identify women at risk for an adverse outcome in an IVF embryo transfer programme. Therefore, it is suggested to include the determination of thyroid antibodies in the evaluation of women with recurrent IVF failure."

CRITICS OF REPRODUCTIVE IMMUNOLOGY

Dendrinos, S. et al.: *Gynecological Endocrinology*, **Aug; 14(4):270-4, 2000**
30 women with recurrent miscarriages were tested for thyroid antibodies and compared with 15 matched controls. The frequency of those with ATAs was 37% versus 13%. "This may represent an additional marker for impaired regulation of the maternal immune system."

Poppe, K. et al.: *Journal of Clinical Endocrinology & Metabolism*, **Vol. 88, No.9, 4149-4152, 2003**
234 women were screened for thyroid peroxidase antibodies before their first IVF cycle and 14% tested positive. The miscarriage rate for this group was 53% compared with 23% for women without thyroid antibodies.

Stagnaro-Green, A. et al.: *Thyroid*, **Jan; 11(1): 57-63, 2001**
This review of the research papers on thyroid antibodies and miscarriage concludes: "The majority of the studies (67%) reported a statistically significant increase in the incidence of thyroid antibodies in the recurrent abortion group as compared to controls."

Further supporting studies can be viewed in the Notes section.

The 2003 RCOG Opinion Paper says the prevalence of ANAs (antinuclear antibodies) varies from "similar" to "increased" among women with recurrent miscarriage compared with normal women, but the presence of ANAs has no effect on pregnancy outcome. It also says that there is no data to suggest that the presence of ANAs influences future reproductive outcome in women with infertility and IVF failure.

Comment. The report recognizes the association between elevated levels of ANAs and recurrent miscarriage, yet it maintains that their presence is not related to pregnancy outcome.

Professor Clark: "If one looks at the general population of women, testing positive for the presence of a single autoantibody does not appear to translate into an increased risk of reproductive problems.

However, in patients with reproductive failure, the situation is very different, since it is in this group that an autoantibody has an increased probability of being pathogenic. For example, patients with positive ANAs may have clinical lupus, which has a reputation for reproductive wastage. A positive ANA can therefore signify the increased frequency of various autoantibodies in women with reproductive failure. This has been called the "Reproductive Autoimmune Failure Syndrome."

There is much data to show that the presence of ANAs is associated with negative pregnancy outcome. Here are some examples:

Geva, E. et al.: *Fertility & Sterility,* **Oct; 62(4):802-6, 1994**
Researchers investigated the role of autoimmune factors in implantation failures after embryo transfer. Anticardiolipin, anti-double stranded DNA, antinuclear antibody, lupus anticoagulant, and rheumatoid factor serum levels were tested in 21 IVF failure patients and compared with a control group. The incidence of circulating autoimmune antibodies in the study group was 33.3%. Autoimmune antibodies were not detected in any members of the control group.

Geva, E. et al.: *Fertility & Sterility,* **Apr; 67(4):599-611, 1997**
Over 300 original and review articles were evaluated, after which it was concluded: "When abnormal autoantibody levels are present in women with reproductive failure, the reproductive failure alone should be considered as one of the possible clinical expressions of autoimmune disorders."

Hasegawa, I. et al.: *Fertility & Sterility,* **Dec; 70(6):1044-8, 1998**
In this study involving 307 women undergoing IVF embryo transfer, 10 mg daily of prednisolone and 81 mg daily of aspirin were given to women with antinuclear antibodies (with and without antiphospholipid antibodies). The administration of prednisolone and aspirin significantly improved both pregnancy and implantation rates.

Kikuchi, K. et al.: *American Journal of Reproductive Immunology,* **Oct; 50(4):363-7, 2003**
In 108 infertile women, the implantation rates per embryo transfer in the first IVF cycle were 14.8% for women with untreated ANAs and

32.4% for women without ANAs. The subsequent pregnancy rates were 28% and 54% respectively. The study concludes: "This indicates that the mechanisms of implantation failure by ANA could be solved, and effective and safe medication should be developed for better implantation rates, especially in the first treatment cycle."

> **"Studies examining the role of antisperm antibodies in women with recurrent miscarriage have reported no association. More recent prospective studies report that antisperm antibodies do not appear to influence reproductive outcome following IVF."**
>
> *RCOG 2003 Opinion Paper*

Comment: The RCOG opinion paper bases this statement on the findings of a 1996 study, which also includes the recommendation: "Further work is necessary to determine whether IgA antisperm antibodies truly are associated with pregnancy loss or whether antisperm antibodies play any role in repetitive aborters."

Before 1996, a clear association between antisperm antibodies and recurrent miscarriage had been established. Subsequent studies have confirmed that their presence also affects IVF outcome:

Beer, A.E. et al.: *Fertility & Sterility*, Feb; 45(2):209-15, 1986
173 women with a history of three or more recurrent consecutive abortions were analyzed for circulating antisperm antibodies. No pregnancies were gestated to term in women who were antisperm antibody-positive unless they were inoculated with their partner's leukocytes as a treatment for an immune basis (not related to antisperm antibodies) for their recurrent miscarriages. This increased their ability to carry their fetuses to term.

Rossato, M. et al.: *Human Reproduction*, Aug; 19(8):1816-20, 2004
This study concluded: "...infertile subjects with ASA (antisperm antibodies) have a reduced sperm plasma membrane functional integrity that could explain, at least in part, the low fertilization and pregnancy

rates observed in these subjects during assisted reproductive procedures."

Witkin, S. and David, S.: *American Journal of Obstetrics & Gynecology*, **Jan; 158(1):59-62, 1988**
109 infertile couples were studied to establish if there was a relationship between antisperm antibodies, conception and miscarriage. During 18 months, 30.3% of couples conceived. Antisperm antibodies were present in 43.8% of women who miscarried and in 38.2% who did not conceive.

Witkin, S. and Chaudhry, A.: *Journal of Reproductive Immunology*, **May; 15(2): 151-8, 1989**
The presence of antisperm antibodies in women with recurrent spontaneous abortions was examined. These antibodies were detected in 36.4% of 44 women with recurrent abortions.

Yan, J.: *Zhonghua Fu Chan Ke Za Zhi*, **Nov; 25(6):343-4, 1990**
686 aborting patients, including 285 couples, were tested for circulating antisperm antibodies. 241 fertile couples served as controls. The positive rate of ASA in repeatedly aborting patients was significantly higher than that of the fertile control group. It was concluded: "ASA ...play an important role in the development of recurrent abortions."

"Increased Th1 cytokine expression may be the underlying immune aetiology for some cases of reproductive failure...There is no evidence of a correlation between peripheral blood and uterine NK cell populations... no peer reviewed clinical applications are available."

RCOG 2003 Opinion Paper

Comment: To agree that Th1 cytokine expression is significant and then to dismiss the idea of testing NK cell levels makes no sense. NK cells are prolific secretors of Th1 cytokines. Furthermore, in a study at St. Mary's Hospital that involved Professor Regan, increased numbers of CD56+ NK cells were seen only in the endometria of women with recurrent early miscarriage. The study concluded: "These findings suggest a possible role for NK cells in the pathogenesis of recurrent early pregnancy loss."

Professor Clark: "The term 'peer reviewed' is usually applied to published papers and grants. One does not review an application of a technology. There are definitely peer reviewed papers showing a correlation between increased circulating NK cell levels and an increased risk of reproductive failure. There are also peer reviewed papers showing that treatment increases the chance of successful pregnancy in such patients by suppressing circulating NK activity.

Professor Regan's own study mentions the presence of uterine CD56+ cells but does not indicate whether they were CD16+ (peripheral) or CD16- (uterine resident), or if they had CD3, suggesting they could be natural killer T cells of either the alpha-beta or gamma-delta type. This indicates a lack of knowledge of the literature. I believe her comment about peer reviewed applications concerned the peripheral blood testing, rather than uterine NK testing. If you want your own report to stand out as significant a common strategy is to disparage what others have done."

Examples of peer reviewed data from an extensive collection:

Beer, A.E. et al.: *American Journal of Reproductive Immunology,* **Aug; 34(2):93-9, 1995**
35 pregnant and 81 non pregnant women with recurrent miscarriage were compared with 22 pregnant and 17 non pregnant controls. CD56+ NK cells were elevated in non pregnant women with recurrent abortion. Pregnant women with recurrent miscarriage had significantly increased NK (CD56+, CD56+/CD16+) cells compared with the control group.

Emmer, P. et al.: *Human Reproduction,* **May; 15(5):1163-9, 2000**
43 women with subsequent pregnancies after recurrent miscarriage, 37 healthy controls and 39 successful IVF patients were included in this study. Lower NK cell numbers were strongly associated with a full-term pregnancy. When the pregnancy was lost, higher numbers of CD56+/CD16+ cells were seen in early pregnancy.

Polgar, K.: *Gynecological & Obstetric Investigations*, 53(1):59-64, 2002

Blood samples from 32 women with a history of at least three spontaneous abortions of unknown etiology were evaluated. The authors concluded that the white blood cell populations responsible for the destruction of the embryo were T cells and NK (CD56) cells that produced a typical Th1 cytokine response.

Yamada, H. et al.: *American Journal of Reproductive Immunology*, Aug; 46(2):132-6, 2001

66 pregnant women with a history of miscarriage were assessed for peripheral NK cell activity. NK cell activity in women with subsequent live births was significantly decreased compared with that in women who subsequently aborted chromosomally normal fetuses. The researchers concluded: "High NK cell activity at 6 to 7 gestational weeks correlates to subsequent abortion with normal chromosomes."

Further supporting studies can be viewed in the Notes section.

"There is no clear evidence to support the hypothesis of human leucocyte antigen incompatibility between couples, the absence of maternal leucocytotoxic antibodies or the absence of maternal blocking antibodies. Hence, they should not be offered routinely in the investigation of couples with recurrent miscarriage."

RCOG 2011 Opinion Paper

Comment: Similar or matching HLA tissue types between partners have been associated with an absence of maternal blocking antibodies and subsequent fetal abortion. There are many reports of improved pregnancy outcomes after paternal lymphocyte immunization, a procedure which helps to treat the immune problems associated with HLA sharing and reduces peripheral NK cell cytotoxicity. The contradictions between study findings (where testing and treatment protocols often vary) do not alter the basic premise that for most women, improving maternal immunotolerance towards the fetus is an effective means of preventing recurrent miscarriage.

CRITICS OF REPRODUCTIVE IMMUNOLOGY

A selection of studies that show HLA sharing is a predictor of pregnancy outcome:

Beer, A.E. et al.: *Journal of Reproductive Immunology*, **Dec; 25 (3): 195-207, 1993**
HLA compatibility was examined in 40 abortuses and 31 liveborn children of 68 couples with a history of unexplained recurrent spontaneous abortion. Significantly more couples with recurrent abortion shared two HLA-DQA1 alleles compared with fertile control couples.

Gerencer, M.: *Fertility & Sterility*, **Apr; 31(4):401-4, 1979**
In this study, a greater degree of HLA compatibility was found between women and their partners in cases of unexplained recurrent spontaneous abortions.

Ober, C. et al.: *Human Reproduction*, **Jan; 13(1):33-8, 1998**
In a 10-year study of 251 pregnancies in 111 Hutterite couples, significantly increased fetal losses were seen in couples who were matched for HLA.

Thomas, M.L. et al.: *American Journal of Obstetrics & Gynecology*, **Apr 15; 151(8):1053-8, 1985**
21 couples with two or more unexplained fetal losses were HLA typed. "...there was a strong indication that aborting couples shared a greater portion of the chromosome that contains the major histocompatibility complex (MHC) than would be expected in random matings."

"A Cochrane systematic review has shown that the use of various forms of immunotherapy, including paternal cell immunization... provides no significant beneficial effect over placebo in preventing further miscarriage."

RCOG 2011 Opinion Paper

Professor Clark: "Professor Regan is citing a reference to a 2006 version of an old Cochrane systematic review which was flawed. These flaws were clearly set out in the peer reviewed paper (Clark DA,

Coulam C et al, *Human Reproduction Update* 7: 501-511, 2001) which critically reviews clinical trials, updates the meta-analysis and comments on new approaches. This paper concludes that according to the results of double-blind randomized and unblinded trials, 'LIT does appear to increase the chance of a livebirth if given to the appropriate patients.'

The author of the Cochrane review, Dr Jim Scott, included one randomized controlled trial where one would not have expected to get a positive result. He knew from a previous study in which he was involved (the Ober trial) that a negative effect would be expected from the patient population that was selected. Women who tested positive for antinuclear or positive antiphospholipid antibodies were included in the trial and some may not have had testing to exclude autoantibodies. These factors possibly reduced the success rates with LIT because such additional immune problems would have required additional treatment.

The Ober trial in which Scott participated claimed to have excluded anticardiolipin antibody positive patients. However, others familiar with the results of the lab testing have since written that entry criteria were too lenient and women in the trial actually had many other complicating autoantibodies. Despite repeated requests, it has not been possible to see the data, so I cannot confirm what autoimmune testing the patients did or did not have."

Dr Beer: "I was involved in the meta-analysis that definitely showed an effect of LIT in preventing abortions. Subsequent work showing LIT also dramatically reduces the killing activity of NK cells has focused interest on LIT as a viable alternative to IVIG, which is so expensive."

Comment: Professor James Mowbray, a colleague of Professor Regan at St. Mary's Hospital Medical School, carried out a "paired sequential double-blind, randomized trial" of LIT. The results were published in the *Lancet* in 1985. 22 women with prior recurrent miscarriage were injected with purified lymphocytes from their partner's blood. 17 had successful pregnancies compared with just 10 of 27 control subjects.

There are numerous other reports that also support the use of LIT as a treatment for recurrent implantation failure and the prevention of miscarriage after repeated losses. Here is just a small selection:

CRITICS OF REPRODUCTIVE IMMUNOLOGY

Mengyuan Liu. et al.: *Reproductive Biology and Endocrinology, 15: 95, 2017.*
64 recurrent miscarriage patients received low-dose lymphocyte immunotherapy and 35 women did not. 5 of 43 patients miscarried in the immunotherapy group. 8 of 23 pregnant patients experienced a miscarriage in the control group. "The proportion of Th1 cells was significantly decreased while the proportions of Th2 cells... were significantly increased in immunotherapy group."

Check, J.H. et al.: *Clinical & Experimental Obstetrics & Gynecology,* **32(1):21-2, 2005**
Women failing to deliver a live baby, despite at least two previous embryo transfer cycles, were offered LIT prior to their next transfer. The clinical and viable pregnancy rates were 70.3% and 51.3% for the LIT groups versus 45.9% and 16.2% for the controls.

Adachi, H. et al.: *Clinical Immunology,* **Mar; 106(3):175-80, 2003**
26 women with unexplained secondary recurrent abortion were treated with LIT. Blocking antibodies appeared in their blood (prior to immunization the level was insufficient). 22 became pregnant and of these, 20 continued. The success rate with LIT was 90.9%. In 11 pregnancies without immunotherapy, only two pregnancies were successful.

Pandey, M. et al.: *Internet Journal of Gynecology and Obstetrics,* **Vol. 2, No.1, 2003**
Lymphocyte immunotherapy was given to 73 women with recurrent pregnancy loss. The pregnancy success rate was 86% in this population compared with 33% for women who declined to enter the trial.

Pandey, M. et al.: *Archives of Gynecology & Obstetrics,* **Mar; 269 (3):161-72, 2004**

Carp, H. et al.: *Archives of Gynecology & Obstetrics,* **248(2):93-101, 1990.**
This paper analyzes the researchers' experience of LIT from 1985-1988, with 207 patients being classified on a clinical basis and by immunological testing. Of these, 143 were immunized and 129 preg-

nancies occurred in 108 patients, the majority of whom had previously experienced recurrent abortions.

Daya, S. and Gunby, J.: *American Journal of Reproductive Immunology,* **32:294-302, 1994**
In this review, the data from randomized controlled trials in eight centers were analyzed. It was concluded that immunotherapy significantly improved the livebirth rate in selected patient groups with recurrent miscarriage. For those without antinuclear or anticardiolipin antibodies and with normal karyotype embryos, the effectiveness of LIT was close to 100%.

When the results of all randomized and non-randomized studies were pooled, it was observed that 67% of women with recurrent abortion who received LIT showed a successful pregnancy outcome compared with 36% of women in the control group. The authors recommended paternal lymphocyte immunotherapy for the maintenance of pregnancy in women with repetitive spontaneous abortion.

"[LIT] is expensive and has potential serious adverse side effects including transfusion reaction, anaphylactic shock and hepatitis."
RCOG 2011 Opinion Paper

Professor Clark: "Side effects such as transfusion reaction and anaphylactic shock sound scary until one realizes that Professor Mowbray at St. Mary's in London administered leukocyte immunotherapy to thousands of patients without any problems and without the transmission of infection, which is usually preventable by screening. Since the FDA, as I understand it, will only accept data generated on There is ample data to indicate that leukocyte immunotherapy can do more good than harm. Furthermore, it is the patient who has the right to make the informed choice."

Comment: In 2006, the results of a survey of over 4,500 women who had been treated with LIT confirmed, "Specific risks for anaphylaxis, autoimmune or graft versus host disease were not detected."

CRITICS OF REPRODUCTIVE IMMUNOLOGY

A recent report on the results of a 2 to 3 year follow up of 2,687 IVF couples who received LIT has also concluded, "Based on micro-biological, immunological and hematological testing, the risks of intradermal LIT are low." (More about LIT and the controversies that surround it can be found in Chapter 13.)

"Intravenous immunoglobulin in women with previous unexplain-ed recurrent miscarriage does not improve the live birth rate... A 2010 meta analysis confirmed this..."

RCOG 2011 Opinion Paper

"There is insufficient evidence to recommend IVIG administration as part of IVF to improve IVF outcomes."

ASRM 2018 Guidelines

Professor Clark: "I dealt with this 2010 meta analysis by Stephenson et al. in a letter to *Human Reproduction* (Vol.26, No.9 pp. 2586–2591, 2011). Her study was rubbished due to a variety of serious method-ologic flaws. 1. Her analysis included just 87 women with the fewest details concerning their health history, selection/testing and how the randomization and blinding was performed. 2. It was not determined if the subjects had any detectable immune abnormalities that would benefit from treatment with IVIG. 3. If these patients did have immune issues then the Gaminume they received was inferior. Eight times more of the IVIG product used by Stephenson is required to achieve the same level of suppression achieved with Gammagard. 4. Stephenson then excluded trials with women with immune abnormalities. If she had included these trials it would have conclusively proved that IVIG is clearly associated with a successful pregnancy outcome in this category of patient. Only patients with immune test abnormalities show a statistically significant treatment benefit."

Dr Stricker and his colleagues also provided formal documentation of this problem. Trials that select patients with immune problems and gave them IVIG at the time of ovulation were positive. Trials that did not select and gave treatment late were negative. In assessing a trial result it is common sense to consider if the design of the study was likely to have shown the desired effect."

The following studies show a strong, positive correlation between treatment with IVIG and a successful pregnancy outcome in women with recurrent miscarriage caused by immune abnormalities:

Han A and Sung K: *Reproductive Medicine and Biology*, Apr; 17(2): 115–124, 2018.
In this review, the authors concluded, "It is obvious that IVIG is effective in recurrent pregnancy losses and repeated implantation failures with immunologic disturbances... including a high natural killer cell proportion and its cytotoxicity or an elevated T helper 1 to T helper 2 ratio."

Virro M, Winger E, Reed J: *American Journal of Reproductive Immunology*, Sept;68(3):218-25, 2012
229 women with multiple IVF failures and/or unexplained infertility received IVIG on the day of egg retrieval. The pregnancy success rate was 60.3% and the live birth rate was 40.2% which is significantly higher than the Canadian average of 30%. Where high quality day 5 blastocysts were transferred nearly a 100% success rate was achieved using IVIG.

Yamada H et al: *ISRN Obstetrics and Gynecology,* **Article ID 512732, 2012.**
60 pregnant women with recurrent miscarriage underwent IVIG therapy. The live birth rate was 73.3% (44/60). When the 11 pregnancies with abnormal chromosome karyotype were excluded, the live birth rate was 89.8% (44/49).

Winger E, Reed J et al: *American Journal of Reproductive Immunology*, Nov;66(5):394-403, 2011
202 IVF cycles were divided into four groups. Group 1 with high Th1:Th2 ratios and/or elevated levels of CD56+ cells received preconception IVIG, Group 2 with similarly elevated immune cell levels did not, Group 3 with normal immune cell levels received IVIG, Group 4 compared to Group 3 and did not receive IVIG. An average of two embryos were transferred. The implantation rate was 45% for

Group 1, 22% for Group 2, 54% for Group 3 and 48% for Group 4. The clinical pregnancy rate was 61%, 26%, 69% and 71% respectively. The results show that in women with Th1:Th2 and/or CD56+ elevation IVF success rates were low without preconception IVIG.

Stricker, R.B. and Winger, E.E.: *American Journal of Reproductive Immunology,* **Dec; 54(6):390-6, 2005**
72 women with recurrent miscarriage (average age 37) were treated with IVIG. Once conception was achieved, treatment was continued on a monthly basis up to 30 weeks of pregnancy. Of the 50 women who became pregnant, 84% had a successful term pregnancy. Of the 27 women who refused IVIG, 20 became pregnant but 18 miscarried.
Batorfi, J. et al: *Orvosi Hetilap (Budapest),* **Nov 6; 146(45):2297-302, 2005**
IVIG treatment of recurrent miscarriage patients with a clear allo-immune background was successful in 88.5% (23/26) cases.

Christiansen, O.B.: *Journal of Reproductive Immunology,* **Jun; 62 (1-2):41-52, 2004**
The author states recurrent miscarriage clinics in Denmark have used LIT and IVIG in placebo controlled trials since 1986. The results show that the correct immunization protocol on the right groups of patients is effective and both treatments are now used routinely.

Christiansen, O.B.: *Human Reproduction,* **Mar; 17(3):809-16, 2002**
When data from this trial and a previous placebo controlled trial of the same treatment were combined, 58% (15/26) of those with secondary miscarriage who received IVIG had successful outcomes compared with 24% (6/26) in the placebo group.
Stricker, R. et al.: *Clinical & Applied Immunology Reviews,* **2:187-199, 2002**
IVIG was given to 40 women with recurrent miscarriage and abnormal immune reactivity. 40 conceived and 35 continued with a successful pregnancy. Of 43 untreated women 15 conceived and 13 miscarried.

Stricker, R. et al: *Fertility & Sterility,* **Mar; 73(3):536-40, 2000**
47 women with up to four previous miscarriages were included in this study. 36 received IVIG preconception and 24 became pregnant. 20

continued IVIG treatment and 19 had a successful term pregnancy. Of the 11 women who refused IVIG therapy, 7 became pregnant and all 7 miscarried.

Beer, A.E. et al: *Early Pregnancy*, **Apr; 4(2):154-64, 2000**
33 women with recurrent abortions and autoimmune abnormalities received preconception anticoagulation and prednisone treatment. 9 patients had anticoagulation and prednisone in addition to IVIG treatment and their livebirth rate was 100%. In 6 women without IVIG treatment, the livebirth rate was 33.3%.

Beer, A.E. et al.: *American Journal of Reproductive Immunology*, **Apr; 35(4):363-9, 1996**
73 women with recurrent miscarriage and elevated NK cells received IVIG and anticoagulation treatment. Controls were 95 women with recurrent miscarriage and normal NK levels who received anticoagulation treatment only. 86.3% of women with elevated NK levels who received IVIG and anticoagulation therapy had a successful pregnancy outcome.

"The only treatment or treatment combination that leads to a significant increase in the live birth rate among women with antiphospholipid syndrome is aspirin plus unfractionated heparin."
RCOG 2011 Opinion Paper

Comment: Incidences of preterm delivery and of fetal and maternal morbidity can be the result of other undiagnosed and untreated autoimmune conditions that may manifest themselves more acutely during pregnancy. As Dr Norbert Gleicher and his colleagues stated in 1998, "Abnormal autoimmune function may lead to reproductive failure at different stages of the reproductive process, depending on the quality and possibly quantity of the abnormal autoimmune response."

A diagnosis of antiphospholipid syndrome is not all encompassing with regards to implantation failure in IVF and recurrent miscarriage. Many women with APAs have activated NK cells that can only be detected through a comprehensive panel of tests, and it is likely that

CRITICS OF REPRODUCTIVE IMMUNOLOGY

they will also require corticosteroids, IVIG and/or LIT and/or anti-TNF-alpha treatment.

A limited approach to reproductive immunotherapy will produce less than optimum results. For example, in 37 of Dr Beer's patients who refused optimal immunotherapy, an ongoing pregnancy success rate of 54% (20/37) was achieved with anticoagulant therapy and aspirin. When LIT and IVIG were included, a 75% (24/32) ongoing pregnancy success rate was achieved in a similar patient population.

Therefore, the question becomes not "do steroids work?" but which group of patients would benefit from them the most, which are safest and most effective, how should the dose be structured and how should steroids be combined with other treatments?

There is good evidence to recommend against the routine use of corticosteroids during stimulation to improve the outcome of live birth in ART cycles in the general population."

ASRM 2018 Guidelines

This statement by the ASRM is correct: Corticosteroids should only be prescribed where appropriate after the necessary evaluation has been carried out and antinuclear have been detected.

Reports that suggest steroid therapy is of benefit when treating women with autoimmune reproductive failure:

Triplett, D.A. and Harris, E.N.: *American Journal of Reproductive Immunology*, **Nov-Dec; 21(3-4):123-31, 1989**
Reviewing study outcomes, the authors observe "...preliminary data suggest the use of prednisone in combination with aspirin significantly improves the probability of delivery of a viable infant."

Geva, E. et al.: *American Journal of Reproductive Immunology*, **Jan; 43(1):36-40, 2000**
52 recurrent IVF failure patients with autoantibodies, including those against cardiolipin, ANA, rheumatoid factor and lupus anticoagulant, received 10 mg per day of prednisone and 100 mg per day of aspirin

before ovulation induction. After treatment, the clinical pregnancy rate per cycle was 32.7%. There was no increase in pregnancy complications, including premature labor, gestational diabetes mellitus, or pregnancy induced hypertension.

Hasegawa, I. et al.: *Fertility & Sterility*, Dec; 70(6):1044-8, 1998
Prednisolone plus low dose aspirin given to women with positive antinuclear antibodies, with or without antiphospholipid antibodies, undergoing IVF between January 1996 and December 1997 resulted in a "significantly improved" cycle outcome.

"There is good evidence to recommend against the routine use of low-dose aspirin to improve the outcome of live birth in ART cycles." *ASRM 2018 Guidelines*

The following study is one in which Professor Regan was involved:

Regan, L. et al.: *Human Reproduction*, Vol. 15, No.10, pp.2220-2223, Oct 2000
367 women with unexplained recurrent miscarriage plus 438 controls and 189 women with unexplained late pregnancy losses plus 61 controls were studied. In the groups with unexplained miscarriage, the livebirth rate was 68.4% for those who took aspirin compared to 63.5% who did not. In the group with late pregnancy losses, the livebirth rate was 64.6% compared to 49.2% who did not take aspirin.

Comment: Low dose aspirin seems to be quite beneficial according to this trial. Even better results are achieved when a broad spectrum of possible autoimmune factors are taken into consideration. To achieve optimum results, low dose aspirin is usually a single element of a more comprehensive protocol. Yet in IVF patients, even this relatively small addition has been shown to be beneficial, as the following randomized, double-blind placebo controlled trial demonstrates:

Rubinstein, M et al.: *Fertility & Sterility*, **May; 71(5):825-9, 1999**
149 patients underwent controlled ovarian hyperstimulation with the addition of a daily intake of 100 mg of aspirin. Results were compared with a control group of 149 who did not receive aspirin. The number of follicles and quantity of eggs retrieved was up to double that of the control group. The pregnancy rate was 45% versus 28% with an implantation rate of 17.8% versus 9.2%.

> **"Two prospective studies...have shown that combination treatment with aspirin and heparin significantly improves the livebirth rate of women with antiphospholipid syndrome."**
> **"A prospective cohort study has shown that aspirin and heparin was of no benefit in APA positive women undergoing IVF."**
>
> *RCOG 2003 Opinion Paper*

Comment: Antiphospholipid antibodies cause thrombosis in the placental vessels and impair embryonic implantation. Therefore, it follows if a treatment is effective in reducing miscarriage it should also be helpful for women with APAs undergoing IVF. In fact, recent studies demonstrate that heparin may also modulate trophoblast cell death and improve blastocyst adhesion to the endometrium. However, women with APAs usually need additional treatment, as at least 50% will have elevated NK cells or other immune problems.

Research that demonstrates that heparin and low dose aspirin may increase conception and ongoing pregnancy success rates includes:

Fiedler, K. and Wurfel, W.: *European Journal of Medical Research*, **Apr; 30; 9(4):207-14, 2004**
"...Heparin not only reduces the abortion rate but also lowers the risk for developmental retardation, premature birth and preeclampsia. The effects of heparin are not restricted to anticoagulation. It is directly or indirectly involved in the adhesion of the blastocyst to the endometrial epithelium and the subsequent invasion."

Bose, P. et al.: *American Journal of Obstetrics & Gynecology*, **Jan; 192(1):23-30, 2005**

In this in vitro study, the authors state that heparin and aspirin appeared to modulate trophoblast apoptosis (cell death), "…thus providing an additional mechanism to explain the clinical benefits of heparin and aspirin on recurrent pregnancy loss."

Sher, G. et al.: *American Journal of Reproductive Immunology*, **Aug; 40(2):74-82, 1998**

This study involved 687 APA positive women younger than 40 years who had failed up to three consecutive IVF/embryo transfer cycles within a 12 month period. The livebirth rate for those treated with heparin and aspirin was 46%. In the untreated group, it was 17%.

Professor Lesley Regan interviewed by Norman Swan for Radio National in 1997:

"We followed a group of women through pregnancy with proven phospholipid disease and we gave them no treatment apart from support and general tender loving care. Their miscarriage rate was 90% so they had a 10% livebirth rate. In the trial, we had an aspirin arm and an aspirin and heparin arm. The aspirin arm did much, much better than no treatment alone, and their livebirth rate was 40%. Looked at the other way, we reduced the miscarriage rate to 60%. But when we analyzed the women on the aspirin and heparin, they had made another very significant improvement in the livebirth rate, which went up from 40% on aspirin alone, to 71% with the aspirin and low dose heparin."

"There are no published data on the use of anti-TNF agents to improve pregnancy outcome in women with recurrent miscarriage."

RCOG 2011 Opinion Paper

"There is insufficient evidence to recommend adalimumab treatment to improve IVF outcome."

ASRM 2018 Guidelines

Jane Reed and Edward Winger have performed many (toughly vetted) peer reviewed and published studies at the Assisted Reproduction and Gynaecology Centre (ARGC) in London which confirmed the value of Humira in IVF.

The ARGC was getting the highest IVF success rates in the UK at the time of these publications according the UK HFEA website. These publications gave credibility to the ARGC, allowing them to sue their detractors. They won a lawsuit against the BBC TV program, "Panorama," which was trying to discredit the ARGC for using "dangerous and unproven" therapies. The ARGC sued the BBC for slander and won. They were awarded substantial damages as well as compensation for their legal costs.

Winger E, Reed J et al: *American Journal of Reproductive Immunology*, **Jul:60(1):8-16, 2008.**
75 pregnancies in patients with a history of recurrent miscarriage were retrospectively evaluated. The live birth rate was 19% (4/21) in those using anticoagulants alone, 54% (20/37) in group using anticoagulants (AC) and IVIG, and 71% (12/17) in group using anticoagulants, IVIG and Humira (TNF inhibitor) combined.

Winger E, Reed J et al: *American Journal of Reproductive Immunology*, **Feb;61(2): 113-20, 2009.**
75 sub-fertile women with Th1:Th2 cytokine elevation undergoing IVF were retrospectively evaluated. There was a significant improvement in implantation, clinical pregnancy and live birth rates for the group using IVIG and Humira combined versus the group using IVIG alone,

Winger E, Reed J et al:. *American Journal of Reproductive Immunology*, **Jun;65(6):610-8, 2011.**
In this retrospective study of 76 women undergoing IVF, it was found that the degree of preconception TNF/IL-10 elevation correlated with an increased risk of IVF failure and this problem could be reduced with Humira (TNF inhibitor) resulting in higher IVF success rates.

Winger E, Reed J et al: American Journal of Reproductive Immunology, Nov;68(5):428-37, 2012.

In subfertile women undergoing IVF, the oocyte quality measured can be measured by Die Off ratio (the ratio between the number of eggs retrieved or the number of quality embryos on Day 3). This specific measure of poor egg quality could be treated successfully with preconception Humira.

Sudhir N et al: *Journal of Human Reproducive Sciences,* **Apr-Jun; 9(2): 86–89, 2016.**
In a study of 115 women aged 21–44 years with history of recurrent miscarriage, the authors concluded, "The current study supports the concept of TNF-a 308G/A variant in particular with reproductive failure…"

Azizieh F and Raghupathy R: *Medical Principals and Practices* **24:165-170, 2015.**
Levels of tumor necrosis factor in 128 women with pregnancy complications were compared to women with normal levels. The authors concluded, "Along with other inflammatory cytokines, TNF-a may play critical roles in causing pregnancy complications, such as recurrent miscarriage, preeclampsia, premature rupture of the membrance and intrauterine growth retardation."

Comment: Dr Beer studied the effect of anti-TNF-alpha therapy on over 400 patients and tracked over 250 IVF cycles. For Dr Beer's "most difficult immune cases" whose average age was 37 and who had failed approximately four previous IVF cycles, the success rate, as of December 2005, was 53% using anti-TNF-alpha treatment.

In a 2006 lecture, Dr Beer reported that the livebirth rate for women with poor NK cell IVIG suppression who did not receive anti-TNF-alpha medication was 55% (6/11). With TNF-alpha therapy, it was 100% (8/8). For women with endometriosis the livebirth rate was 45% (9/20) without medication and 73% (16/22) with medication.

Since then, many peer reviewed papers have been published confirming similar findings. It appears that anti-TNF -alpha therapy offers new hope for select immunologic populations that have been traditionally the most difficult to treat: those with endometriosis, poor egg quality, and poor NK suppression, an elevated preconception TNF-alpha:Il-10 ratio, and/or a prior history of failure with LIT and IVIG.

CRITICS OF REPRODUCTIVE IMMUNOLOGY

Further supporting studies can be viewed in the Notes section.

"A significant proportion of cases of recurrent miscarriage remain unexplained despite detailed investigation. These women can be reassured that the prognosis for a successful future pregnancy with supportive care alone is in the region of 75%."

RCOG 2011 Opinion Paper

A few studies seem to support this view, but they are not very convincing. One of these spanned a period of nine years, during which the pregnancies of 61 women with three or more miscarriages were handled in one of two ways. The control group of 24 received no treatment and the remaining 37 were given psychological support and weekly medical checks. In the control group, a third of the women delivered their babies. In the "treated" group, 29 carried to term, which equates to an average of three births a year: not exactly a statistically robust conclusion.

Similar outcomes have been seen in studies where psychological support is given after the time the woman would usually miscarry and she is out of the miscarriage "danger zone." Furthermore, TLC trials tend to include groups that emerge through a process of self selection, or that have been preselected such as Regan's in 1997 and Liddell's in 1991. It is very unlikely these populations had the same frequency of autoimmune abnormalities found in Dr Beer's patients.

In Professor Regan's 1997 trial it is claimed that nearly 70% of 119 women with between three and 13 miscarriages carried to term "without any interventions to prevent miscarriage." However, during the selection process, patients who tested positive for antibodies to phospholipids or had polycystic ovary syndrome (PCOS) or luteinizing hormone imbalances were eliminated. As the researchers admitted, "Women in whom no abnormality was detected... formed the study population."

Considering that a large percentage of Dr Beer's miscarriage patients who tested positive for APAs (about 50%) had coexisting NK cell and/or cytokine issues, and that PCOS patients often have immune problems, Professor Regan and her associates excluded those who probably required immunotherapy. Three years later, a study at St. Mary's Hospital produced a livebirth rate among 253 women of just 58.5%. Another trial the same year quoted a livebirth rate of 58% for 81 women with unexplained recurrent miscarriages and no known abnormality. How, after the success of their TLC study can these relatively poor results be explained?

Tender loving care is unquantifiable and cannot be administered in a standardized way. Moreover, the implications of this theory are worrying for women who have repeatedly miscarried. Did emotional neglect, a lack of empathy or support from their partner or their doctor mean they lost their pregnancy? Turn the hypothesis around and you get guilt and blame, the not so appealing flipside of the TLC theory.

Professor Clark, who has assessed many thousands of clinical trials, identifies another fundamental problem associated with this debate. In his opinion, "The role of all health care providers should be to offer care and support to all patients. Tender loving care is not a luxury, it is a basic human right. Therefore, a double-blind, placebo controlled trial that compares one group that does not receive emotional support with a group that does would be unethical and virtually impossible to deliver in a controlled way.

"If tender loving care is so important, why does IVIG in controlled trials seem to work in recurrent miscarriage and IVF failure patients with autoimmune features? The data does not support the belief that TLC is equally as, or more effective than, immunotherapy. Patients in Chicago with recurrent spontaneous abortions received optimal psychological support and close monitoring after the FDA prohibited the use of lymphocyte immunization therapy. Yet the success rate for this group still fell significantly soon after LIT prohibition took effect."

Professor Clark also adds, "The odds of success with IVIG are higher when used to treat cancer or cardiovascular diseases. No one would suggest these patients should only be given psychological support. Couples with reproductive failure should be able to make a sensible decision regarding their treatment, rather than having the emotion based opinion of someone else imposed upon them."

Dr Kwak-Kim states in her 2009 paper, "Recurrent pregnancy loss: A disease of inflammation and coagulation," that there are two major concerns regarding women who repeatedly lose their babies. First, half of these cases are unexplained or clinically under diagnosed. Secondly, potential treatment should provide pregnancy success rates above the success rate of supportive therapy.

She comments, "Women with recurrent pregnancy loss have systemic inflammatory immune responses and increased vascular thrombosis and combination treatment should be considered." An uncontrolled inflammatory response or an untreated blood clotting disorder during pregnancy can harm placental growth, negatively impact the baby's development and can be a threat to the mother's own health.

While there is no doubt that stress reduction can be of some benefit to those with autoimmunities it is very dangerous to consider it as an exclusive therapy for the treatment of reproductive failure.

IS YOUR BODY BABY FRIENDLY?

"When a thing was new people said it was not true. Later, when the truth became obvious, people said it was not important. When its importance could not be denied, people said it was not new."

William James, 19th century philosopher

IS YOUR BODY BABY FRIENDLY?

17

Trials on Trial

In his 2002 article, "Wars of the Roses: Disagreements Among Reproductive Immunologists," Dr Norbert Gleicher said newcomers to reproductive immunology often look at questions in isolation, whereas seasoned reproductive immunologists and professional societies call upon a broader circle of experts before publishing clinical theories. He also draws attention to the fact that for years, reproductive immunologists have been "split into feuding camps, with different factions accusing each other of poor science, bad will and more recently, unethical behaviour."

This is not good for medicine, for reproductive immunology or for women who need help. Such antagonistic debate also reflects something of a double standard, an opinion that is voiced by Dr Geoffrey Sher, who says, "If only those therapies that have previously been proven by placebo controlled, prospective, randomized clinical trials were deemed appropriate for routine usage, then the practice of reproductive medicine would be vastly different today. In fact, virtually none of the clinical treatments used for IVF would be available because virtually none has met this 'gold standard.'

"In the IVF arena for example, where are the randomized controlled trials documenting a definitive benefit from gonadotropins over clomiphene? Virtually no one questions the benefit of using gonadotropins in this setting. Where are the trials for assisted hatching (widely used throughout the IVF world), nuclear/cytoplasmic transfer, ICSI versus other methods of assisted fertilization, blastocyst versus day-3 embryo transfer, or even IVF versus IUI? No one would question the benefit of IVF over the latter procedure in most cases." According to the U.S. Congress Office of Technology Assessment only 10 to 20% of all procedures currently used in medical practice have been shown to be efficacious by controlled trial.

Dr Sher continues, "This does not mean to imply that we should not continue to strive for the gold standard. However, it must also be remembered that randomized controlled trials are themselves imperfect, when a very large number of variables influence the endpoints being measured (e.g., as with recurrent miscarriage and IVF). Simply because the literature is discordant does not mean there is no merit to treatments that are not based on randomized controlled studies. It would be more constructive to determine why the success rates between the recurrent miscarriage studies are so different.

"It is somewhat hypocritical to single out immunologic treatment of recurrent miscarriage and IVF failure for criticism. The thousands of women with immunologic problems who had multiple pregnancy losses and after selective immunotherapy went on to have healthy babies would argue with the position stated in the 2011 RCOG report."

Professor Clark also argues philosophically, "One does not offer treatment on the basis of a theoretical mechanism. It is offered because it works consistently. There is an anecdote about an engineer who visited a factory to view a marvellous new machine churning out widgets. He turned to his host and said 'I see it works in practice but does it work in theory?'

"Why have the regulators not banned IVF pending the supply of data from a National Institutes of Health funded trial? One baby seems to be evidence enough that it works, yet the same principle is not applied to immunotherapy. Maybe this is because IVF involves relatively straight-forward procedures and is conceptually easier to grasp. Reproductive immunology, by contrast, involves complex and changing gobblede-gook theories that even immunologists can't understand."

"Perhaps resistance to this field has been created by the difficulty that statisticians have in explaining their results, bearing in mind that 'figures lie and liars figure.' That is why one must learn the key princi-ples and technology of statistics and re-examine the data oneself. More and better data is always needed, as utopian perfection only exists in the Aristotelian heavens and not in the real world, where there is variation and uncertainty. It would be unfortunate if that which was useful to patients was lost because of failure to properly re-examine the data we already have."

Dr Beer was not so equivocal, having spent many years in the front-line of hostility. He threw down the gauntlet to those who doubted his theories: "Patients should demand that the 'doubting doctor' supplies articles and evidence that support their views instead. When a baby dies or a pregnancy fails, something is wrong. The data speaks for itself; I did not dream it up. Reproductive endocrinologists must start reading the literature and stop being so critical before they have digested it."

He added, perhaps more tellingly, "By sticking to a standard approach, REs and fertility doctors receive all of a couple's IVF insurance benefits. If couples had a better alternative, this arrangement would be threatened. Reproductive immunology is getting a bad press and many doctors in the United States would like it to go away because it cuts into their business. It's as simple as that."

The Suspension of LIT
A Miscarriage of Justice?

The British immunologist Peter Medawar, who was knighted in 1965, was the first to discover that a mother could have an immunological reaction against her own fetus. He observed how, after delivering a stillborn baby, a 25-year-old woman reacted very badly to a blood transfusion from her husband who shared her blood type. This led Dr Medawar to speculate that the fetus had triggered a similarly aggressive immune response. It later transpired that the woman's blood lacked the Rh factor, whereas her husband was Rh-positive and it was likely that their baby was too. As Dr Medawar had suspected, a severe antibody reaction had killed their child.

In 1953 Dr Medawar introduced the idea that the immune system could be responsible for reproductive failure. His description of the fetus as a graft, akin to a transplanted organ, opened up possibilities for generations of researchers to follow. These included his own graduate student, Dr Rupert Billingham, who later demonstrated that immune factors clearly passed between the mother and fetus via the placenta in both directions and that in a successful pregnancy the mother's immune system responded non-aggressively to the fetus's foreign cells.

His explorations helped shape the entire field of reproductive immunology. In recognition of Dr Billingham's involvement, when Dr Medawar was awarded the 1960 Nobel Prize in physiology and medicine for his work on immunological tolerance and cellular immunity in organ transplantation, he shared the prize money with his former student.

Yet the questions remained. Why did some pregnancies end in miscarriage and how could it be prevented? It was not until the early 1970s that Dr Billingham and Dr Beer, who had joined Southwestern Medical School in Dallas as a faculty member, finally provided some answers to these challenging questions. They spent the next ten years working jointly to unravel the mysteries of the immune tolerance of a normal pregnancy and produced over 20 articles on the subject.

They noticed that when male and female tissue types were dissimilar there was a greater likelihood of successful reproduction. Dr Beer explains their observations: "When animal brothers and sisters were mated in experiments to produce an inbred strain, the mother produced runts and soon she was infertile. So there was something about pregnancy compatibility that led to a type of rejection that was totally different from the rejection of a kidney or heart."

In the same experiments, they also demonstrated that the female could be immunized using lymphocytes from the male partner to create antibodies that would stop her immune system from attacking her future offspring. The publication of these discoveries in *Science* in 1973 marked the beginning of the lymphocyte immune therapy (LIT) story.

In 1979, Dr Beer tested their theories in real life and found three couples all of whom had lost between five and seven pregnancies. Tests revealed genetic compatibility was a problem for each couple and the women were suitable candidates for paternal lymphocyte immune therapy. All three became pregnant that same year and had children (who are now approaching their 30s).

The first of the women to give birth had previously endured seven miscarriages. She recalled her experience as Dr Beer's first successful LIT patient: "My husband and I were frustrated, exhausted and emotionally drained from so many pregnancy losses. There were no explanations just countless days filled with every imaginable test. I was not infertile; I just couldn't stay pregnant. We agreed that this would be our last try as I had just turned 40.

We were reaching the end of a long journey that had started with an online search where I located and read all that was available on the subject of recurrent miscarriage and in the process, discovered Dr Beer. I knew he would be our last chance to create a family of our own.

"Our first visit with Dr Beer was indeed memorable. Here I sat with a gentle, caring man I had met just moments before, telling him my story. I was crying, yet still attempting to appear normal and emotionally capable of handling any process or tests. Dr Beer provided the strength, knowledge, trust, understanding and competence, which at that point we so desperately needed.

"I began a series of immunizations and shortly afterwards I conceived. Throughout the following nine months, Dr Beer was always available by phone and he was the first person I called after giving birth to our son Michael, who was a healthy 6 lbs 8 ozs. He was the first ever 'Beer Baby.'"

Around the same time, the London based physician Dr W. Page Faulk found four couples with recurrent miscarriage and similar HLA types. He used white cells pooled from unrelated male donors to immunize the women. He reported successful pregnancies in all cases in an article in the *Lancet*. Although the evidence from these small, uncontrolled trials was compelling, there were demands for a large, double-blind, randomized controlled study.

Professor James Mowbray of St. Mary's Hospital Medical School, also in London set up a trial in 1982 involving 105 women with unexplained recurrent miscarriages. 49 became pregnant. 22 were immunized with their partner's lymphocytes and 27 received placebo injections of their own white blood cells. 78% of the treatment group had live births compared with just 37% of the untreated group. The researchers announced, "A successful outcome of the next pregnancy was significantly more common in women injected with purified lymphocytes prepared from their husbands' blood." Since then many studies have reinforced these initial findings with success rates approaching 100% for selected patient groups.

The results of this groundbreaking treatment attracted considerable media attention. Dr Beer was invited to take part in radio and TV interviews and in 1996, *People* magazine ran an article about his revolutionary therapy entitled "Injection of Hope." It described how he was treating women who had endured multiple IVF failures and numerous miscarriages and became pregnant with LIT.

Indeed, this remarkable therapy is still making headlines today. In 2005, a national U.K. newspaper reported how a 33-year-old specialist at the CARE fertility clinic in Nottingham had suffered a series of miscarriages, but went on to deliver a daughter after receiving white blood cells from her partner. Sadly, similar achievements are no longer being announced by IVF centers in the United States. Although LIT can be obtained in many parts of the world, including England, Canada, Australia, South America, the Philippines, Japan (approximately 70% of Japanese university hospitals still provide this therapy), the Middle East and other parts of Europe, it is no longer available within the U.S.

In 2002, the Food and Drug Administration (FDA) suspended the use of lymphocyte immunization therapy pending the results of FDA-approved, randomized, multi-center clinical trials. Their decision was made largely in response to the findings of the controversial five-year-long Recurrent Miscarriage Study (REMIS) that began in 1992 and was organized by Dr Carole Ober at the University of Chicago Hospitals.

In this trial, paternal lymphocyte therapy was found to cause more miscarriages than it prevented. "We began the study to determine if immunotherapy was effective in preventing recurrent miscarriage, but it's surprisingly ineffective," declared Dr Ober after the results were published. In her trial, 73% of 179 women became pregnant over a year. 45% miscarried and the livebirth rate for immunized women was 36% compared to 48% in the control group. Given LIT's previous track record, this shockingly poor outcome seemed quite unbelievable, until you look at the way the study was organized.

To construct a meaningful study one must first understand the requirements of the treatment. There are defined parameters to determine how LIT should be administered and who should receive it. For example, it is important to determine the woman's leukocyte antibody detection levels before LIT is given to find out whether the treatment is needed and how effective it will be. LIT is more suitable for certain subsets of patients, primarily those who have never had a live birth. If a woman experiences recurrent miscarriage after having a baby, she will probably need other treatments like IVIG.

In the Recurrent Miscarriage Study, the majority of participants had already given birth to at least one child. In Dr Beer's opinion, "Women with one liveborn child who then repeatedly miscarry have immune problems caused by abnormal NK cell activity. I would not have included this subset of women in the trial." However, this was not the only unsuitable patient group to receive treatment.

Those who were involved in the lab testing for the Recurrent Miscarriage Study reported that the entry criteria were relaxed to include women who were positive for antinuclear or anticardiolipin antibodies, allegedly to increase the number of patients taking part.

It was already known from the 1991 American Society for Reproductive Immunology Ethics Committee study, that LIT did nothing to improve pregnancy success rates in patients with these kinds of autoantibodies. Women who test positive for antinuclear antibodies or anticardiolipin antibodies need additional treatments such as corticosteroids and heparin.

Dr Beer explained the dangers of such poor patient selection: "LIT is not a magic therapy for all the immune factors that may underlie recurrent loss. If a patient has wide ranging immune dysfuntion and is given only LIT, the success rate is 60% below that of women who receive LIT and are also treated with aspirin, heparin, corticosteroids, IVIG or anti-TNF medication. When all the categories of immune problem are treated, the reproductive outcome is over 80%. Untreated autoimmunity will result in many losses, even if LIT therapy is administered."

In the Recurrent Miscarriage Study, only 26% of women who received LIT developed blocking antibodies, which led to questions about the way the serum was prepared and administered. In Dr Ober's trial, patients allegedly received far less of an initial dose than they needed which meant the success rates would never be optimal. In addition, the lymphocytes used to treat the women were prepared from blood samples that were usually stored overnight. The failure to use fresh donor cells would render the treatment useless.

To prevent abortion the cells need a paternal antigen and a molecule called CD200, which is a tolerance signal. With overnight storage the CD200 molecule is lost. The serum containing the paternal cells was also stored at room temperature which meant that the cells lost all their anti-abortive effect.

So disappointing were the results that the trial was halted. In late 1997, the board of the University of Chicago asked the researchers not to immunize any more patients and those who needed follow up immunizations were not treated.

To date, Carole Ober has refused to allow anyone access to any trial material, despite the fact it was a state funded study and as such, information should have been made publicly available. In 1999, Professor Clark asked her for the raw data for the ASRI Ethics Committee database. Dr Ober informed him that there were "confidentiality issues" and that she intended to write up the results herself and publish them in the *Journal of Reproductive Immunology*. Professor Clark sent a second request, reassuring her about confidentiality and the preservation of her ability to publish independently. The database remained unforthcoming.

Finally, there was an appeal to the National Institutes of Health (NIH) asking them for assistance in releasing the data. The verdict was that the data belonged to Dr Ober. It has been reported that $2.2 million of taxpayers' dollars was spent on an abortive trial whose details remain unavailable to the public.

In July 1999, this severely flawed Recurrent Miscarriage Study was referred to in an article entitled "Mononuclear-cell Immunization in the Prevention of Recurrent Miscarriages: A Randomized Trial," published in the *Lancet*. The article concluded that more women miscarried with LIT than without. Although Dr Beer was listed as a co-principal investigator in the application for the NIH grant, incredibly he did not see the report until it had been published. However, he had seen the trial records, which did not impress him at all. "The post immunization data was dismal," he recalled, "with less than 30% of women showing a post immunization response and only two of those were sufficient enough to be cleared for a cycle of conception."

He expressed his concerns to Professor Clark in August 1999 saying, "Many of the patients included in the study were very autoimmune and were tested for abnormal NK levels and activity. This study is about inoculation not immunization. We must do everything possible to expose these misdemeanors."

Dr Beer wrote to the *Lancet* explaining his concerns and told them he had not been consulted regarding the interpretation or analysis of the results. He also outlined some of the report's flaws: the suboptimal standards of immunization and the fact that karyotypically abnormal pregnancy losses had been included in the final statistics, which had further decreased the success rate. (LIT does not guard against chromosomally abnormal pregnancies.)

Professor Clark, Dr Coulam and others produced an analysis of the discrepancies which was also published. Professor Mowbray also questioned the trial's integrity, saying that storing the father's cells overnight might have been the problem. "It *does* work," he confirmed, "I've seen 5,000 couples with repeated miscarriages and have had a very high success rate and a very low abnormality rate." Rupert Billingham played no part in the debate; he retired in 1986 and died shortly after the results of the Ober trial were published.

All these rebuttals were later to be overshadowed by the publication of a 2003 Cochrane Review written by Dr Jim Scott, a colleague of Dr Ober, who was also involved in the Recurrent Miscarriage Study. This official sounding paper comprised a collection of small, disparate studies with two main features in common: faulty methodology and a damning verdict on white cell therapy. For example, insufficient doses of LIT were administered, or cell concentrations were not specified. In Professor Clark's opinion, "The Cochrane review was flawed and this problem would remain even if it had been written on stone tablets on high and carried down from Mount Sinai."

The FDA's decision to suspend the use of lymphocyte immunization therapy in 2002 was also precipitated by pressure from an Atlantic Monthly journalist who, according to an FDA government official, regularly called the department insisting that action should be taken in view of the Ober trial's findings. The journalist issuing these warnings was Jon Cohen, author of *Coming to Term: Uncovering the Truth About Miscarriage*, published in 2005.

In his book, Cohen casts doubt on the validity of immunotherapy and suggested that miscarriage, in many cases, cannot or should not be prevented because the fetus is probably genetically defective. To add weight to his argument Cohen presented the views of an Ob/Gyn named Dr Joseph Hill III, author of the 1997 article, *Immunotherapy for Recurrent Pregnancy Loss: 'Standard of Care or Buyer Beware*, a critique that was praised by Professor Regan in her own book on miscarriage written in 2001.

Currently working for the Fertility Centers of New England, Dr Hill was probably the most outspoken critic of lymphocyte immunotherapy on the lecture circuit. Among those who heard him talk was Dr William Matzner, a board certified internist and immunologist. Dr Matzner recalls, "When Hill was talking he would speak like a preacher, not a scientist. He didn't talk a lot about scientific data because he really didn't have a lot, whereas there is quite a bit of scientific data to back up LIT. The whole idea of blocking antibodies has been known by transplant immunologists for years. And to rheumatologists, the whole approach of using paternal white blood cells to build a female response that protects the pregnancy makes perfect sense."

Dr Hill's verdict that the Recurrent Miscarriage Study was "the best trial to find that the therapy does not work," was echoed by Cohen who lobbied the FDA until they conceded "lymphocyte immune therapy should have had their approval but it had never been sought or granted." Finally, in January 2002, the FDA sent out a letter saying that Dr Beer and others required permission to test this "investigational new drug" (IND) and would need to apply for a license before they were allowed to use it.

Whole blood and its byproducts are only considered drugs when they are manufactured by a facility for mass distribution. In such cases licensing is required, particularly if the material is sold or transported across borders. As lymphocyte immunization involves a single blood sample that is processed and given to a single recipient it hardly falls into this category. With modern screening methods, it is not at all difficult for this vaccine to meet strict safety standards (as is routinely done by most blood banks) and to be produced in accordance with stringent regulations.

Nonetheless, the use of LIT in the United States was suspended. At the Chicago Medical School's Finch University of Health Sciences, (since renamed the Rosalind Franklin University of Medicine and Science) the ongoing pregnancy success rate dropped from 84% to 64% the year after the directive was imposed.

The FDA usually requires two positive randomized controlled trials before it can endorse the use of a specific clinical treatment. Determined to revalidate LIT, Dr Beer and his close colleague and former student Dr Joanne Kwak formed *The Society for Immunotherapy and Investigation*. Along with others, including Professor Clark, they worked on finalizing proposals for a further study of LIT, this time with 2,432 patients. The society's mission statement indicated their confidence in the outcome: "There is no better scientific and clinical retort to the published work than an adequate, well designed and controlled trial... The results still stand on their own to support continuance of this important therapeutic program."

Unfortunately, their hopes were dashed with the arrival of a new President at the Chicago Medical School at the end of 2002. He had no interest in pursuing the idea despite the fact that the FDA was keen for a further trial. The society's application for an IND license for lymphocyte immunization therapy was brought to an abrupt and frustrating end.

As Professor Clark relates, "Initially we had two Phase 3 randomized controlled trials: one for repetitive spontaneous abortion and one for IVF failure patients. The FDA had asked that we develop and execute a Phase 2 dose response study, but this was not to be."

Coming so close to having the proposal accepted only for it to be withdrawn by his own School was a huge blow to Dr Beer, who reflected, "You can imagine my disappointment when the FDA had our proposal in its hands and was already asking for Phase 2 studies only to have all our efforts taken away."

During his 16 years with the School, Dr Beer had worked with four Deans and four Presidents. Recognizing that it would be too arduous to continue to renegotiate his position on LIT he decided to set up his own private practice in California, "The Alan E. Beer Center for Reproductive Immunology and Genetics." One mission was at the forefront of his mind: to restore the reputation of lymphocyte immune therapy and take back control of his program.

But he was yet to face another hurdle. Dr Beer discovered he could not apply for a new IND license because the original application from the Chicago Medical School had to be submitted. Despite several requests to the School, they refused to release the documents to him.

Without the original IND application papers his center could not apply for the license that would have allowed him to generate the data needed to return the therapy to U.S. patients. "Only then," Dr Beer said, "will it once again be possible to reduce the death toll of unborn babies for women with immune mediated miscarriage."

In the meantime, Dr Beer he opened a state of the art testing laboratory in California with Edward Winger, a leading immunopathologist. He also continued to collect LIT data from Europe, Asia and South America. In Mexico, the treatment is still achieving an excellent 78% ongoing pregnancy success rate in patients with a history of losses.

Despite all these setbacks, Dr Beer remained hopeful that a further trial of lymphocyte immune therapy would take place saying, "I think the FDA would approve a proposal from David Clark, Edward Winger and myself. The question is, will someone allow us the opportunity to prove what we believe to be the truth."

Sadly, Dr Beer passed away before he was given the chance.

18

Hope

By Alan E. Beer, M.D.

I know I can make a difference in the lives of many couples struggling, hurting, seeking and experiencing repeated disappointments. In good faith, many of you have listened to advice that has not served you well and the cycle of failure goes on.

I have four grown wonderful children who are beautiful, bright and healthy and in committed relationships. It would kill them and me if they were bruised and abused with infertility and loss of hope that they may never become parents. I weep inside when I see a message composed at 3:00 am by someone's wife and companion, unable to sleep, seeking answers at the computer, on a mission, knowing there is a problem, silently blaming herself, feeling sadness, feeling guilt, fearing to hope because disappointment stands outside the nearest door...and yet she never gives up.

I have a mission to provide the data that I know I can trust about this problem and share it with all of you in a manner that can be understood, taken to heart, and applied to each emerging case. With understanding of the problem comes healing, partial hope is restored and what courage is remaining surfaces...and you try again. This time I can quote statistics of changes of failure or success; this time you have names and addresses of patients who have walked before you; this time it is different because I exist.

To travel the world as I am privileged to do and to meet couples in their own environment, to view their growing families, to see their businesses thriving, to see a totally new look to their posture and the aura of their faces, to see their need to tell me all about what it has done for them, to receive their thanks in thousands of different ways is a tribute few on this earth ever receive and I receive it often.

To work any other way would not work for me. I am a "giant" in my field but I know the work place. I could have colleagues answer many of these questions appropriately disguised and signed by me. I could lighten my load but the time might be filled with other activities that do less good. If I did not do it the way I do it now, everyone would know and be less satisfied. Real people and committed people work hard because their spirit dictates this. These are a few words on why I do what I do.

...and Inspiration

Cherylann

When I was a little girl I would dream of the day when I would marry a wonderful man, have four perfect children, live in a perfect house, have the perfect life and live happily ever after. Then my life happened.

Mr. Wonderful had yet to show up, man, I kept wasting wishes on him every birthday. So when I was 42 I decided I had to do something on my own. As a professional nurse one would have thought I would have known that our fertility decreases rapidly after age 35. But no, I never knew that. With all the celebrities having babies I assumed I would have no problem either. Maybe a few months tops and I would be pregnant and well on my way to "almost perfect land."

Well, I ran into some pretty bad doctors. One actually told me she once knew a RE who said he wanted to make the exam room doors smaller to discourage the "really fat women" from trying to get pregnant with IVF. This was as I was walking through the door to my first intrauterine insemination aka IUI where they inject sperm directly into the uterus. Oh, did I mention I was one of those "really fat women"?

This doctor blamed my failure month after month on the fact that I was "morbidly obese" (that's an attractive label isn't it?) and did no testing to see if anything was wrong.

The strange thing about the times when I was trying IUI every month was that I would get peculiar symptoms. Not pregnancy symptoms but my allergies would act up as if I was coming down with a cold every time. My asthma even kicked in a few times. This is important to remember. I also had panic attacks and restless legs.

At the age of 45, three years and many thousands of dollars later, I was still nowhere near my dream. Eventually I made my peace with not having a genetic child of my own and began my search for donor eggs.

Since I was using donor sperm, the decision wasn't as difficult as one might think. My family history includes everything from cardiac disease to diabetes, so it wasn't too much of a crisis for me to forgo my genetics if I could make sure I had a healthy child.

I found my donor and had my fresh transfer. No way could I fail with 26 year old eggs. I was sure to become pregnant! Well I did. I got a positive pregnancy test for the first time in my life. I was ecstatic until I was told it was not meant to be. Oh, mind you, I was told I lost the baby because I was fat and obviously liked being that way or I would have done something about it. Man, I could write my own book about rude, unethical doctors.

I was heartbroken, depressed, sad, mad, hurt, confused, irritated, you name it I had the emotion. I didn't know where to turn. Realizing that my childhood dream might never come true, I briefly thought that life wasn't worth living. If I couldn't be a mother what would become of me? Would I die alone with a bunch of cats?

Maybe it was my Irish stubbornness, but I decided to fight for what I wanted. I wasn't going to abandon my life long dream because some jerk in a suit had told me I was fat. Plenty of fat people get pregnant every day. There was a reason why I wasn't getting or staying pregnant and I was going to find out what it was if it was the last thing I did.

Now the story takes a very serendipitous turn. My allergies had been so severe that I went to see an allergist. I showed him my list of ailments and medications and past medical history. He said, "Wow, you have been really sick here!" I said, "Yeah, I keep getting sick all the time, pneumonia, bronchitis, sinusitis." I also told him I was trying unsuccessfully to get pregnant.

He did major testing of my immune system and told me he knew exactly what was wrong with me. I finally found out I had a genetic disorder called Common Variable Immune Deficiency. This meant I had very little resistance to most viruses and some bacteria. I was a basically a walking germ bomb. The treatment for this was IVIG every two weeks to keep me healthy.

At the same time as this, I was looking up immune problems on the Internet and found the Yahoo Reproductive Immunology Support Group. After much debating whether I should invest a lot of money I really didn't have, I decided to fly out to California. I had nothing to lose and only my dreams to gain.

I met with Dr Beer and my life changed. He was the kindest, most intelligent human I have ever had the privilege to meet. I was immediately drawn to him as a person and a doctor. I knew innately that he could help me. I felt the tears flowing as he explained that yes, he knew what my problem was and he was confident he could fix it.

He said that while my immune system really bad at killing off germs, it tried very hard to kill off anything it saw as an intruder. Every embryo I put into my body it destroyed, thinking it was a cancer or something that would harm me. Mind you, it didn't do it in the normal way. Nope, my body enlisted the special forces: the eosinophils, NK and CD57 cells. By the time I got to Dr Beer they had invaded my uterus and taken up residence there.

Remember how I said I was getting allergy symptoms every time I had an IUI? That was my eosinophils popping into action and killing off my embryos. For this I required some Enbrel as well as the IVIG I was already receiving.

I learned through Dr Beer's testing that I also had a gene mutation called MTHFR that can cause clotting problems as well as a folic acid absorption deficiency. Plus I had some suspicious APAs, which meant I needed heparin to maintain a pregnancy. I also had some autoimmune problems, namely insulin resistance and Hashimoto's thyroiditis. Nobody ever told me any of this before because nobody had ever bothered to test for these things.

Sure I brought up these test results with my RE. He pooh poohed them and even called Dr Beer a quack and warned me I would be risking my life if I continued seeing him. I said to myself that this RE had not done anything for me, whereas Dr Beer had tested me and what's more, he could provide me with real treatments.

The IVF center gave me a 30% chance of getting pregnant with frozen embryos. They transferred three and I became pregnant with twins! I was in shock and very happy, but still very unsure I would be able to carry my babies to term. But with Dr Beer's careful monitoring of my natural killer cells and cytokines and the assistance of my allergist, I delivered my two precious sons in March 2004.

They are my life, my breath and the reason why I get up in the morning. Never in my life have I felt so much love as when I first held my tiny sons in my arms. It was if my world suddenly went from black and white to wild, vivid Technicolor. I saw life in a whole new way, as something actually worth living. I had joy for the first time in many, many years.

I could never have achieved my lifelong dream without Dr Beer. To me he is a miracle worker. My babies would not be here if it were not for his therapies. So when I hear of a doctor speaking negatively of his treatments or saying there is no data on his work, I want to tell them, and believe me I do at every opportunity, "Here, look at these two gorgeous boys, is that enough data for you?"

Elizabeth and James

Elizabeth: Both my daughters were both born as a result of the treatment I received from the Zouves Fertility Center and the help of Dr Beer.

My husband and I were told for years that I was too old and we should just go home or think about adoption. My problem was that I had scar tissue in my tubes. I could get pregnant with IVF but kept on losing the baby. In addition to the two definite miscarriages that I knew of, over the years I must have lost quite a few others. Looking back, I was having late periods and many other symptoms that all pointed to chronic immune related implantation failures.

We kept asking questions and continued doing our own investigations. Then one evening, my husband and I caught the tail end of a TV program about a doctor who treated women with the same kind of problems I was experiencing. We also learned, very fortunately for us, that he visited a clinic near us once a month. If only we had discovered him earlier.

Dr Beer carried out a series of tests, which revealed I had high levels of natural killer cells that needed to be brought down and I had problems with low levels of blocking antibodies. I was put on a cocktail of drugs and responded well. In addition to heparin and baby aspirin, I had IVIG and was inoculated with a serum made from my husband's blood.

On the first cycle, Dr Zouves put back four embryos. I was scared that more than one would take, but he must have known what he was doing as just one implanted. The second time, when I was 44, he put back six. He must have worked out the odds because again, just one took. Both pregnancies went as smooth as clockwork. All this was after

HOPE AND INSPIRATION

we had been told by other doctors that there was virtually no hope and that immune therapy was useless.

James: We talked to so many doctors about immune testing and found there is a lot of disagreement about the procedure. It's the same with the IVF people. After one failed cycle, we were told immune treatment was useless and Dr Beer was a snake oil salesman spreading misinformation around the Internet. A couple of years later this same clinic is promoting Dr Beer's therapies because of consumer demand and because it gets results.

Looking back, the propaganda against Dr Beer and Dr Zouves was tremendous. In my opinion, the medical establishment is too conservative and inbred. It hates pioneers and it hates people asking questions they can't answer because they don't know anything about the subject because it's complicated and new and they can't be bothered to read up about it. Instead they say that people like Dr Beer are idiots and they just go back to their tried and trusted old ways.

We could have saved ourselves thousands of dollars if we had gone to the right doctors in the first place, but all the way down the line we were sent off in the wrong direction by these people. Now when I think of the hundreds of couples sitting there in these clinics I just think that so many are destined to failure because they will only be given the standard procedures. When they don't work they'll be given the brush off like we were and told to go home.

As for Dr Beer being a salesman, whoever says that is just ignorant. Dr Beer was a dedicated medical doctor who took his protocols very seriously. We met him when he was in his 60s, traveling around the world at his own expense. He didn't get reimbursed for a lot of what he did. It's many years since he pioneered his treatment and the results today show that he was right. But still they keep on asking for a huge population study. How could one man do that with the select few patients he had? Because of this, the establishment has written him off as some kind of crank.

We were in our 40s and given less than a 3% chance of success. We had been to many so called "specialists" and spent years doing things their way. All we got was chronic failure.

Yet when we did immunotherapy and IVF with Dr Zouves, it worked first time, both times. That's not luck. It's all about finding the right

Mike and Jodi

Mike: It was seven years and four specialists before we found Dr Beer. During this time we had had two miscarriages and several other early losses. Everything was going fine with our first baby until it just stopped growing at eleven weeks.

While we were having blood work done in relation to the first miscarriage we found out that Jodi was pregnant again. What happened next was a total nightmare. We discovered our baby was dead when we went in for a high definition scan at twelve weeks. That was a terrible experience. We just flipped out. A D&C showed the pregnancy had been molar, where two sperm fertilize one egg. It was quite a while before we could try again, but then we just couldn't get pregnant at all.

The doctor told us that before we could have tests done to see if anything was wrong they usually waited for three miscarriages. After about six months, we went to see a fertility specialist. As I was taking Jodi's notes over to our new doctor I noticed a message stuck to her file that said, "Call patient about thyroid problem." Unbelievably, not only had they not called us, but nobody had told us that Jodi had also tested positive for antinuclear antibodies, antiphospholipid antibodies and an abnormal thyroid, which turned out to be Hashimoto's disease.

It seemed that my wife's immune problems flared up even more when she was pregnant and her NK cell count reached extremely high levels. Unfortunately, our fertility doctor outright rejected the idea of immune problems. He told us that Jodi's test results were nothing to worry about and said immunology wasn't something they believed in.

So I decided to do a bit of research of my own and looked online. I found some websites and discussion boards and a fertility doctor called Dr Jonathan Scher who wrote the book, *Preventing Miscarriage: The Good News*. He seemed to agree with immune testing and treatment. We went to see him and he told us we definitely needed IVIG and heparin. When I mentioned this to our fertility doctor, he said, "Don't go to Dr Scher, he's a quack who'll take your money!" He also warned us, saying, "IVIG's a human blood product. Who knows, in the future you could get mad cow disease!" I replied, "What are all the hormones you are giving us; aren't they human blood products?" The doctor had nothing to say, except, "You're right."

But once more, we listened to him, as he seemed so sure we would be okay. We tried IVF again without immune treatments, which didn't work at all. I figured we had given him enough chances and his way wasn't getting us anywhere except closer to bankruptcy.

We went back to Dr Scher and on our next try at IVF Jodi got pregnant again with twins. By this time, my wife was 35 and I was 37. We weren't taking any chances, so I called Dr Beer who collaborated with Dr Scher to make sure that we kept our babies. The blood work up with Dr Beer found all the things that none of the other specialists could find.

During the pregnancy Jodi's numbers went whacky. Her NK cells were sky high and her ANAs were totally abnormal. Dr Beer told us we that we needed LIT as well as IVIG so we went to Nogales in Mexico and made a vacation out of it. (That was a surreal experience, sneaking over the border as if we were drug smugglers or something!) But we followed what Dr Beer was advising every step of the way. Jodi needed folic acid and prednisone as well as the heparin and IVIG. He also recommended we have blood tests every three weeks to keep the pregnancy in check.

It was then we found that NK cells can jump within two weeks, to triple or quadruple the number they were. IVIG therapy worked very well for my wife. Twice we had to do double doses of IVIG in one week. It must have worked, because for the first time in seven years the pregnancy went beyond the first trimester. Previously, not only could we not get pregnant on our own, but we couldn't keep it after Clomid, artificial insemination and in vitro fertilization.

Dr Beer made sure that our beautiful little boy and girl arrived safe and well. Without his help, the outcome would no doubt have been very different.

Maryann

I got married when I was 33 and we didn't start trying for a baby until I was 35. Nobody back then said, "Oops, you'd better hurry up," so I had no idea that it got more difficult the later you left things. My mother had me at 27 and kept trying for another but only managed to get pregnant one more time at 41 and then she had a miscarriage.

Just to make sure we wasted no time, I bought an ovulation monitor and believe it or not the first month I used it we got pregnant. This is so easy, I thought, but right from the beginning I was spotting. I had suffered from quite bad hair loss from the age of 21, but when I became pregnant, it stopped falling out. In addition, I had extreme sensitivity to smells and everything tasted like a chemical, even chocolate! These became "my signs" that I had conceived.

We saw a heartbeat at six weeks and then we went for another ultrasound a few weeks later. I remember that my husband and I were kept totally in the dark as they looked at the screen. I kept on asking what was wrong but nobody said anything. Then we were told that we had to wait for the doctor to speak to us. So we were left sitting in the reception area for an hour until she called us on the phone and said, "Maryann, there's no heartbeat." "What does that mean?" I asked frantically. She just replied, "Well, it died."

My husband and I were crying and distraught while everyone stared at us. I will never forget that moment. I later had a D&C and asked if the fetus could be tested for genetic problems. But they said they didn't usually test the first miscarriage so I will never know for sure what went wrong with that pregnancy. I was shocked they didn't take the loss of my baby seriously. I felt they just dismissed it by saying it was a "bad egg." It was then that I realized how common miscarriages were.

As we were moving house we decided to wait a while before trying again, but would you believe it, I got pregnant again four months later.

My hair stopped falling out as usual, the chemical taste was back and the spotting started again. This time my HCG levels were not quite doubling and it was eventually determined that it was a blighted ovum. Eight weeks later, I had another D&C and this time they found the embryo had trisomy 2 chromosomal abnormalities.

After this, we made a real effort to try to conceive for six months but nothing happened. However, after the second miscarriage my cycles changed dramatically. Instead of being like clockwork, the usual 28 to 32 days long, they ranged anywhere from 18 to 35 days. I would also spot for 7 to 10 days before the actual flow came which had never happened before. Finally, when my period did arrive it would be very clotty and dark and the flow was short lived.

I knew in my heart that something was very wrong and that the pregnancies and miscarriages had changed my body in some way. Yet my Ob/Gyns told me that my disordered cycles were absolutely no problem and that we should just keep on trying.

Trusting our doctors like most people do, we tried to conceive for six months but nothing happened. This shocked and frustrated me, because it had been so easy to get pregnant twice before. Nearly every month I felt as if something was starting and then it would just stop and my period was delayed. Later I discovered that these were implantation failures and very early miscarriages.

My Ob/Gyn suggested that I go to an infertility specialist, but I also knew I needed someone to tell me what was wrong with me so I could get treatment. I scoured the Internet, searching for answers, and posted my story on countless infertility websites. Eventually I found INCIID (pronounced "inside") and that was the beginning of the rest of my life. Someone reading my story suggested that I posted it on the immune board, where Dr Alan Beer was answering questions.

My husband and I had our blood tested and found we were a complete match for both DQ alpha 3 and 4.1. I also tested positive for APAs and antithyroid antibodies and had elevated levels of NK cells in my blood and my uterus. Dr Beer put me on anti-TNF-alpha therapy, LIT, IVIG, dexamethasone, aspirin and Lovenox.

After a month, my period returned to normal and our first IVF cycle was a success. However, once again, my immune problems reared their ugly heads. I spotted right from the beginning and had several hemorrhages during the first and second trimesters. I continued IVIG every three weeks and had LIT every five weeks throughout the pregnancy.

At the age of 38, seemingly against the odds, I gave birth to my beautiful son. I never actually met Dr Beer face to face, but I am sure that my little boy would not be here today if it had not been for his diagnosis, therapies and vigilance.

Janine

I worked with Professor Regan at the St. Mary's Recurrent Miscarriage clinic a couple of years ago as a nurse and I have only good things to say about them, *but* I have to admit, they are very conservative in their approach. They did not believe in treating miscarriages with anything other than Clexane and aspirin, which I know was not enough for me because I had these twice in IVF cycles and still miscarried. They said that it was "bad luck" and that there must be something wrong with my uterus. I had a hysteroscopy, but it showed no uterine problems. Clearly, something else was going on.

After several more emotionally painful chemical pregnancies and one miscarriage using their conservative therapies, I decided to see Mr. Taranissi in London who heads the Assisted Reproduction & Genetics Centre and uses similar treatments to Dr Beer. Here they did the full blown panel, including the NK cell assay, which is not done at St. Mary's. In fact, the tests recommended by Professor Regan had all come back negative.

With a complete immune evaluation, I finally had some answers. I was positive for NK cells and needed immunotherapy. I had two loads of IVIG in addition to Clexane and aspirin throughout my cycle, which resulted in a successful pregnancy.

I don't think I would have had my baby with the conservative approach they have at St. Mary's. I don't hold it against them, I just feel they should "get real" and recognize that not everyone has antiphospholipid antibodies/sticky blood syndrome.

With miscarriage there is often a wider picture and patients do not have time to wait. The Recurrent Miscarriage Clinic has helped many women and I do respect their work, but perhaps it is not the best place to go to if you need that "little bit more."

Pam

I got my first period just before my thirteenth birthday and blacked out as the blood gushed out of my body. It felt as if I was being pulled inside out. My periods were always the same: painful and long. So began 25 years of physical anguish and psychological suffering.

I became pregnant for the first time a month before I was to get married. Several weeks into the pregnancy I had a miscarriage and a D&C. The doctors' office called to tell me the pathology revealed no "products of conception." I had two independent blood tests, which both showed very low levels of HCG. The doctor reassured me I was no longer pregnant and sent me on my way without an ultrasound.

A few days later, I went on a trip out of town with my fiancé to spend Easter with his family. I woke just after midnight in excruciating pain. My abdomen seemed to be growing by the minute and blood was trickling out of me as we rushed to the hospital. They poked and prodded and eventually I had emergency surgery to remove an ectopic pregnancy which had burst inside my left fallopian tube. The surgeon removed the tube but was able to save my left ovary.

When I woke up he said, "We almost lost you little girl." He explained to me that I was filled with endometriosis. Finally, there was a reason for all my years of pain. A few months later, I had further surgery to remove the adhesions. Now with only one tube left, my chances of getting pregnant were cut by half.

A year passed without me getting pregnant. My husband whom I had known since fifth grade became impatient and angry. He told me he no longer loved me since I couldn't give him a family. My marriage was annulled by the Catholic Church because I was apparently unable to bear children. It was a very low point in my life and depression crept in like a thief. Infertility was stealing my life.

In my late 20s, I met my second husband. At this time, my periods were as regular as clockwork although I suffered with raging PMS and behaved like a crazy woman at times. I began to feel pain during ovulation as well as during my period and sometimes intercourse was excruciating. Each doctor I saw recommended a hysterectomy but I was not willing to give up the dream of becoming a mother.

We started building a new house and a new life together. Unexpectedly, my husband gained full time custody of his two children aged six and seven, when it became apparent their mother was neglecting them. I quit my job to care for the children, who had been emotionally damaged by their experiences. These years were very painful for me. Time was passing me by, our household was in constant crisis and we didn't have money for infertility treatments. It was all being spent on attorneys and therapy for the children.

Over the years, I had many more surgeries to remove the endometriosis, which found its way to my remaining fallopian tube, ovaries, abdomen, bowels and rectum – it grew everywhere. When I was 35, my remaining fallopian tube was surgically removed. It was filled with clusters of endometriosis and had been the cause of most of my pain.

By the time I was 36, my stepchildren had reached their teens and my husband and I were able to save some money for IVF. With the first cycle, our embryos were textbook perfect: spherical and well divided, nearly blastocysts. We were so confident of the result we didn't think about not getting pregnant. We were even talking about selective reduction. So we were astonished two weeks later when my pregnancy test was negative. There had to be some mistake. My fertility doctor sent me to a different lab for another test, but the results were the same. We waited just over four months to try another IVF cycle and again to our disbelief, it was negative.

After this second failure I fell into a depression so dark I asked my husband to hide the shotgun. I was obsessed with putting it in my mouth and pulling the trigger. I imagined slamming my car into an oncoming truck or wall. I could not rid myself of these thoughts.

My stepchildren were acting out and I lost my beloved cat and dog within three months of each other. I wanted to collapse inside myself and not emerge. Then I got on the Internet and started searching until I could find someone to help us. Finally, we arranged an appointment to see Dr Beer.

He explained his theory about the immune system turning against itself and how this was the probable cause for my failed IVF cycles. The information flowed like a tidal wave. He drew pictures of my uterus and poked at them with his pen, emphatically driving home his point. This man believed so strongly in what he was saying we found it impossible to ignore his ideas. Dr Beer immediately recognized my depression and gave me a prescription and samples of Prozac. Then he ordered blood tests for antibodies to neurotransmitters as well as his standard work up.

The lab report showed I had very high NK cell counts. I was diagnosed with Hashimoto's thyroiditis, antibodies to neurotransmitters and extremely low serotonin levels. My treatment program included Synthroid, heparin, LIT and IVIG preconception with follow up testing and more medications upon a positive pregnancy test.

Our third IVF cycle was done in a clinic that accepted Dr Beer's immune protocol. My FSH levels were elevated by this time and I responded poorly to the stimulation medications despite a very high dose. Only seven follicles developed, containing five eggs.

Several days after retrieval the doctor told us our embryos were very poor grade and my chances were less than 2%. This was devastating news. Two weeks passed and as always. My mother in law passed away the day we got our news: another negative. We planned her funeral and grieved our own private death at the same time. It was a horribly sad time.

Weeks passed and it was very strange, I felt pregnant. Having been through IVF cycles before I knew my body went through changes from the large doses of meds and steroids. Still, I couldn't help feeling different. My family thought I was painfully obsessed and crazy with grief and my husband even sat me down and told me I needed to move on.

I phoned a friend who I had met in the infusion room at Dr Beer's office. We were both in cycle at the same time and she too had failed her IVF. We met up and I asked her if she had started her period yet and she said, "Yes, just."

On the way home, I stopped at the drug store and bought a pregnancy test. It was clearly positive which meant I was over six weeks pregnant! My Ob/Gyn told me to come in right away for a blood test. An ultrasound revealed a tiny beating heart. I was told the fetus was small for six plus weeks, but the heartbeat was strong. Instead of being overjoyed, I was consumed with fear. I had stopped taking all my immune support drugs when the pregnancy test was negative. It was after six o'clock on a Friday and too late for an IVIG infusion.

On Monday, I had the IVIG and requested an ultrasound, but the machine was completely booked for the day. The next available appointment was Wednesday. That morning it did not take long for me to see there was something wrong. My doctor had a solemn face as he moved the wand inside me. The heartbeat was gone. I had a D&C and the tissue was sent to the lab to determine the cause of the miscarriage. My grief was immeasurable.

Two weeks later, we received a fax from the lab. The baby's placenta had been attacked by tumor necrosis factor and she was a baby girl. My own immune system had choked off her lifeline. I was horrified, but my husband kept telling me gently, "But you got pregnant, you got pregnant and that's something."

In weeks that followed, I was upset and angry my fertility doctor had missed the pregnancy. Dr Beer was very sympathetic and encouraged his colleague to give us a free cycle of IVF. The doctor refused citing two legitimate negative pregnancy tests and the fact that my embryos were poor quality to begin with. He believed that even with adequate immune therapy I would have lost the pregnancy. There is no way we will ever know.

Dr Beer tested me for antibodies to HCG and I tested positive. I may have been pregnant many times and never have realized it. I was exhausted, emotionally and physically and spent time healing. I took long walks, meditated, prayed and exercised. After a few months I felt well enough for our final try. We decided to start afresh at a new clinic.

By now, I was 38. Our new fertility doctor was familiar with Dr Beer's program but didn't support his views. Regardless, he was willing to work with him. I told the new doctor I had previously been given a 2% chance of getting pregnant and after reviewing my records, he agreed that those were my chances.

I met with Dr Beer many times to review my previous cycles. It was during these weeks I began to see Dr Beer not just as a physician or a scientist. I felt his sincere compassion and sensitivity. I spent so much time doing IVIG infusions and in the office for blood draws I got to know him outside of the "doctor to patient" mode. Dr Beer is a funny, funny man. His wit is lightning quick and our repartee was something I looked forward to each visit.

My killer cells had skyrocketed after the miscarriage so I needed several pre-cycle IVIGs and two LIT's. Despite a high dose regimen of follicle-stimulating medications, again I responded poorly but I was still optimistic. Our eight-celled and seven-celled embryos looked perfect to me. I had another IVIG just after embryo transfer for insurance.

About a week after the transfer, I felt a sharp digging feeling in my uterus. I could feel three separate embryos implanting and grabbing into me. Two were stronger than the other. I called my husband and told him three embryos had taken hold inside me! The feeling was extraordinary. My pelvis was vibrating. I knew I was pregnant even if no one else did. I lay in my bed and smiled myself to sleep.

A home pregnancy test showed a faint line, so I went in for another IVIG infusion. Of course, this time it was positive. On the way to the first scan, I told my husband I knew there were two babies for sure, maybe three. In fact there were three sacs and two had heartbeats. My fertility doctor was astonished and I left the office as happy as anyone could be.

The third heart never started beating but the sac continued to grow along with the twins. It may have been what kept driving up my killer cells as I needed an IVIG infusion every ten days throughout my pregnancy. I was so fortunate that Dr Beer practiced in the same building and was present at many of my scans and saw our babies grow.

At 30 weeks, I delivered my children: a girl and boy. They were tiny but perfect. Dr Beer and his assistant Chris came to the hospital to see our babies just after they were born. Willie and Katie have transformed our lives. All my pain has been replaced with joy and our household is filled with laughter and love.

Karin

At the age of 32, you don't expect to have a mini stroke, but that's what happened to me. I had no idea it was related to antibodies to phospholipids. The year before, I had been tested at a fertility clinic in Australia because I'd had a miscarriage and wanted an overall assessment of my health. That's when they discovered I had antibodies to cardiolipin but I did not appreciate that this was a serious problem or that it was related to the loss of my baby.

For the next 18 months, I was oblivious to the risks until I had the suspected stroke and another miscarriage. Then alarm bells started to ring. I knew low dose aspirin would help, so I started taking that and immediately looked on the Internet for information. A friend of mine told me about Dr Beer so I filled in a form and registered with him for immune evaluation.

A few days later I called him to say, "I'm sorry, there's a spanner in the works. I'm pregnant!" Of course, I was excited, but I was also very scared. I knew I wasn't prepared and could easily lose yet another baby. Dr Beer told me to take heparin immediately. It was a fight to get it as all the doctors said, "You haven't had three miscarriages yet, so I can't tick the box to prescribe it for you." Eventually I got the blood thinners privately, after quite a struggle.

Then my NK cell test results came in. The numbers were sky high. Dr Beer said I needed IVIG, which he arranged right away. I am convinced that this emergency measure saved my pregnancy and enabled me to give birth to a healthy, beautiful boy.

I was then told by Dr Beer that I had an eighteen month window of opportunity after having my baby to get pregnant again. This is because the immune system "reboots" itself and is less of a threat to the growing fetus. He also put me on low dose aspirin and Folgard indefinitely.

Now I know about the antiphospholipid syndrome I can do something about it. You don't think that miscarriages can be a symptom of a life threatening health condition, but this is what I now know. Dr Beer was the only one that listened to me and the speed of his emails was fantastic. I must have been on some kind of rapid response list because he replied almost straight away and gave me the answers and the help I needed. He was my savior."

Shawn

Soon after I was married in 2000, we started trying for a baby. To make a long and painful story short, we went through five heartbreaking miscarriages. So I was given infertility shots which I didn't need as I easily became pregnant. My problem was staying pregnant. My reproductive endocrinologist (RE) said the shots would "help the good eggs fertilize" and fix the problem. That's just a bunch of boloney. I never conceived with the shots or with intrauterine insemination. Then this same RE told me I needed to consider IVF, a surrogate or adoption.

At the hospital for the D&C after my fifth miscarriage, I told my Ob/Gyn that there must be something we were missing. She said, "You know, I heard a doctor in Chicago is using some experimental drugs and he might be able to help you." While I was in the operating room I asked my husband to get a medical record release form and find this doctor's details from the receptionist. That afternoon I called Dr. Beer's office. It was the answer to all of my prayers.

During my initial consultation Dr Beer said, "I have no doubt in my mind that in a year from now, you will be a mom." I cried with relief to have met someone who understood my problems and could help me. He was right too. I went to Mexico for LIT, took blood thinners and other medications daily and had IVIG every three weeks. Then I gave birth to a healthy baby boy in February 2005, exactly a month shy of Dr Beer's prediction.

The second time around, after my period didn't arrive I called Chris at Dr. Beer's office and told her I was cramping and felt like I was going to start my period. She told me to take a pregnancy test the next morning. Lo and behold, it was positive!

During week five I started to spot and thought, "Oh no, the dreaded miscarriage." I just knew the pregnancy was destined to fail and was heartbroken. After two weeks of bed rest I was referred to a high risk doctor who told me that that the bleeding was due to the fact that I had been pregnant with twins and had lost one of them. I was saddened and scared, but with a lot of faith I got through it and successfully delivered our longed for baby girl.

Sharon

My husband and I had suffered four miscarriages all between seven and nine weeks within a nine month period from 1994 to 1995. After the first three losses, extensive testing showed no obvious genetic hormonal or structural problems so we sought the opinion of our local Ob/Gyn. He agreed that we had immune issues and should probably use IVIG and recommended that we work with Dr Beer. We had read about him and were completely intimidated by the aggressiveness of his treatments so we didn't take things any further.

Our Ob/Gyn managed us long distance through our next pregnancy, which took 16 months to happen. We had preconception LIT and once the pregnancy was confirmed I also used heparin, baby aspirin and progesterone. Sadly, we never saw a heartbeat with this pregnancy and I had a D&C performed at eight weeks. I had been doing immune treatments but not with the thoroughness that Dr Beer would have recommended.

After this fourth loss, we knew it was time to get serious. I contacted emailed Dr Beer and he responded promptly from Europe and told us to get slides from my D&Cs and send them to his lab for testing along with blood samples. Two weeks later, he gave us the ray of hope we had been searching for. We will never forget his words in that phone conversation. He said, "I know what your problem is and I know how to fix it."

I was diagnosed with elevated natural killer cells and low blocking antibodies and needed IVIG, LIT, prednisone, progesterone, heparin and baby aspirin all starting preconceptually. We tried for eight natural cycles on this regimen and after expending emotional and financial resources we asked Dr Beer to recommend a fertility doctor. He told us that without doubt Dr Christo Zouves in San Francisco had the highest success rate with his immune patients.

We consulted with Dr Zouves by phone and were immediately impressed. So much so, that we decided it was worth the expense and trouble of traveling across the country to work with him. Our first attempt was a success. Out of the five embryos transferred, four implanted. It was completely overwhelming to us, but we cheered them all on with every weekly ultrasound scan.

Finally, after it was clear that my body was not going to reject any of our beautiful babies we had to make the painful decision to have a reduction to give the remaining fetuses a chance of success. It was the most painful day of my life but I was left with thriving healthy twins.

The rest of the pregnancy was quite uneventful. I was monitored all the way and my natural killer cells stayed in check. I stopped the immune treatment in the second trimester and was put on bed rest. At 37.5 weeks I gave birth to two beautiful, perfect baby girls. We still cannot believe how incredibly blessed we were to have them.

Two years later we traveled to San Francisco to work with Dr Zouves again to transfer two of our remaining frozen embryos. Dr Beer's tests showed that my immune system was still under control ("rebooted" he described it) and I didn't need any preconception IVIG. I squeezed in one LIT booster before the U.S. restrictions took effect and took heparin, baby aspirin, prednisone and progesterone. I also had acupuncture before during and after the IVF cycle which helped me to relax.

The transfer was more successful than I expected and at the age of 37 I conceived twins. Sadly, one of them failed to thrive and was lost at six weeks. Dr Beer ordered one infusion of IVIG just as a precaution and no more was required. The pregnancy was otherwise uneventful and resulted in our precious son, Euan.

There is no doubt in our minds that our children would not be here today were it not for the tireless efforts of Dr Beer. He was always there for us and responded promptly to each of my messages with reassurance, calmness and compassion. We corresponded almost entirely by email. In fact I never met him in person until after my daughters were born.

He was a wonderful doctor with a passion for what he did and he genuinely cared about his patients.

I hope that my story inspires those of you who are still struggling. Parenthood, although it has its challenges, is well worth the effort and worth fighting for. I wish all of you the very best and wish that you too are some day soon holding your own miracle baby in your arms.

Jane Reed

I always knew I wanted a large family and had no other great goals in life than to be a mother. Having children meant the world to me. Nobody would have guessed that after three "picture perfect" healthy pregnancies I would ever have an immune problem, least of all a severe one. I was certainly not the typical example of an immune patient. Maybe this is why some deeper chord was struck in me that would later change my calling for the rest of my life.

The birth of my third child was the beginning of the end of my fairy tale. Just seventeen weeks into my fourth pregnancy, without warning or any symptoms or signs, the heart of the beautiful baby inside me just stopped beating. My precious baby was gone. I was devastated that she had been so brutally stripped away from me. How a mother cries for her first pregnancy loss, in a way she can only cry for the first.

I was told that miscarriages rarely repeated themselves, so I cloaked myself in false hope and told myself it would never happen again. We tried once more and I became pregnant. Although I had cramping and there were growth issues with this pregnancy in addition to low amniotic fluid and fetal distress at delivery, my baby was born alive and well. Life was still happy...life was still good. I was blissfully ignorant of the silent issues going on inside my body.

The first ultrasound of my next pregnancy revealed that it had happened again. There was no heartbeat, not even a fetal pole; nothing except a circular shape on the ultrasound screen – an empty looking mass they called a "blighted ovum." I was grief stricken. Two lightning strikes against me this time. Still it never occurred to me that there was a cause for these random losses after my live births.

Then the joint pains came. I went to an orthopedist after the miscarriage complaining of strange aches in my foot. Next, I experienced all-over body pain that I naively thought was caused by tendons stretching back from the previous pregnancy. I started developing hives and food allergies, so I saw an allergist and changed my diet. Then migraines entered my life and I found myself unable to think straight at times and my brain turned into a fog at random intervals. When my grandmother came to visit that summer, I looked at her with her arthritis and failing memory and thought I was getting old faster than she was! Something about my health was deteriorating within me...

My next pregnancy was doomed from the start. When the dreaded bright red spotting started a couple of weeks later, it almost felt like I was waiting for it. The bleeding worsened and then came clots. The whole choreography of a classic textbook miscarriage took place seven weeks into the pregnancy. My losses were coming earlier and earlier – another classic symptom of immune related loss.

I remember asking the doctor, "Can something about the mother's body actually cause a pregnancy to miscarry?" I felt a chill when he told me, "Sometimes miscarriages are caused by conditions of the mother, not just the baby." Maybe this was not a chromosomal problem I thought; maybe something was indeed wrong with me. But nobody suggested diagnosis or a treatment. Nobody gave me any direction, recommendations or leads. They all simply patted me on the back and sent me home with those same old words "try again."

I went to the library and searched through faded books on miscarriage written back in the 1970s. Again and again I read the words "miscarriage is a natural, random event and extremely common. Best treatment – simply to try again." But among these dusty books was a fresh, new title that intrigued me: *Preventing Miscarriage: The Good News* by Dr Jonathan Scher.

In this book was talk of antiphospholipid antibodies and lymphocyte immune therapy. It all seemed rather obscure. I thought there was no way these situations could apply to me. Instead of investigating further, I contacted a reproductive endocrinologist who ran some tests. Everything came back normal. He simply said I had a luteal phase defect (a cycle length issue) and progesterone would solve the problem for me.

However, once again I was to experience that deathly feeling of losing a pregnancy. Another dear baby embryo passed naturally one night. Oh, that feeling of losing that pregnancy again...that beautiful crystal embryo in a white gel sac: a gem of a baby, amazing perfection in so much detail in such small size. I wanted to take my precious one down to the river to let her swim into a better place, but I could not let her go. I held her tight that night and cried and cried. The lonely sadness of the memory of that day cannot ever be relived...my fourth loss.

I remember asking my doctor about the immune therapies that had been invented by a doctor named Beer. He promptly replied, "There are thousands of doctors in this country and the only doctor that believes in what Dr Beer does is Dr Beer. Nobody believes in that treatment; it's extremely expensive and simply does not work, plus you've had many liveborn children already. This problem could not apply to you."

I became pregnant again that summer. I had the full progesterone treatment and did everything I was supposed to do to resolve the luteal phase defect. I went in for the dreaded first ultrasound and the results sounded hopeless. A fetal heartbeat was seen but it was too slow and the crown to rump length was too small. "Does this pregnancy have a chance?" I asked, pleading for a glimmer of hope. "The prospects with a heart rate this slow are not good. I give this pregnancy a 5% chance," the doctor announced. I lost the baby later that week. My fifth loss.

The darkness of that day simply cannot be described. I descended into a miserable, oppressive place where no living being can ever enter. Life seemed to end for me. I was lost in a netherworld where you can no longer think or feel because there is nothing more to think or feel for. Looking back on it now, I was in a dangerous state of depression and seriously needed help.

Recurrent miscarriage can do this to a person – rip the soul and spirit away from your being. You take the beating again and again, until finally, at that last breath you stop feeling hope, and when you stop feeling hope you stop feeling life. I was at that point of losing a grip. I was falling fast. If there truly was a God, how could He be so cruel and allow a fellow being to suffer so much and kill her babies one after another after another?

It was during this moment of great darkness that I had an inspiration that was to rescue me. A notion came to my mind to email the doctor who treated immune caused miscarriages with therapies my local doctor had called "dangerous and unproven." I'm not really sure why I contacted him that day, maybe it was random luck, or a larger force of fate, all I know is after I sent that message Dr Beer's reply changed everything. I asked, "Does the fact I've had so many pregnancies make it unlikely I have an immune problem?" His very simple answer was, "It makes it *more* likely you have an immune problem."

I cannot explain the feeling that came over me with this idea. It was not like a sudden revelation, I was far too deep in depression to think clearly like that. It was rather like a crack of light was slowly shining

HOPE AND INSPIRATION

on me again: a warm feeling of hope and possibilities. If I did have an immune problem, why had nobody ever mentioned this? The rage and anger at this question drove me along my journey of discovery – and more and more pieces began to fall into place.

Tests revealed I was a standard textbook case of an immune miscarriage patient after livebirths. I had antiphospholipid antibodies and a high natural killer cell count of 23%. Apparently, over time, my body had acquired sensitivity to pregnancy and each loss had made my immune problems worse. This explained why my miscarriages were getting earlier and earlier and why I had autoimmune colitis, strange aches and pains and fevers only with my pregnancies.

I followed Dr Beer's program with IVIG for my elevated NK cells, prednisone for my positive ANA, heparin for my APAs, extra progesterone for my luteal phase defect and carried my first pregnancy under Dr Beer's treatment to term. My first "Beer Baby," Jessica, was born in 1999 and was perfect and healthy in every way. Can I say what it is like to be brought from the depths of total depression to the heights of glory and beauty? To have the worries of my past tamed with clarity and science is too powerful a feeling to convey in words.

Over time, I have learned not only about the greatness of this medicine, but of the greatness of Dr Beer's work. He is truly a man on a mission to push science ahead. I learned it does not matter how many children you have had or lost, or whether the losses are interspersed or in a row, immune problems can still develop anyway. No, miscarriages are not "bad luck" or "Nature's way." Miscarriages are often immune mistakes that should not have happened – and yes, they can be treated.

The tremendous reward of running the Yahoo Immunology site has been eye opening for me: connecting with women all over the Internet, following the great example set for me by my friend, my comrade and my mentor, Dr Beer. It is so heart warming to see women who have been through the darkest suffering, finding answers to their problems, receiving immune therapy and having beautiful babies and success.

I have learned that from great pain can come great meaning and after great suffering can come great mission. It has been my honor to share my personal story in the hope it might inspire others.

The Reproductive Immunology Support site, hosted by Jane Reed, can be found at: http://health.groups.yahoo.com/group/immunologysupport

IS YOUR BODY BABY FRIENDLY?

ADDENDUM

ADDENDUM

I
Fertility under Fire

"There is no question that environmental toxins have a negative effect on the immune responses. This area has been under study for many years through the National Institutes of Health. It appears that many of the toxins that enter our body need to be cleared by phagocytic cells that prepare antigens for normal processing by the immune system. Diverting themselves to fill their bellies with pollutants can alter their function, which creates a dysfunctional rhythm within the immune system. I am amazed each day when I see perfectly healthy, exercised, trim males who are producing mutant sperm of the kind I did not see years ago. Is this a warning that we are exposed to a degree that is damaging us? Yes, I have great fears..."

Alan E. Beer, M.D.

The increasing population of the planet is not due to humankind's ability to reproduce with ease. It is because people are surviving longer due to improved hygiene and better disease control. In reality, human fertility is on the decrease. Fewer babies are being born per couple and more couples are resorting to fertility treatment. As this reduction in fertility has taken place within two generations, genetic causes are unlikely as these problems evolve over many thousands of years. The increased number of chromosomal changes that are being seen today coincide with the introduction of chemical products into the environment.

In the U.S., over five and a half billion pounds of neurotoxins and carcinogens are produced every year. Worldwide, over 400 million tons of chemicals are manufactured annually. Of the several thousand that are produced in volume, reproductive toxicology data exists for only a hundred or so which means we are all unwitting participants in a massive global scientific experiment.

A 2006 Canadian report revealed that everyone who took part in their study was contaminated by more than half of the 88 chemicals that were tested. A further investigation found over 500 potentially dangerous manmade chemicals in a fat sample from a seemingly healthy British 30-year-old female, whereas a fat sample taken from an Egyptian mummy contained none. In fact, it has been estimated that each of us consumes around four and a half pounds of pesticides and herbicides and nine pounds of artificial additives every year.

Since the introduction of industrial, agricultural and household chemicals in the 1960s and 70s, fertility problems have risen relentlessly. In the U.S. the estimated number of visits to private physicians' offices for infertility related consultations in 1972 was almost a million. By 1983, the figure had doubled. This number has increased year on year, resulting in a $2 billion per year fertility industry today.

As of 2018, infertility is estimated to affect 15% of the population and in some countries it has exceeded 25%. According to a 2005 report, the rate of infertility in Europe and other developed nations is set to rise to 33%. Effectively, infertility could be classified as an epidemic.

Over the past fifty years, women have been subjected to a dramatic rise in health problems never seen before in history. In the U.S. endometriosis afflicts upwards of 10% of women of childbearing age. Around 30% suffer from premenstrual syndrome and by the age of fifty, up to 80% of women have uterine fibroids. Breast cancer now affects around one in eight women and evidence is mounting that exposure to harmful chemicals is the common factor in all these conditions. In infertility treatment too, the detection of toxins in the follicular fluid surrounding the egg has been associated with increasing levels of fertilization failure.

The sexual development and fertility problems that are seen in both men and women are strongly linked to substances called endocrine disruptors or "gender bending" chemicals which mimic human reproductive hormones. Endocrine disruption can occur at extremely small doses which is of concern because these substances accumulate in and are stored within our body's fat and tissue.

Petrochemical compounds have molecular structures that are similar to estrogen and act like estrogen in the body. They are found in a whole range of products including everything from body lotions, hair spray, air fresheners, shampoos and perfume to birth control pills, till receipts, plastic containers, cooking pans, fresh fruit preservatives, cleaning products and pesticides.

In addition to falling sperm counts, male health problems that are associated with endocrine disruption include undescended testicles, poor sperm motility, malformed urinary tracts and reduced penis size.

Sperm levels are falling dramatically throughout much of the world and according to a review of thousands of studies by Hagai Levine at Icahn School of Medicine at Mount Sinai, sperm concentration fell by 52 percent between 1973 and 2011. It now stands at just 47.1 million per milliliter. This is alarming because anything below 40 million per milliliter is considered below normal and can impair fertility especially when it is estimated that up to 85% of these sperm will be defective. Some carry the wrong chromosome while others have bits and pieces of genetic material out of place, such as a tapered head, two heads or two tails. It is now considered "normal" that between 4% and 14% of sperm display a healthy morphology.

The incidence of testicular cancer has also risen by a third over the past five years in industrialized countries, with a leading French cancer specialist speculating that "some 75% of cancers are due to mutations induced by environmental factors, mainly chemicals."

Trying to avoid environmental toxins is virtually impossible, but we can minimize our exposure and that of our children before, during and after their birth when they are most vulnerable to physical and neurological damage. In all, just 275 (of the thousands of mostly untested chemicals out there) have proven to be toxic to the reproductive system and/or fetal development. A few of the most harmful that we know about are:

Organic Mercury

This toxic heavy metal is consumed via food and is easily absorbed by the body. Mercury is the most extensively documented environmental pollutant associated with adverse reproductive events. It interferes with cell division in the developing fetal brain and binds to DNA to disrupt the copying of chromosomes.

This toxin is absorbed through the maternal gastrointestinal tract and passes into the brain of the developing fetus where it can cause cerebral palsy, mental retardation, seizures, blindness and delayed development.

In 2003, the FDA estimated that 1 in 12 U.S. women of childbearing age had potentially hazardous levels of mercury in their blood due to the consumption of contaminated fish. The FDA recommends that pregnant women and women planning to become pregnant should not eat farmed salmon, swordfish, shark, king mackerel, tilefish or ahi and albacore tuna, avoid them while breastfeeding and not feed them to young children.

Dioxins

Sources of dioxins come from the manufacture of pesticides and paper and the incineration of materials that contain chlorine. As dioxins are not broken down in the soil, they pass up through the food chain and accumulate in fat tissue. More than 90% of our exposure comes from food, including fish, meat, poultry and milk.

Popularly known as endocrine disruptors, the dioxin chemical family (with 30 dioxin like members) has the potential to harm human life at every stage of its development. Laboratory studies have shown that dioxins can adversely affect fertility, pregnancy and fetal growth. Such is their toxicity that they are measured in the parts per trillion, i.e. one drop in enough water to fill 300 Olympic sized swimming pools.

These hormone altering substances can change genetic material, cause miscarriage and give rise to birth defects. Exposure during early pregnancy has been associated with abnormal male testosterone levels in the fetus. Dioxins make males more "female-like" and reduce sperm production in adulthood.

Dioxins also have a particularly powerful hormonal impact on the ovary and are associated with infertility, cancer, diabetes and autoimmune disorders. In a study of German women, elevated levels of dioxins were measured in those with endometriosis, fibroids, miscarriage and persistent infertility.

Alkylphenols

Alkylphenols are another group of endocrine disrupting chemicals linked to sexual deformities. Male fish near sewage outlets are feminized and have genitals of both sexes. There is currently no research to show the effects of these chemicals on humans, but in animals alkylphenol are associated with reduced sperm counts and testicular size and cause estrogen sensitive cells to grow in the uterus.

Found in sunscreens, detergents, paints, pesticides, plastics and cling-wrap to name but a few products, hundreds of thousands of tons of these chemicals are produced every year and mostly end up in sewage works where they infiltrate water supplies.

Bisphenol A is a type of alkylphenol that is found on the inside of food cans, in flame retardants on soft furnishings and carpets and in epoxy resins. It is also used in the manufacture of hard polycarbonate plastics for drinking water bottles and food containers. This massively produced compound is one of the top 50 production volume chemicals in the U.S.

In experiments on mice, this chemical induces a similar chromosomal defect to the one that results in Down's syndrome. Female offspring were also seen to grow faster, weigh more and enter puberty earlier. Other studies have reported elevated levels of Bisphenol A in women with antinuclear antibodies and a history of three or more pregnancy losses. Prenatal exposure of the fetus to alkylphenols has also been shown to increase the Th1 immune response in adulthood.

A 2005 review of the literature revealed that of 115 published studies involving Bisphenol A, 94 reported "significant effects" at doses below the "safe" level (although industry funded studies disagree with these findings). The authors of the review recommended that a new risk assessment for this chemical is needed.

Phthalates (Plasticizers)

Phthalates are one of the most abundant manmade chemicals in the world. One of their main uses is as a plasticizer in plastic containers, from which they can leach out into food and drinks. They are also found in many skincare products, clothing, toys, baby bottles, baby mattresses, packaging, medical products and thousands of other household items.

Individually, phthalate levels in cosmetic products are low, but their concentrations in the body can be cumulative. The Centers for Disease Control and Prevention reported the highest levels of phthalates were found in the urine of women aged between 20 and 40, probably because they use more perfumes and skincare products.

In animal studies carried out by the U.S. Environmental Protection Agency (EPA) and other groups, a common type of phthalate called DEHP, which is found in many food products interfered with male and female fertility, particularly during early life. It is clear that all pthalates undergo hydrolysis in the body to produce compounds which rapidly reduce fetal testosterone production in the cells of the testes, resulting in profound "feminizing" effects on the male reproductive system. High blood levels of phthalates have also been detected in women with endometriosis.

Based on amounts ingested by animals in studies, young children far exceed "safe" levels of exposure for this toxin. For this reason, the European Union banned the use of phthalates in baby toys and related baby products in 1999. In the U.S. and Canada, they have also been removed from milk bottle nipples and other products designed to go in a baby's mouth.

The Cosmetics Toiletry and Fragrance Association, the trade group representing the industry in the United States, says phthalates present no health risk and the U.S. Cosmetic Ingredient Review panel (an industry-sponsored watchdog) has voted to allow their continued use. U.S. regulators are still waiting for clear evidence that these chemicals are harmful to humans. In the meantime, the European Union has banned the use of two types of phthalates: DBP and DEHP.

DEHP is still widely used in the U.S. A study of 256 women at Massachusetts General Hospital Fertility Center from 2004 to 2014 found concentrations of 11 phthalate metabolites in their urine. Women with the highest concentrations of DEHP, were 60% more likely to lose a pregnancy prior to 20 weeks than those with the lowest concentrations.

Being only loosely chemically bonded in plastic products, DEHP can easily leach out via plastic water bottles and food containers. Because it is lipophilic it is more easily absorbed by fatty foods like cheese and meat.

Pesticides

This group of chemicals includes organophosphates and organochlorines such as DDT, DDE, PCP, PCB, methoxychlor and lindane. Originally produced as poisonous nerve gas agents during World War II, organophosphates are less toxic than in previous years, but are still very potent. In animal tests, they have been shown to cause disruptions to estrogen, androgen, prolactin and thyroid hormones.

Organochlorine compounds are known to affect female human reproduction by shortening the menstrual cycle and decreasing progesterone levels: factors that can influence other endpoints such as fertility, pregnancy and reproductive cancers. An analysis of men undergoing IVF has also shown that pesticides may affect sperm quality, resulting in significantly lower fertilization rates.

Furthermore, a 2001 report has uncovered a strong association between exposure to commercially applied agricultural pesticides and fetal death due to congenital defects when the mother lived within a mile of the spraying. Researchers have discovered a "window of vulnerability" for birth defects, between the 3rd and 8th week of pregnancy when the fetal organs are forming and the fetus is most susceptible to the effects of these chemicals. Regular exposure (both indoors and outdoors) to pesticides before pregnancy has also been linked to a 300% greater incidence of cleft palate, cleft lip and stillbirth. The use of home pesticides during the first two months of pregnancy has also been associated with a risk for stillbirth due to congenital defects.

It is estimated that 90% of U.S. households use at least one pesticide product indoors (e.g., ant powders and fly sprays). However, up to a dozen different pesticides have been found in the air inside some homes. Other possible sources include contaminated food, water, soil and airborne dust.

Developed in the 1930s, DDT was banned in the United States because of its effects on wildlife reproduction. For example, male animals developed abnormally small penises and undescended testicles. However, this chemical is so persistent that even today a major metabolite of DDT has been identified in the follicular fluid of women undergoing IVF, with high levels being associated with fertilization failure.

Methoxychlor was developed as a substitute for DDT and has an estrogenic effect on birds and mammals, disrupting sexual development and reproduction and stimulating the growth of cancer cells. In animal studies, methoxychlor "feminized" male embryos, with reduced fertility seen in 90% of males over three generations, while vinclozolin blocked the production of testosterone, causing feminization of males and other birth defects. These changes reduced the sperm counts and sperm motility, not only of those in the generation exposed to the chemical, but also of those in three subsequent generations.

Furthermore, the pesticide chlorpyrifos (Dursban) has been associated with increased autoimmune antibodies in tests on animals. The pesticide methoxychlor and the fungicide vinclozolin have also been identified as being partly, or even wholly, responsible, for a number of inherited diseases that had previously been attributed to "bad genes."

The effects of lindane are similar to those of DDT, except that lindane works faster and is more acutely toxic. It is readily absorbed by the skin and can easily cross the placenta. A Class 2B carcinogen, lindane has been linked to breast cancer and has been shown to accumulate in the ovarian follicles, fallopian tubes and uterus of animals, causing reproductive failure. Data from other laboratory tests have shown that it also retards testicular growth and reduces sperm quality. Repeated exposure (e.g., the use of head lice shampoos on children) may also cause neurological damage and compromise the immune system. Lindane can be found in some household pesticides and wood preservatives.

Pentachlorophenol (PCP) is another pesticide linked to immuno-deficiencies. In animal studies, PCP dramatically reduced levels of thyroid hormone and levels of thyroxine uptake in the fetal brain. An investigation in the mid-1990s found that around two thirds of the U.S. population had PCP residues in their urine.

Polybrominated Diphenyl Ethers (PBDEs or fire retardants)

Banned in Europe since the 1990s, these compounds are still widely used in the U.S. in fire retardants on mattresses, bedding and furniture. PBDEs are also found in plastics, clothing, building materials and electrical goods, including TVs. As these chemicals pass through the placenta, they are easily absorbed by the fetus.

PBDEs mimic thyroid hormones, which can affect the baby's neuro-logical system. Exposure, even at low levels, appears to disrupt brain development, reduce learning ability and cause hyperactivity and hearing problems that worsen with age. PBDEs have also been implicated in reduced conception rates, increased abortion rates, menstrual abnormalities and developmental defects of female reproductive tissue.

Perfluorochemicals (PFCs)

PFCs were developed to take the place of PBDEs. They are found in fabrics, carpets, food packaging (e.g. microwaveable popcorn bags, plastic bottles and pizza boxes), Teflon and non-stick coatings, shampoo, insecticides, fire- fighting foam, and other household products. High blood concentrations are associated with irregular periods, longer conception times and infertility. The EPA asked manufacturers to reduce PFC emissions and product content by 95% by 2010 and to eliminate the chemical by 2015. These substances break down very slowly in the soil, air, and/or water they will remain in the environment for decades. They also accumulate and remain in the body for years.

Benzene

As a component of gasoline, benzene is found in high concentrations along roadsides. This tasteless, odorless compound has also been detected in soft drinks, especially sugar free varieties (benzene is created by a combination of sodium benzoate and ascorbic acid). Other sources include aerosols, fragrances, air fresheners and many types of spray on household cleaning products. Because this substance has been classed as "inactive," it is not required to be included in a product's list of ingredients.

However, environmental exposure studies have shown that it can cause chromosomal damage and affect the fetal blood producing cells, leading to bone deformities and low birthweight babies. Benzene has also been linked to neural defects and childhood cancers including leukemia, lymphoma, and brain and urinary tract cancers.

Solvents

Organic and industrial solvents (such as methanol, ethylene glycol, acetone, carbon disulfide, n-hexane, methyl-butyl ketone, trichloroethylene, perchloroethylene, toluene and xylene) are neurotoxic and are associated with a greater risk of miscarriage. Solvent exposure is also thought to be a trigger for autoimmune disorders including connective tissue and other rheumatoid diseases.

These substances are used in waterproof sealants, lubricating oils, ironing and dry cleaning products, disinfectants, paint and varnish removers, vinyl flooring, adhesives, paints, varnishes, dyes, cosmetics, perfumes, nail polish and remover, glues, carpet shampoo and other cleaning products.

A Canadian study found that women who were exposed to solvents during the first trimester of pregnancy were approximately 13 times more likely to have a baby with a major health problem (including spina bifida, clubfoot, a heart defect or deafness).

Research has shown that children born to women exposed to solvents through their work (e.g., in nail salons, factories, laboratories, graphic studios, print works and dry cleaning companies) for at least eight weeks during pregnancy had learning difficulties and an increased incidence of hyperactivity. This was despite the use of protective equipment to reduce exposure. The gap between the exposed and unexposed children was described as "huge" and showed that, as a class, solvents are more hazardous than previously understood.

ADDENDUM

Electro Magnetic Field (EMF) Radiation

Although not technically a chemical, electro magnetic field (EMF) radiation has been included here as it has now been recognized as a serious public health challenge. EMF radiation is emitted from power lines, transformers, microwave ovens, wireless networks, smart meters, cell towers, routers and Bluetooth and Wi-Fi wireless operated devices such as laptops, ipads and cell phones. All humans are now being exposed to this invisible, man-made health threat with ever increasing intensity.

Multiple studies have confirmed a link between EMF radiation and diabetes, heart disease and autoimmune disorders. The International Agency for Research on Cancer also classifies it as a possible carcinogen and several observational studies have shown that EMF exposure during pregnancy is associated with abnormal fetal development and an increased risk of miscarriage.

5G (short for "fifth-generation") is the next evolution of wireless networks and will be in all the major U.S. cities by 2020. It uses very high frequency pulsed radiation, which is more biologically active and because transmitters will have to be erected every 500 feet, even if you don't use a cellphone, you will be in an EMF zone. According to Dr. Martin Pall, an expert in this field, "The impacts on the outer one to two inches of our bodies will be massive."

Information for the majority of this chapter was adapted with kind permission of Noah Chalfin, coauthor of the 2002 report: "Identifying Toxic Risks Before and During Pregnancy." – A Report to the March of Dimes by Marc Lappe PhD and Noah Chalfin B.A. at the Center for Ethics & Toxics, California, U.S.

II

The Legacy of a Toxic Pregnancy

"In reproduction we depend too strongly on newer and more effective medications. If the environment has damaged those carrying the future generations, then nothing may be able to help."

Alan E. Beer, M.D.

The embryo relies on its mother's blood for survival. If that blood is polluted, chemicals can flow into the developing baby's body and interfere with its natural growth patterns. The baby's central nervous system is especially sensitive to toxic substances. Agents of small molecular weight cross the placenta by passive diffusion, the rate of which depends on the concentration and type of the chemical. Water soluble chemicals are also retained longer in the body of a pregnant woman, which further increases their toxicity. With a body that is ill equipped to rid itself of manmade chemicals, the developing baby is extremely vulnerable to toxic exposure. Indeed, in 2003 the EPA concluded that carcinogens have around ten times the potency for babies compared to adults.

Pesticides and fertilizers in food and water, and chemicals in drugs and household products can all diffuse down through the placenta. A 2005 survey of unborn U.S. babies reported that they were "soaking in a stew of chemicals, including mercury, gasoline byproducts and pesticides." The report by the Environmental Working Group was based on tests of samples of umbilical cord blood, which were found to contain 287 chemicals.

In 2011, researchers found traces of dozens of harmful chemicals in 99% of urine samples from 268 pregnant women in the U.S. Among them were organochlorine pesticides, perchlorate, phthalates and cancer causing compounds found in vehicle exhaust and smoke.

Although most workplace regulations set chemical safety standards according to their hazard to adults, they are not necessarily set to safety levels appropriate for the developing fetus. Concentrations are thousands of times higher in the tiny frame of a growing baby compared to that of an adult body and the damage often occurs at doses that do not harm the mother.

3 to 5% of babies in the U.S. are born with birth defects, which are now the leading reported cause of infant mortality according to national health statistics. Over 3,000 types of congenital defects have been identified. These are thought to be responsible for around 13% of deaths in children under four, and for many permanent disabilities and behavioral problems later in life. Early puberty, obesity, and. attention deficit disorders, the feminization of boys and the masculinization of girls have all been linked to the effects of toxins during pregnancy and the child's early years.

For example, scientists in the Netherlands have discovered that, with exposure to PCBs during gestation, boys tend to engage in more "feminine" behavior and girls become more masculine. Studies have shown that fish (i.e. those caught in contaminated lakes and rivers) as well as high fat meat and dairy products are the main food sources of PCB exposure.

Dioxins also have a feminizing effect on both sexes. Again, the main source of human exposure is via food. Female babies subjected to excess estrogen from hormone mimicking chemicals may appear normal at birth, but any damage to their ovarian follicles will also put them at greater risk of experiencing ovulation problems. They may also be prone to developing breast cancer later in life

In male babies, an increased blood level of estradiol stimulates the excessive release of TGF-alpha (transforming growth factor) that can lead to endocrine mediated cancers. Other related disorders include male genital defects and a reduced sperm count, which are associated with low testosterone levels. Indeed, so many interrelated diseases and abnormalities of the male reproductive system can be initiated in the first months after conception, that scientists have given them the generic name of "testicular dysgenesis syndrome."

In the United States, cancer is the leading cause of death in those aged between 1 and 20. According to the EPA's "Guidelines for Carcinogen Risk Assessment," children receive 50% of their lifetime cancer risks during their first two years of life. Since very young children don't make lifestyle choices that promote their risk of developing the disease, most childhood cancers are thought to be linked to involuntary exposure to environmental agents before birth and shortly after.

Confirmation of the harmful effects of pollution on children's health was published in January 2005. In this U.K. report, Professor John Knox of

Birmingham University compared birthplaces of young cancer victims to maps showing air pollution caused by heavy industry and traffic. The report concluded: "Children born near sources of atmospheric industrial pollution are about 20% more likely to die of leukemia and non-blood cancers, before they reach adulthood." It appeared the cancer began when the mother inhaled these substances and they passed through the placenta.

After the baby is born, it is subjected to a further barrage of toxins administered via lotions and oils, creams, talcum powder, shampoo and body washes, food, drinks, cleaning products and perfumes. As their skin is thinner and more permeable than an adult's, more toxins are able to pass through it.

Baby care products are often applied head to toe on a daily basis and even when they are labeled "natural," "organic" or "hypoallergenic," they can contain synthetic preservatives and softening agents. This is because only a small percentage of the ingredients need to be classified as natural or organic to qualify for an organic label, unlike food, where at least 95% must comply. So once again, potentially damaging substances can be inhaled or absorbed through the skin where they accumulate in tissues such as myelin (the nerve sheath) and the fatty areas of the body, including the brain.

The seeds for many adult diseases, including cancer and reproductive failure, can be sown in childhood. With their reduced ability to metabolize and excrete environmental toxins, many children are unable to escape the long term effects of the chemicals that they harbour in their bodies. A 2004 report by the wildlife charity WWF has found blood samples of children as young as nine contained 75 hazardous chemicals, with higher concentrations of certain newer chemicals than their grandparents. Some of these substances were even banned before the children were born. They included pesticides, PCBs, flame retardants, phthalates, artificial perfumes and other industrial chemicals linked to cancer, birth defects, low fertility and neurological damage.

A spokesperson from the organization said, "Without our knowing about it or sanctioning it, the indiscriminate use of hazardous chemicals in our modern way of life is contaminating the present generation and the next."

EMF Radiation Exposure During Pregnancy

Wireless radiation can cause DNA breakages in the developing fetus even at low levels. The fetus's brain absorbs radiation at a greater rate as it has relatively little bone protection. To give an idea, even young children absorb 60% more electro magnetic field (EMF) radiation than an adult.

In 2014, Dr Devra Davis launched a campaign called "BabySafe Project" to raise awareness about the effects of EMF radiation during pregnancy and how women can take steps to protect themselves and their unborn child. He commented, "Right now, we are treating our children like experiments in a subject with no controls."

Several laboratory and human studies have demonstrated that EMF radiation can damage the neurons in the prefrontal cortex of the developing brain, causing tumors and developmental problems. Exposure to wireless radiation in pregnancy can produce offspring that are more likely to be anxious, hyperactive, unable to focus and display other traits within the autistic spectrum.

There is also a three times greater risk of miscarriage with high EMF exposure. Anti-radiation "belly bands" and other types of maternity wear claim to reduce exposure by up to 100%. It is worth investing in an EMF detection monitor to measure the before and after effects of these products which are available online.

III

The Toxins Eating at Our Health

Before the advent of ready meals and processed packet foods, people generally knew what they were eating and where it came from. Today much of what we consume is the result of chemical experimentation involving a vast range of manmade substances whose effects in combination are mostly unknown.

Two flavorings that have attracted particular attention are monosodium glutamate (MSG) and aspartame. MSG is a white crystalline flavor enhancer that is added to Chinese takeaway food, chips (potato crisps), packet soups and other processed foods. Interestingly, it is used to create obese rodents in the laboratory (they are not naturally fat) by making their pancreas produce three times more insulin than normal.

MSG has been linked to many health problems including nervous system and neuro-degenerative diseases and hormonal and metabolic disorders. It has also been shown to cause infertility in animals. The amounts of MSG added to foods have doubled every decade since the 1940s. Because it is used in several ways (e.g., in hydrolyzed vegetable protein and yeast extract), it can be difficult to identify.

Aspartame (Nutrasweet is a brand name) is an artificial sweetener found in soft drinks, food, medicines and confectioneries that are labeled "diet" or "sugar free." When ingested, certain ingredients turn into formaldehyde and then into formic acid, which is highly toxic. A regular intake of aspartame has been linked to brain tumors, migraines, epilepsy, chronic fatigue syndrome, diabetes and joint pains.

Exposure to food additives during a child's development has also been associated with behavioral problems such as attention deficit hyperactivity disorder. Industry funded studies have all suggested that aspartame is safe for consumption, whereas the vast majority of independently funded research programs have identified a problem. For example, the results of a two-year independent study suggest that aspartame may interact with other common food additives (including monosodium glutamate and brilliant blue E133 and quinoline yellow E104 food colorings) to interfere with the development of a child's nervous system. In combination, these additives can have a more potent effect on nerve cells than they do individually.

Dr Vyvyan Howard, Head of the Development Toxic-Pathology Research Group at the University of Liverpool and editor of the journal *Nanotoxicology*, conducted the research. Commenting on its findings he warned, "Although the use of single food additives is believed to be relatively safe in terms of development of the nervous system, their combined effects are unclear. There are no basic methods for analyzing complex mixtures of toxic substances and the 'cocktail' effect of synthetic chemicals that each one of us carries in our body. We think there are signs that when you mix additives, the effect might be worse."

Thousands of different kinds of additives are used in food processing, but only a small proportion are listed on the label. Some additives have even been approved without having been fully tested. Added to this quota of synthetic ingredients are the drugs, nitrous compounds, fertilizers and other toxins that are used in industrial farming.

Antibiotics, which are known to upset the human endocrine system, are often fed to livestock, particularly poultry. Dairy cattle are given high-protein feeds made from genetically modified crops, and injected with estrogen-like and growth hormones. Up to two thirds of beef cattle in the U.S. are also given hormone injections or implants (primarily containing estradiol, testosterone and progesterone) to boost their development and speed their maturity. Such interventions are banned in Europe.

Endocrine disrupting pesticides are also found in fruits and vegetables, especially those grown in developed countries. Indeed, the U.S., the Environmental Working Group has found commercially grown fruits and vegetables contain the highest levels of pesticide contamination. Traces of pesticides were found in 34% of the 1,089 food samples tested in 2004 according to the U.K.'s government backed Pesticides Residue Committee. In some fruit and vegetables, levels were up to three and a half times over the safe limit for children.

Altogether, it is estimated that our daily diet contains the residues of at least 30 different artificial chemicals, growth hormones, colorants and genetically modified ingredients – traces of which can pass through the placenta to the developing fetus.

Dr Howard, who is a member of the British Government's Advisory

Committee on Pesticides, points out: "We don't have the tools to analyze how mixtures of these chemicals work in the body and we probably never will. To test just the most common 1,000 toxic chemicals in combinations of three would require at least 166 million different experiments. However, when we do look, we find some surprising interaction. The only logical way forward is to reduce exposure as much as possible. Eating organically grown food is an efficient way of applying precaution on a personal basis."

The medical industry cannot be relied upon to produce an antidote to all the problems that are being created in our environment. As far as possible, we must take responsibility for preserving our own health and that of our offspring. There are many books and online resources to help people establish a toxin reduced lifestyle.

Using chemical free cleaning products, toiletries and cosmetics and eating organic, unprocessed food are basic measures that we can all take. Guidelines to help reduce the burden on the immune system and improve reproductive functioning are presented in the next chapter.

ADDENDUM

IV

Natural Immunotherapy for Life

"Although holistic medicine is not my area of expertise, many of my patients choose to adopt natural therapies alongside my medical treatments. In my opinion, it is unlikely that natural therapies alone can completely solve the problems of immune mediated reproductive failure. However, it is important that patients know about these approaches and are provided with a reliable reference.

We are living in a dirty world and there may soon come a day when we will need to be chelated to 'car wash' our chemistry in preparation for pregnancy. Holistic therapy and special dietary advice can often work to supplement the baby friendly treatments that my program promotes."

Alan E. Beer M.D.

Many of Dr Beer's patients have sought the advice of a London based holistic therapist who is very familiar with his immune treatments and provides his patients with specially tailored programs to help enhance protocol effectiveness and counterbalance any side effects.

Zita West adopts a realistic and "workable" approach to health, which she explains in her books: *The Zita West Pregnancy Program* and *Fertility and Conception.*

Her program addresses the fact that we live in a stressful, toxin filled world and our bodies need to be flushed free of these pollutants as part of a preconception plan. Here is Zita's advice for maximizing the chances of a healthy and successful pregnancy for women going through immune therapy, IVF or both.

A Baby-Friendly Diet and Lifestyle:
for Optimal Health and Fertility

By Zita West

My knowledge and experience is within the field of diet and natural therapies, but having collaborated with Dr Beer, whose patients were also my clients, I soon realized the significance of scientific intervention in the IVF journey and how it was producing much higher pregnancy rates. So in 2011 I opened a holistic fertility clinic in London to cater for couples who had failed to become parents though conventional fertility treatments.

Dr George Ndukwe, a former student of the late Dr Beer, manages the tests and treatments that are necessary for those couples who have immune problems. The results have been astounding and we now have one of the top success rates in the country, especially among difficult cases who have come to us as a last resort.

There is no doubt in my mind that the immune system needs to be modified to accept a pregnancy, in more cases than you would think. Immunotherapy provides a temporary state of immune suppression during the vital weeks of conception or embryo transfer when using IVF. However, some of the drugs that are used can have a detrimental effect on your gut microbes so they should not be used indefinitely. The high doses of hormones used in IVF can also create an inflammatory effect. A long term solution that will assist your body as it undergoes treatment is to eliminate known hyperactivators of the immune system and modify the pattern of your daily life.

Our routines can become very rigid: we have the same thing to eat and drink at breakfast and set ideas for lunch and dinner. We have our favorite type of alcohol for stress relief and take vitamins to counteract our "vices." For years, without knowing it, we are gradually undermining our health and fertility. This doesn't just apply to women; I often see the same problem with men too.

Fertility is a whole body event and your nutrition, lifestyle and even your mindset can tip the balance in favor of a successful pregnancy.

Food and Immune Connection

Many women that come to me for help have bad eating habits, drink too much alcohol and have chronic stress in their lives.

Our fertility, our hormones and our immune system are governed by the food and drinks we consume. Please read that sentence again so you "get it." There are several important aspects that I focus upon when treating patients with infertility:

1. Restoring proper digestion and gut flora
2. Detoxification or "detox"
3. Establishing the correct acid/alkaline balance

Some of my clients have asked why they should eat healthy foods that will make their immune system robust and even more combative. I think the best way to answer this is to re-define the idea of what "healthy" food is and describe how the immune system actually deals with the things you consume.

We now know that certain kinds of foods that can inflame the immune system, activating cravings, food intolerances and allergies and ultimately leading to a lack of energy, weight gain, infertility and other serious health conditions. The foods I am talking about are not the substances our bodies were designed to eat or even tolerate, namely plant proteins called lectins. These are toxins that plants emit to repel insects and stop other animals from eating them. In reality we are all just another form of animal that evolved millions of years ago, whose body is struggling to adapt to the demands of a modern day diet.

The body doesn't like strange proteins in the gut. They are tagged as "foreign" which elicits an immune response to clear them away. When our body is forever overproducing inflammatory cytokines, a disease state is not far away. This can manifest as anything from fatigue, hormonal disruption, depression, obesity and infertility to autoimmunity, diabetes and heart disease or in my 30 years' of experience, a combination of all of the above.

You have probably read about modern farming methods and are aware that cattle these days are speed-fattened on a diet of corn and grains, instead of the grass their stomachs were designed to process. They commonly have digestive problems such as "feedlot bloat" and acidosis and are very disease prone because their guts are not built to cope with such a lectin heavy diet. Huge amounts of antacids are added to their food and they're given antibiotics, probiotics and vitamin shots to keep them alive for a year or so before they're slaughtered.

Humans too are eating this same lectin heavy, carbohydrate loaded corn, grain based diet as well as the animals that are fattened up with it and our collective health is being similarly compromised. Most of us are overweight or obese and endure bloating, nausea and other digestive problems on a daily basis. We take heartburn pills, stomach acid neutralizers and laxatives, probiotics and vitamin supplements in an effort to counter the effects of this toxic diet. If you think I'm being overly dramatic, look at the statistics.

In 2015, 70% of American adults were overweight and more than half of this group was obese. 74% of the population reported living with digestive symptoms like diarrhea, gas, bloating and abdominal pain in 2013. It is predicted that 40% of Americans will develop Type 2 diabetes and a third of this group will lose their lives to cardiovascular disease. To stem this tide of disease, doctors write an average of twelve drug prescriptions per year for every US citizen.

Here in the UK it's a similarly depressing picture. British people are officially the fattest in Europe. Almost 60% of women and 65% of men are overweight and 26% of this group is obese. 86% of Brits have reported experiencing some form of gastrointestinal problem in the past year. And doctors write an average of eighteen prescriptions annually per person. Now can you see why I think feedlot cattle and people have a lot in common?

Given this quite alarming information, we must re-evaluate the whole idea of what constitutes a "healthy" diet. We need to find a food plan that our bodies can cope with: food that calms our gut environment (pain and bloating are not something you should live with) and the destructive immune activity that goes with it.

By cutting out the substances that trigger inflammation, weight gain and disease our immune system can work at a calm, steady pace and you'll be giving your digestive tract a well earned rest. Basically this is what Dr Beer's treatments do within a short time frame. They regulate the activity of the white blood cells creating a temporary immune cease fire, allowing your cells to heal and natural hormonal rhythms to be re-established.

For those who have the time – three months and beyond – and the self discipline, you can achieve a much more sustainable and healthful balance by modifying your diet to create your own blueprint for health and longevity.

Dr Beer once told me that he'd seen hundreds of patients with elevated NK cell activity and endometriosis that were exacerbated by immune activating foods. When they were removed, their cytokine ratios went back to normal baby friendly levels and these women were able to become pregnant and successfully deliver a robust, full term baby.

A New Perspective on "Health Foods"

When I was asked to revise this chapter I felt a slight sense of trepidation. I knew I was going to have to "eat my words" to some extent, if you'll pardon the pun. My understanding of what constitutes a healthy diet has been overhauled in the light of the results of decades of research and analysis by an American cardiac surgeon who has treated tens of thousands of patients suffering from a range of diseases including cancer, diabetes, cardiovascular disease and autoimmune disorders.

When he realized precisely what was wrong with certain types of foods at a cellular level, he gave up his lucrative surgical career to convey his knowledge to a wider audience. After meticulously reviewing his patients' histories as well as numerous lab results and tests on the flexibility of their blood vessels, he observed that heart disease and cancer, which are both inflammatory conditions, can be avoided and even reversed simply by eating the right things.

The doctor I am referring to is Dr Steven Gundry, who I believe is ahead of his time and just like Dr Beer and other proponents of reproductive immunology, he has received his fair share of criticism from the mainstream medical establishment. When the pharmaceutical industry calls you a "quack" and anti-holistic doctors vigorously argue against your data you're probably on to something!

At this point, the best thing I can do is recommend that you read his book, *The Plant Paradox*. It guides you through the scientific principles of a gut microbiome and what constitutes a pro "good bacteria" anti-inflammatory diet. A number of foods (especially beans, seeds, cereals and legumes, including soybeans and peanuts) have been shown, with substantial scientific evidence, to increase inflammation in the body due to their high lectin content.

Lectins are part of a plant's defense system to keep insects away. For the most part our immune systems protect us from their adverse effects. However, in lectin sensitive individuals with certain blood types, these indigestible proteins stick to the cell membranes in the digestive tract and cause bloating, gastric discomfort and even chronic illnesses such as heart disease, cancer, diabetes and rheumatoid arthritis. Lectins have also been shown to cause red blood cells to cluster together, which is a particular problem for women who already have inherited blood clotting disorders.

Another book that I recommend is *Eat Right for Your Type* by Dr Peter D'Adamo which also explains how you can tailor your diet to minimize immune hyperactivity. For example, those with blood group O are susceptible to an inflammatory reaction to lectins. And of course, there is my own book, *The IVF Diet* which contains several immune calming recipes to optimize the health of the eggs and sperm and prepare the body for pregnancy.

Going Gluten Free to Help Calm Your Immune Response

In patients where there is immune involvement of pregnancy rejection, I recommend a gluten free diet. Gluten is a protein found in wheat, barley, rye, spelt and oats. It's in pizza crusts, pasta, bread, wraps, rolls and most processed foods and it can cause health problems for many. American wheat has a higher gluten content than European wheat. It is needed to make light, fluffy white bread and giant bagels. This "super gluten" was recently introduced into the food supply and is now present in nearly all American wheat varieties. Gluten sensitivity can create inflammation throughout the body, affecting all the systems in your body including your brain, heart, joints, digestive tract and reproductive organs.

Because exposure to lectins and proteins such as gluten can create an inflammatory state that is not antibody mediated, it can fly under the radar of conventional testing.

Any new eating plan will require effort as you will have to prepare a lot of what you eat. It will also involve willpower, as many of the foods that have been fixtures in your life have an addictive quality and will be difficult – but not impossible – to give up. So before you attempt to do so, make sure you have some tasty "immune friendly meals" planned using recipes from the books I have recommended.

Bad Habits and Poor Reproductive Outcomes

One thing I ask all my clients to rethink is their dependence on coffee. More than one cup a day can increase the time it takes to conceive by up to 50% and in pregnancy caffeine has been linked to increased rates of miscarriage and low birth weight. Pharmacologically caffeine belongs in the same category of stimulant drugs like cocaine and amphetamines. It makes the body produce cortisol which raises stress levels and competes with receptor sites of progesterone causing a deficiency of this vital pregnancy hormone.

Caffeine can also limit the absorption of iron and magnesium, which are needed for conception. I believe that decaffeinated coffee may be just as bad because of the way it is made. Indeed, research has linked it to the onset of rheumatoid arthritis. You can replace it with any one of the huge choice of refreshing herbal teas that are available today.

Obviously, recreational drugs and cigarettes are a definite "no." This may seem like basic common sense, but it is surprising how many couples still believe that a line or two of cocaine at the weekend won't affect their fertility. It will. It can cause changes in the fallopian tubes, stop sperm binding to the egg and even result in birth defects.

Cocaine can significantly increase the body's inflammatory immune response. In addition to cocaine's strong association with infertility, women who use this drug during the first three months of pregnancy are at twice the risk of placental abruption and premature delivery.

Cigarettes contain at least 30 chemicals that can deplete fertility and reduce the thickness of the endometrial lining and the amount of oxygen in the blood. Smoking is directly linked to a disruption of hormone levels, which can inhibit ovulation. Did you know that the fertility of smokers is up to 30 to 50% lower than that of non smokers and that smoking can increase your reproductive age by more than 10 years?

The chances of a successful IVF cycle are also severely reduced as exposure to toxic hydrocarbons cuts the number of viable eggs, lessens the likelihood of implantation, and increases the risk of chromosomal abnormalities in the fetus. Smoking can also have a pro-inflammatory effect leading to thrombophilia, which may be another reason why smokers have far more pregnancy complications compared to non smokers. If you are serious about having a baby, you will stop smoking.

There is bad news too for those who think marijuana (also called cannabis) is a "safer" alternative to cigarettes. The THC (tetra-hydro-cannibol that produces the "high") in marijuana is known to be toxic to the developing egg and can cause chromosomal damage. Pregnant women who smoke this drug also risk inflicting severe harm on their unborn child.

Finally, think about your alcohol intake. A couple of glasses of wine after a stressful day may soothe your nerves, but in terms of your fertility and general wellbeing, it is best to be restrictive, or think about saying "no" altogether. Alcohol stimulates the production of TNF-alpha, which, as you know, can adversely affect fertility and pregnancy outcome. One drink a day for a year prior to an IVF attempt has been associated with fewer eggs and lower pregnancy rates.

Remember that our body reacts to foreign substances as intruders to be wiped out. This inflammatory response can lead to all kinds of health problems including infertility and pregnancy loss.

Finally, do your gums bleed when you brush your teeth? Are they red and swollen? If so, you probably have gum disease which is usually caused by poor dental hygiene (in other words, forgetting to brush your teeth!). This can delay the achievement of a positive pregnancy test by, on average two months or more according to an Australian study. Swollen gums and deep pockets around the teeth breed bacteria, which enter the bloodstream and trigger inflammation which potentially reduces an embryo's chances of implantation. Other research has also linked gum disease in men to poor sperm quality.

Make sure you visit your dentist for 6-monthly check ups, brush and floss regularly and keep up the regimen when you're pregnant to avoid bacteria-triggered inflammation which, in severe cases, can result in late miscarriage.

Non-Baby Friendly Foods

Unfortunately, if you have developed a sweet tooth and enjoy more than the odd plate of steak and fries this next section will come as bad news. According to research, on average we consume around 66lbs of refined sugar a year (via candy, pastries and even foods like ketchup and soup) with soda and energy drinks being the single biggest source in the

American diet. Sugar also comprises ingredients ending in "ose," like sucrose or glucose. All these products should be enjoyed occasionally or avoided if possible.

However, this is often easier said than done. Eating refined sugary confections like cakes and cookies elevates our mood and induces a sense of relaxation because the insulin that is released to lower blood sugar levels also promotes the release of serotonin in the brain. So it is easy to literally become addicted to things made from a combination of sugar, fat and white flour, as these contain simple carbohydrates and have the greatest impact, although the effect will only last one or two hours. Then, as in all addictions, there is a downside to their feel good effect because these simple carbohydrates also produce crashes in serotonin levels as well as insulin levels.

In addition, sugar acidifies the blood. As the body's cells are slightly alkaline, they must remain that way to keep functioning properly. High consumption can also lead to the loss of the trace mineral chromium, which further fuels the craving for sugars. Altogether, a diet laden heavy in refined sugar can promote immune dysfunction and lead to hormonal disruption and mineral deficiencies. If you can break your dependence on these so called 'irresistible' foods, you will be taking a major step towards improving your health and fertility.

It is also now known that eating too much red meat can aggravate an inflammatory response. Red meat is taken to mean beef, pork, lamb and processed meat such as hot dogs, bacon, sausages and hamburgers. A study involving 25,000 people has shown that consuming large amounts of steak, burgers and lamb may be an independent risk factor for arthritis. The high collagen content of meat may lead to collagen sensitization and the production of anti-collagen antibodies in certain susceptible individuals.

A high intake of red meat, especially processed meat, is also linked to a greater incidence of bowel, breast and pancreatic cancer. Barbequed beef is particularly bad as it combines burnt meat with oxidized sugar which further increases the risk of cell mutation in the body.

Choosing the right kind of fat is essential. Today's diets are often low in omega-3 essential fatty acids (EFAs) and have excessive amounts of "bad" omega-6 EFAs. This imbalance can lead to many disorders including inflammatory autoimmune diseases. Omega-3 EFAs are vital for good health and there is strong evidence to show that they can help moderate inflammatory immune activity. The best sources come from unrefined vegetable oils (especially organic extra virgin olive oil and avocados) and oily fish.

Organic dairy produce, including cheese, cream and butter all contain more omega-3 EFAs than non organic varieties, however, they should still be consumed sparingly. A diet that is heavy in saturated transfats or hydrogenated fats can have a pro-inflammatory effect and is linked to a host of chronic diseases.

Finally, a word about diet foods. Packaged products including frozen ready meals, nutrition bars and other so called healthy alternatives labeled "low fat," "sugar free," "reduced calorie," "lean" and "lite," are often packed with artificial sweeteners, sugar, preservatives and other additives. Anything you eat or drink that has been highly processed is likely to contain man-made ingredients that will stress your immune system.

What to Limit or Avoid:

Alcohol
Coffee
"Diet" foods and drinks
Smoked or preserved meats
Vegetable oils (omega-6 polyunsaturated oils such as sunflower, corn and safflower) and any hydrogenated or partially hydrogenated oil
Hard margarines
Fried foods
Salt
Refined sugar and high fructose corn syrup
Dextrose (corn sugar, glucose)
Corn and corn based products
Refined grains (e.g., white flour and white rice)
Cookies, cakes & pastries

Boosting Fertility by Balancing the Immune System

OK, so what can you eat and drink? There are several guidelines I suggest, but the one that sums them up best is to eat nutrient-rich "real" foods (foods that exist in a natural form). Your daily intake should include five portions of fruit and vegetables plus plenty of water. The aim is to eat a range of proteins, carbohydrates and "good" fats to produce a steady stream of energy without creating the peaks and troughs in blood sugar levels, which lead to hormonal and autoimmune problems that can disrupt fertility. This is particularly important for anyone who has been diagnosed with a blood sugar imbalance.

Many women today avoid carbohydrates and are turning to high protein low carb diets. However, a protein dominated diet can harm fertility by producing toxins that disrupt the development of the embryo. Slow release or complex carbohydrates like vegetables, beans and whole grains contain fiber and phytoestrogens which can lower blood cholesterol, regulate bowel movements and stabilize blood sugar levels. However, these must be peeled and prepared properly and cooked thoroughly to reduce their lectin content, preferably using a pressure cooker in the case of beans.

Complex carbohydrates that are more resistant to digestion, also referred to as "resistant starches" enable the body to produce the mood-boosting hormone serotonin more consistently, so they will make you feel better physically and emotionally. Certain vegetables and fruits also contain antioxidants and folate, which help regulate immune responses and guard against thrombosis.

Protein should form around 10 to 15% of a person's food intake. It is needed to repair and renew cells, produce hormones, make antibodies to fight infection, grow new tissue for muscle and transport oxygen and nutrients around the body. In moderate amounts, it also helps women produce better quality eggs.

Good sources of protein are A2 milk, cheese, plant based meats, grass fed meats, fish, eggs, pasture raised poultry, nuts and seeds. For a complete list of low lectin, immune friendly foods and recipe ideas please refer to Dr Steven Gundry's book, *The Plant Paradox*.

Water: A Powerful Life Force

Being dehydrated negatively impacts your health and definitely impedes your chances of getting pregnant. Being dehydrated is associated with poor egg quality and reduced cervical mucus which is vital for transportation of sperm to the fallopian tubes.

Please try to make an effort to drink water, not coffee or canned drinks. Just plain, filtered tap water or glass bottled water (out gassing from plastic can pollute the water and unfiltered tap water contains chlorine by-products and possibly fluoride). Aim to drink around two liters or eight glasses daily. The danger with low level dehydration is that it stops the brain letting you know you are thirsty, so the problem just gets worse. Your urine should be straw colored (not clear, which indicates over consumption).

If your urine is orange, you are dehydrated and the more caffeinated or alcoholic beverages you drink, the more severe this condition becomes, triggering all kinds of hidden side effects. For example, more cholesterol is used to surround each cell to conserve the water within it which stops nutrients from entering and toxins from escaping.

Those with blood clotting tendencies should be especially mindful of the dangers of drinking too little water. Dehydration can make the blood more viscous, which is not just a problem when it comes to pregnancy, but it can also present a very serious health risk by increasing the likelihood of blood clots and thrombophilia. Being dehydrated also diverts what little water there is to the essential organs, such as the heart and brain and away from the ovaries and testicles. Dehydration in men also leads to decreased sperm quality and lower semen volumes.

Adding more pure water to your daily routine effectively flushes your body clean and reduces the demands on your immune system. Herbal teas and pressed fruit and vegetable juice are also very effective hydrators and detoxifiers. Pure fruit juice drinks should be limited to 6 to 8 ounces daily and preferably diluted with water because of their high sugar content.

Adding lemon to your water provides your body with vitamin C, magnesium, calcium and potassium in a readily available form. You may also want to try taking two tablespoons of a good quality organic cider vinegar three times a day with a little honey mixed in. Drink it through a straw and rinse your mouth several times afterwards to avoid damaging the enamel on your teeth. Many of my clients have found this greatly reduces the symptoms of inflammation.

Women I have treated with autoimmune conditions have found that increased water intake together with an immune friendly, organic diet and a good quality multi-vitamin and mineral supplement are helpful in managing the symptoms of their disorder and preventing flares.

Significant improvements to health and fertility can be experienced relatively quickly simply by substituting good habits for bad ones and eating meals that you have made yourself using fresh, natural ingredients.

Food for Special Thought

Omega-3 Essential Fatty Acids (EFAs)

Research has established that oily fish is a highly effective immune modulator because it contains anti-inflammatory essential fatty acids (EFAs) like omega-3, and a derivative known as docosahexaenoic acid (DHA). Eight out of ten women have a shortage of omega-3 fats in their diets. This deficiency is linked to many diseases, including autoimmune conditions.

A diet rich in omega 3 EFAs can significantly decrease natural killer cell activity and suppress the production of TNF-alpha cytokines to moderate the symptoms of rheumatoid arthritis, endometriosis and psoriasis and even depression. Omega 3 fish oil is also a good choice for women with blood clotting tendencies who have suffered recurrent miscarriage, as it can help increase uterine blood flow and a recent Cochrane review has shown that taking a daily fish oil supplements during pregnancy can reduce the chance of a premature birth by up to 42%.

Omega 3 fish oil is a great supplement for patients with elevated NK activity and elevated TNF levels as it lowers both. In pregnancy, low consumption of fish has been correlated with a higher incidence of preeclampsia, preterm delivery and low birthweight. Even small amounts of omega 3 EFAs can assist in protecting against these outcomes by decreasing the production of Th1 cytokines and improving blood flow through the placenta. The benefits of these nutrients are then passed on to the baby (via the placenta and breastfeeding), to promote healthy brain and central nervous system development.

Salmon, trout, fresh tuna, herring, mackerel, kippers and sardines are all rich in omega 3 and some organic varieties are now available. As cooking depletes omega 3 and there are concerns about mercury contamination in some types of fish (shark, swordfish and tuna, especially albacore tuna), you may prefer to increase your intake with pharmaceutical grade fish oil, which has been ultra purified to remove toxins. Choose a variety with between 500 and 1000mg of omega-3 fats and at least 500mg of DHA.

Vegans can obtain omega 3 EFA from flax, hemp, pumpkin and sesame seeds, avocados, walnuts, olives, green leafy vegetables and walnut, olive or flaxseed oils. However, there is some evidence that omega-3s from vegetable sources are not as health promoting as fish oil.

If you are undergoing heparin therapy you must seek advice from your doctor before self medicating, because fish oil has a slight blood thinning effect (1g of fish oil has the anticoagulant effect of one sixteenth of a full-strength aspirin pill). Also, cod liver oil is best avoided during pregnancy because it is extremely high in vitamin A which has been associated with birth defects in pregnancy.

Flavonoids (Antioxidants)

Free radicals are a byproduct of the process whereby oxygen turns food such as fat and sugar into energy. Oxygen combines with hydrogen to make water during this process, however if the oxygen escapes before the conversion is complete, free radicals are formed. They can also be created by air pollution, chemical toxins and smoking.

Because of their chemical instability, free radicals can alter the DNA of cells and the structure of tissues and their functions. Such changes can trigger the production of damaging TNF-alpha cytokines and lead to degenerative diseases like arthritis, cardiovascular disease and cancer.

Over time, oxidative stress can also influence a woman's entire reproductive lifespan, from egg quality and maturation to fertilization and embryo development. For example, free radical activity in the follicular fluid can damage the egg and if levels of oxidative stress are not within a low range, pregnancy will usually not occur. Antioxidant and pro-oxidant nutrients reduce levels of free radicals and modulate the inflammatory response by promoting the production of Th2 cytokines.

Flavonoids are powerful antioxidants found in all fruits and vegetables. They can reverse oxidative damage, slow the aging process and improve overall reproductive health. They enhance the ability of vitamin C to form strong, flexible blood vessel walls and slow the blood clotting process. So far, over 4,000 different types of flavonoids have been identified.

Quercetin, an antioxidant found in grape and cranberry juices has virtually the same clot preventing benefits as low dose aspirin but without the side effects. Resveratrol, another compound found in grapes, has anti-inflammatory, antioxidant, anti-tumor and immunomodulatory properties.

You may be familiar with the probiotic formula Kombucha. Although it's certainly an acquired taste, this fermented drink is high in glucaric acid which is very effective at reducing inflammation according to recent studies. It is also claimed to promote heart health, fight cancer, aid digestion and act as a liver detoxifier.

Fresh ginger is widely used in Ayurvedic medicine to treat auto-immune illnesses by decreasing the activity of pro-inflammatory cytokines such as TNF-alpha. As it interferes with the formation of the blood clots and lowers cholesterol, it can also help guard against thrombosis.

Spinach is another wonderful immune modulator that can help reduce pro-inflammatory TNF-alpha and TNF-beta levels. Avocados also contain ingredients that can help alleviate inflammation and have long been used to treat the symptoms of osteoarthritis, while rosemary, sage and thyme contain compounds called diterpenoids that reduce inflammation. By adding these herbs (fresh, not dried, as a lot of nutrients are lost in the drying process) to your cooking or sprinking them over your food you can increase the flavour of your meals as well as increase their beneficial effect on your health. I like to take a bunch of fresh cilantro or basil and cut it very finely with scissors over the meal before serving.

Citrus fruits have antioxidative and cardio protective compounds. They also contain a substance called nobiletin which has anti-inflammatory properties which, according to one report, are similar to those of corticosteroids such as dexamethasone. Rhubarb, in addition to being a highly effective scavenger of free radicals, can help relax the blood vessels and suppress the vascular inflammatory process.

Onions and garlic are major sources of selenium, which is a powerful antioxidant and immunomodulator. Garlic contains allicin and cysteine, which have been shown to regulate the TNF-alpha immune response. It is also rich in blood thinning compounds, which help keep the coronary arteries clear. When chopped or crushed and added to food garlic helps to decrease platelet stickiness. Indeed, research has shown that eating three cloves of garlic a day, or the equivalent in supplements, reduces cholesterol for extended periods and can guard against blood clots. In addition, garlic is known to reduce elevated blood sugar levels and protect against environmental toxins, bacteria and fungal infection.

Other antioxidant rich fruit and vegetables include asparagus, beets, broccoli, brussel sprouts, Chinese cabbage, arugula, collards, carrots, onions, leeks, parsley, mustard greens, seaweed, fennel, spinach, blueberries, raspberries, peaches, plums, prunes, blackberries, boysenberries and pomegranates. Greens formulas in particular have a very positive effect on egg quality.

Flavonoids lower TNF-alpha and reduce ROS (reactive oxygen species) both of which can have an adverse effect on egg quality as well as immune related pregnancy loss. To ensure you have an adequate intake of these nutrients it is best to try to consume an average of five to eight servings of organic fruit and vegetables every day.

To preserve the antioxidant content of your food I recommend that you avoid irradiating it the microwave. For example, broccoli "zapped" in some water for five minutes loses 97% of its flavonoids, whereas steaming results in just an 11% reduction. To get the maximum health benefits from anything you cook, it's worth investing in a countertop steamer or pressure cooker and using your microwave oven as little as possible.

Giving Your Body a Fresh Start

Patients who come to our center with immune mediated reproductive problems are encouraged to undergo a physical detox alongside manual lymphatic drainage and electro-acupuncture. Detoxification is the process of clearing or neutralizing toxins and ridding the body of excess mucus and congestion. It is also essential in the reestablishment of a healthy gut flora.

Waste products can also be eliminated by massaging the skin in the direction of the lymph flow, a process known as manual lymphatic drainage. Finally, stagnant "energy" (or "qi" as it is called in Chinese medicine) is stimulated with the aid of electro-acupuncture to help restore vitality.

Detoxification and Rejuvenation

Many women who come to see me are desperately in need of a complete internal cleansing process, which I feel can play a key role in dietary immunotherapy. Therefore, in the run up to an IVF or natural conception cycle, I recommend a liver detox program. The liver acts as filter, processing toxins and chemically altering excess or used hormones. If it is under constant stress, it cannot eliminate harmful agents like pesticides, herbicides, food additives and caffeine from the bloodstream effectively.

When these toxins start accumulating, particularly in the colon and fat cells, the body demands that they are diluted. This leads to water retention. Other symptoms of toxic build-up are headaches, low energy and nausea. A daily supplement of the anti-inflammatory herb milk thistle, (also called silymarin), is a good idea because it helps protect the liver from the effects of pesticide residues and works to repair any existing damage.

Another important aspect of a detox is to rebalance the gut's bacteria and drive out the overpopulation of the harmful kinds of bacteria that cause cravings for the unhealthy foods they thrive on. If your gut is damaged you simply will not gain the maximum benefit from eating healthy foods.

An initial three day cleanse can change the type of bacteria that inhabit your gut by starving out the invaders that shouldn't be there and encouraging the proliferation of probiotics, otherwise known as good bacteria. This protocol is part of *The Plant Paradox Program* and can be found in Dr Gundry's aforementioned book. Essentially it contains organic foods like cabbages, mushrooms, greens and seaweed, wild caught fish, pasteurized chicken, avocado plus some selected oils and seasonings. A three-day cleanse meal delivery service featuring these ingredients is available to residents of the USA through www.catalystcuisine.com.

Phase two is a six week repair process with an immune calming detoxification to "chelate" or cleanse your body of harmful chemicals. This process restores the hormonal balance that is needed to make your body baby friendly. Chelation is a process in which a substance binds to certain molecules to remove them from the body. It can rid the body of arterial plaque build-up, excess calcification and toxic metals, such as mercury, which promote autoantibody production.

For example, vitamin C and pectin found in apples, pears and bananas and sulfur rich foods like fresh garlic, onions and eggs can help to remove lead. Other chelating substances include choline or lecithin granules which can be sprinkled over food. Choline is an element of one of several phospholipids (including phosphatidylcholine) that are important for normal cellular and organ functions. It is found in many foods, particularly eggs, fish, nuts and vegetables.

Fresh cilantro (otherwise called coriander or Chinese parsley) is known to be an effective mobilizer of mercury, lead, aluminum and tin that may be stored in the brain and the spinal cord. It moves these substances to other areas of the body where they can be eliminated by metal binding agents such as chlorella. Other green juices, such as wheat grass and spirulina, are also high in chlorophyll that will help chelate out toxic metals.

Green tea, plus vitamins A, C and E are powerfully anti-mutagenic and can help limit damage by pollutants. Green tea has even been shown to reduce DNA damage in human eggs. Drink at least two liters (four pints) of water daily with a dash of lemon juice if you like. This quota can also include herbal (but not chamomile) and fruit teas which also have a cleansing and restorative effect and help flush toxins through the kidneys.

Exercise is a very effective detoxifier as sweat is an important route for the elimination of toxic agents. In addition it improves blood circulation and helps oxygenate the tissues. To limit further exposure to heavy metals, I also advise my clients to use stainless steel cookware and avoid pans with non stick coatings.

Baby Friendly Micronutrients

There are many key nutrients for maintaining a healthy body. However, some are more important than others when it comes to enhancing fertility by improving blood circulation, promoting healthy cell metabolism and controlling unwanted inflammatory responses. Although food should provide us with all the essential nutrients we need, sometimes supplements are required to make up for the minerals that are lacking in today's mass-produced foodstuffs (another reason to buy organic). But please remember, vitamin pills should not be used to compensate for a bad diet.

Research has shown that over a period of 14 months, women who took nutritional supplements conceived earlier than those who did not. Studies also indicate that nutritional supplements such as antioxidants, multivitamins and amino acids can help balance hormones, encourage egg production and improve sperm quality.

A single daily high quality prenatal multivitamin and mineral supplement should contain a well balanced blend of essential nutrients. You may also want to consider taking a lectin blocking supplement to minimize the inflammatory effect of lectin containing foods known to aggravate the colon and intestines, at least until you are able to fully modify your diet.

Women undergoing immunotherapy need particular vitamins and minerals to support the depletion that certain drugs cause. For example, those taking corticosteroids will need extra vitamin C and patients that have been prescribed heparin will need extra calcium, vitamin D and magnesium. Please do not take any supplements or herbal formulas without checking with your reproductive immunologist first, as some of these over-the-counter herbal products can be counterproductive to fertility goals. For example, patients who are taking immunosuppressant medication should avoid chamomile and turmeric, as these compounds are known to interact with these certain immunotherapy drugs and reduce their beneficial effects.

Important: To avoid over treatment (e.g., overly thinning the blood) or creating a conflict and possible hormonal interactions with prescription drugs, dietary supplements must only be taken under medical supervision. High doses of one vitamin can create a deficiency of another and overdosing can be detrimental to the health of both mother and baby. Supplements other than prenatal vitamins should never be taken while pregnant or breast-feeding unless prescribed by your doctor.

Acupuncture

"I'm becoming a firm believer in electrical acupuncture, which is a form of really deep massage. Patients who have this treatment for at least six weeks sometimes see an improvement in their natural killer cell levels. As it also reportedly helps improve blood flow and aids relaxation, it is certainly an option worth considering alongside immunotherapy."

Alan E. Beer, M.D.

Some of my patients have told me that acupuncture has achieved significant results in reducing the clinical symptoms of their autoimmunities. Acupuncture is widely recognized for its ability to balance organ systems, reestablish the proper flow of energy through the body and to help regulate inflammatory autoimmune activity and I strongly advocate its application by a practitioner who is familiar with immune and fertility problems.

In Chinese medicine, the focus of attention is on the various pathways (also called "channels") that run between the major organs. Fine needles are inserted at specific points along these pathways. A very mild pulsing electric current is then passed through them to increase the benefits of the treatment. This subtle, yet intense form of stimulation can improve the function of the kidneys, spleen and liver, all of which are associated with increased fertility.

Different types of acupuncture can also be used to regulate the menstrual cycle and treat other fertility problems such as failure to ovulate, elevated FSH levels and endometriosis. This therapy has proved to be particularly beneficial to those undergoing IVF, reportedly improving follicular development and egg quality, and encouraging implantation. Studies have shown that it also improves blood flow to the ovaries and pelvic area and could be very helpful for women with PCOS.

Manual Lymphatic Drainage (MLD)

"Natural herbs, deep therapeutic massage and acupuncture are often used by my patients as part of their preconception treatment plan. Combining a general detox with stress reduction therapy has physical and psychological benefits. I recommend that patients preparing for a cycle of conception have these procedures twice weekly starting a month before the cycle of conception, twice weekly during the cycle of conception and continuing until the pregnancy status is known."

Alan E. Beer, M.D.

The lymphatic system is a network of organs, nodes, ducts and vessels that both produces and transports excess fluid from the tissue to the bloodstream. Lymph is a clear liquid made from blood fluid that contains mainly white blood cells. If the lymphatic flow stagnates or even stops (for reasons such as fatigue, stress, emotional shock, lack of physical activity or certain food additives), toxins can accumulate which can lead to various physical problems that can compromise fertility.

Unlike the blood, the lymphatic system has no pumps or valves to push it round the body and organs. It relies totally on exercise and other forms of stimulation. Manual lymphatic drainage (MLD) assists the body with this process by encouraging the lymphatic vessels to contract. A daily 30-minute walk or rebounding on a mini trampoline can also encourage healthy lymphatic flow. The fluid with its proteins and waste then passes into the bloodstream and toxins can be eliminated by the kidneys.

MLD can help restore the balance of hormones and neurotransmitters, regulate the monthly cycle, aid digestion and reduce the symptoms of premenstrual syndrome. However, during a conception cycle, this kind of deep therapeutic massage should be avoided at the time of ovulation, (although it can be resumed 48 hours later). It should also be avoided in the 24-hour period before an IVF transfer and around the estimated time of implantation.

Mind-Body Therapy

Wanting a baby and not being able to have one is a huge source of frustration and anxiety for many women. If you are constantly feeling under pressure, your cortisol level will probably remain elevated for some considerable time. Chronically elevated levels of cortisol can set the stage for estrogen dominance as it has the effect of reducing progesterone levels, which can lead to immune dysfunction and disease. Research has linked cortisol defects to many health disorders including raised blood sugar levels, abdominal fat accumulation, insomnia, heart disease, allergies and autoimmune problems.

Mind-body therapy together with healthy nutrition and lifestyle choices can really help to reduce your immune system's stress burden. Hypnotherapy, positive visualization and meditation will enable you to identify and release negative emotions and replace them with a more optimistic attitude. Talking things over with a counselor is another good way to release any self defeating thoughts that may be running around your head.

Physical activity, particularly when combined with deep breathing, has a wonderful anti-inflammatory effect and can elevate serotonin levels. Activities that have a calming effect can be quite simple and pleasurable. A warm bath, a good book or listening to music can all help to soothe your mind and body. Other activities that can greatly enhance feelings of well-being include yoga, tai chi and aromatherapy massage. Even regular deep-breathing sessions, a daily half-hour walk and low impact exercise like swimming can make a real difference.

Being active, feeling positive and being kind to yourself are the basic prerequisites for a baby friendly body as well as a healthier, calmer, happier life.

POST SCRIPTS

POST SCRIPTS

Alan E. Beer, M.D.

My heartfelt thanks to Dorothy, my wife of 47 years, and mother to our four adult children and grandmother to our ten grandchildren. Thank God that she happily busied herself during my long, long hours, days and months at this computer on a mission to help those suffering with immune infertility and losses, many of whom would never become my patients. I thank her for experiencing our life together, knowing the joys of parenthood as well as the trials.

My deep gratitude also to Chris Sanow. Without her help, support and attention to detail, my program would not operate so smoothly. Chris, who is a licensed medical technologist, has been with me since the opening of the California Clinic and is the person who makes the program work. I have known Chris as a patient who suffered so much with repeated pregnancy losses following the birth of a beautiful son, but was able to add to her family thanks to immune treatment.

Our office receives more than a thousand calls a month and Chris deals with every couple in the most competent, sensitive and caring manner. Truly, she is the calm in the storm. When panicked patients, phones and fax machines are demanding her attention all around, she deals with each one with total control and professionalism. There is no other person who knows my immunological mind better than she does. I have never worked with any person so dedicated, intelligent and competent.

When viewing the flag I think of Betsy Ross. When seeing women in politics I think of Eleanor Roosevelt, and when considering reproductive immunology in the public domain, I think of Jane Reed and the Yahoo website that she single handedly constructed and manages hours each day, every day of the year. When I met Jane for the first time, she was not an Internet guru, she was woman whose life had been tortured and turned upside down by repeated pregnancy losses. Both Jane and her husband radiated the picture of health, yet were psychologically crippled by all the sadness and disappointment they had endured. Jane knew in her heart something was terribly wrong and was on a mission to find the diagnosis. Many have read her story in this book. Many have been helped by her Internet site and her words.

She has teamed with Chris Sanow and Julia Kantecki, talking to them daily by phone or email, addressing the questions of old and new patients

POST SCRIPTS

and assisting couples seeking help with the program. I am so proud to have her help coauthor this book. Jane has read every word repeatedly, and has distilled my "difficult to understand words" into words that can be understood and felt by the reader. My appreciation for what she does day and night every day of the year is immense. Thank you Jane, and thanks to your husband and family for sharing you with all of us.

"Knowledge heals." These two words have new meaning for me. Julia is the living example of this. Her son Thomas, her precious gift, has changed her life and inspired her to share her healing, hope and wonderful vitality with all of you. I see pictures of Julia strolling through her beautiful British garden, the small hand of her son in hers, the glow of happiness radiating from them both. I remember her in our home with her son playing happily in the toy box of Beer children long gone and busy raising their own families. I see her behind piles of paper, chapters edited with notes, and I think how big the task was putting this important work together. It is the best product possible because of her devotion, knowing her mission must be completed for the benefit of many.

I am so fortunate to have had such brilliant, hardworking women who know the sadness and joy of reproductive immunology work with me on this project and assist me with my program.

I am grateful and humbled too by the words of the Foreword written by Dr Christo Zouves and I am honored to know this "giant" of a man. No other reproductive endocrinologist has been more helpful, supportive and devoted to my program and its patients than he and his staff. Support like Christo's has buoyed me up through some difficult times in this country. And when Lesley Regan and other leaders in the U.K. were shouting from mountains that reproductive immunology was a hoax, Mr Mohamed Taranissi and Dr George Ndukwe were by my side, formalizing programs in London and Nottingham, England under my direction. Through their efforts, many couples in Europe have enjoyed new lives as parents.

Lastly, I would like to thank an extraordinary and internationally respected colleague of mine, sadly now deceased. It was Dr Rupert Billingham – my mentor, research collaborator and dearest friend – who shared my interest in the immune mechanisms that allowed the survival of the embryo as a transplant. I think of him daily and with reverence. I know for certain that he would have taken great pride in this work.

Thanks "Bill" – your passion lives in me.

Alan E. Beer, M.D.

From the Coauthors

This book has taken years to complete and some special people have helped along the way. Thank you first, to my parents for their wisdom, intelligence and useful critiques. Jane Reed is my sounding board, my educator and a trusted, long standing friend, providing support and direction throughout this long journey. Thank you for making this book the success it is today. .

Working with Dr Beer was a privilege. He impressed and humbled me with his single minded determination to helping those in need.

Finally, thank you to my son Thomas who is now a smart, handsome, musically talented, kind hearted 6'2" 15 year old. All I have ever wanted was to give others who are struggling like did, access to the incredible gift of parenthood. Whenever my son says, "I love you mom" it makes all the time and effort spent writing this book worthwhile.

Julia Kantecki

Thanks to my wonderful children who gave me tolerance and understanding during my long days and nights in front of the computer. My love and appreciation also goes to my talented husband Ed, who meticulously sifted through the book and enhanced it with his fresh and critical insights.

Warmth and respect goes to Dr Douglas Austin who showed me the power of listening with an open mind, you are truly a credit to the infertility field. Much gratitude also, to my Reproductive Immunology Support Group, who taught me the magical ability of knowledge and communication to heal the suffering and touch the soul.

Finally, the deepest thanks to my hero and friend, Dr Alan Beer, whose genius not only gave me the gift of four of my beautiful children: Jessica, Robert, Jonathan and McKenna, but whose passion and vision taught me the great honor of fighting for truth. Thank you, Alan. You are my inspiration.

Jane Reed

POST SCRIPTS

Alan E. Beer, M.D.
1937 - 2006

Dr Beer died on May 1st, 2006 at the age of 69, just weeks before this book went to print: a bittersweet ending to a powerful and influential life. It was a twist of fate that he saw the final draft of his book, but sadly he never held a printed copy in his hand. We know he was so proud of the text and thankful that his life's work had been so faithfully documented. During his final days he would have felt great peace knowing that this book would stand as an important part of his legacy.

In 2006 Dr Beer announced that the laboratory he had always dreamed of was completed and staffed by a team of world leading experts. In addition, patient numbers at his Californian clinic had virtually doubled since it opened in 2003. Yet despite an ever increasing workload he never felt compelled to retire or even rest. When he said, "I will die at my desk," he meant it.

Until his last days, he dedicated himself to his mission of providing explanations, effective treatments and hope for those suffering the misery of failure and loss. It was his ultimate achievement that couples like these, wherever they live, are can now receiving help thanks to his revolutionary protocols. New discoveries within this sphere of science continue to emerge, resulting in the introduction of even more finely tuned treatments.

Dr Beer touched many thousands of patients and doctors with his dedicated soul and pioneering mind. He was a determined warrior and a unique visionary for the reproductive immunology cause.

As a final note, here are some words from President Abraham Lincoln with which Dr Beer identified:

"If I were to try to read, much less to answer all the attacks made on me, this shop might as well be closed for any other business. I do the very best I know – the very best I can; and I mean to keep on doing so until the end. If the end brings me out all right, then what is said against me won't matter. If the end brings me out wrong, then ten angels swearing I was right would make no difference."

NOTES

NOTES

INTRODUCTION

ix   **"Fertility centers using his methods are seeing similar results today."** – Columbia Fertility Associates, *Reproductive Immunology* eBook download: "Once patients are diagnosed with immunologic infertility factors, and undergo the correct treatment protocol, their pregnancy rates are as high as 70% (assuming transferred embryos are chromosomally normal)."

xxvii   **"...a study by a team of psychologists in Australia..."** – Conway K and G: "A report on grief caused by miscarriage." *British Journal of* Russell *Medical Psychology*, 73 Pt 4:531-45. Dec 2000.

xxviii   **"In his 2003 book on miscarriage, Dr Henry Lerner describes them as 'spontaneous, frequent and normal reproductive events.'"** – p.3 *Miscarriage, Why it Happens and How Best to Reduce Your Risks,* by Lerner HM. Perseus Book Group, 2003. ISBN: 0738206342.

xxviii   **"...the figures from the miscarriage societies of the U.K. and U.S. make depressing reading."** – According to the American College of Obstetrics & Gynecology (ACOG), studies show that 10 to 25% of all clinically recognized pregnancies will end in miscarriage. The estimated percentage of chemical or unrecognized pregnancies that are lost is as high as 50 to 75%.

xxx   **"The Royal College of Obstetricians and Gynecologists which sets guidelines..."** – Regan L, Backos M and Rai R: "Royal College of Obstetricians & Gynecologists Scientific Advisory Committee Opinion Paper 5." Oct 2003. See:
http://www.rcog.org.uk/resources/Public/pdf/SAC_Opinion_Paper_5.pdf

2. DEFINING REPRODUCTIVE FAILURE

Chromosomal Abnormalities

30   **"...influenced by mutagenic environmental agents that have the ability to damage genes and chromosomes."** – Ralston A, "Environmental Mutagens, Cell Signaling and DNA Repair." *Nature Education* 1(1):114, 2008.

30   **"Trisomies are more often associated with 'advanced maternal age'..."** – Abdalla MGK and Beattie RB: "Ultrasound markers of chromosomal abnormalities." *Progress in Obstetrics and Gynecology.* See: www.atyponlink.com/RCOG/doi/pdf/10.1576/toag.2001.3.3.147

30   **"Studies have shown that approximately half of all embryos are chromosomally abnormal in women undergoing IVF..."** – Clark DA: "Is there any evidence for immunologically mediated or immunologically modifiable early pregnancy failure?" Journal of Assisted Reproduction & Genetics, Vol. 20, No.2, 64-65, Feb 2003.

30   **"...in non-recurrent spontaneous abortions, around 66% are defective."** – Menasha J et al: "Incidence and spectrum of chromosome abnormalities in spontaneous abortions: new insights from a 12-year study." Genetics in Medicine, Apr; 7(4):251-63, 2005. In tests on tissue samples taken from over 2,000 spontaneous abortions, 66% displayed chromosomal abnormalities.

- 308 -

NOTES

"...IL-8, IL-6 and G-CSF increase in the human cervix during the ripening process indicating their important role in the cervical remodelling. These data demonstrate that cervical ripening is similar to an inflammatory process."

31   **"...multiple D&C procedures or an extreme, inflammatory immune response."** – Sennstrom MB et al: "Human cervical ripening, an inflammatory process mediated by cytokines." *Molecular Human Reproduction*, Apr; 6(4):375-81, 2000.

31   **"Researchers have since observed certain alterations in the immune systems of DES-exposed women."** – Milhan D: "DES exposure: implications for childbearing." *International Journal of Childbirth Education*, Nov-Dec; 7(4):21-8, 1992.
Here the author states that, as well as uterine abnormalities, researchers have observed certain alterations in the immune systems of DES-exposed women. "Altered immune response in adult women exposed to diethylstilbestrol in utero." *American Journal of Obstetrics and Gynecology,* NCBI PubMed PMID: 11483908, 2001 Jul.

31   **"Some women who miscarry repeatedly have an irregularly shaped uterus which may impair fetal growth."** – Homer et al: "The septate uterus: a review of management and reproductive outcome." *Fertility & Sterility*, Jan; 73, 1-14, 2000.
In this review of the literature, it was determined that prevalence of the septate uterus is increased in women with repeated pregnancy losses. A meta-analysis of published retrospective data comparing pregnancy outcome indicated a marked improvement after surgery.

31   **"Large uterine fibroids can affect implantation..."** – Horne A and Critchley H, "The effect of uterine fibroids on embryo implantation." *Seminars in Reproductive Medicine* Nov;25 (6):483-9, 2007.
"Fibroids cause a mechanical distortion of the endometrial cavity-their presence may alter gamete and embryo transport (due to blockage of the tubalostia or by altering uterine contractility and peristalsis) and subsequent embryo implantation (due to compression of the endometrium)."

Infection and Illness

32   **"Toxoplasma gondii...carries a risk for pregnancy."** – Nakano Y et al: "Role of innate immune cells in protection against Toxoplasma gondii at inflamed site." *Journal of Medical Investigation*, Feb; 48(1-2):73-80, 2001.

32   **"...chronic gum disease during the second trimester..."** – Persson GR et al: "Periodontitis, a marker of risk in pregnancy for preterm birth." *Journal of Clinical Periodontology*, Jan; 32(1):45-52, 2005.
A periodontal examination and collection of amniotic fluid was performed at 15-20 weeks of pregnancy in 36 women at risk for pregnancy complications. Periodontitis was diagnosed in 20% of normal births and in 83% cases of premature births. Amniotic cytokine levels were significantly higher in preterm cases.

NOTES

33   **"Chlamydia is the most common sexually transmitted disease in the United States."** – CDC. Sexually Transmitted Disease Surveillance, 2016. Atlanta, GA: Department of Health and Human Services; September 2017.

33   **"[Chlamydia] increases the risk of a tubal or ectopic pregnancy and spontaneous abortion."** – Kishore J et al: "Seroanalysis of Chlamydia trachomatis and S-TORCH agents in women with recurrent spontaneous abortions." *Indian Journal of Pathology & Microbiology*, Oct; 46(4):684-7, 2003.

33   **"Gonorrhea and syphilis are also known to be associated with first trimester pregnancy losses."** – Sciarra J: "Sexually transmitted diseases: global importance." *International Journal of Gynecology & Obstetrics,* 58:107-119, 1997.

Environmental Factors

33   **"Environmental factors have been associated with unusually large clusters of birth abnormalities."** – 2002 report: "Identifying Toxic Risks Before and During Pregnancy," by Marc Lappe PhD and Noah Chalfin BA at the Center for Ethics and Toxics. *See also*:

Sharara F et al: "Environmental toxicants and female reproduction." *Fertility & Sterility*, 70(4):613–622, 1998.
"Published data indicate that chemical exposures may cause alterations in reproductive behavior and contribute to sub-fecundity, infertility, pregnancy loss, growth retardation, intrauterine fetal demise, birth defects, and ovarian failure in laboratory animals and wildlife…"

33   **"In the U.S. about 5 boys out of every 1,000 have hypospadias, making it one of the most common birth defects there is.** – Cara T Mai et al: "Population-Based Birth Defects Data in the United States, 2008 to 2012: Presentation of State-Specific Data and Descriptive Brief on Variability of Prevalence." 2015 study published in *"Birth Defects Research Clinical and Molecular Teratology."*

33   **"In animal studies, some toxic chemicals have even been shown to alter the structure of genes and chromosomes."** – Anway MD et al: "Epigenetic transgenerational actions of endocrine disruptors and male fertility," *Science*, 308:1466-1469, 2005.
In this report, the author concludes: "The ability of an environmental factor (for example, endocrine disruptor) to reprogram the germ line and to promote a transgenerational disease state has significant implications for evolutionary biology and disease etiology."

3. RECURRING NIGHTMARES

Recurrent IVF Failure

37   **"Studies have reported that many couples consider infertility to be at least as, or more stressful than divorce or the death of a loved one."** – Millard M: "Infertility stress syndrome: Trauma exacerbated by gender differences (a study

NOTES

of pre-adoptive and adoptive parents)." Doctoral dissertation, the Professional School of Psychology, San Francisco, California, 1993.

Describing the stress responses they experienced during the acute phase of "infertility stress syndrome," over 25% of subjects had emotional anguish levels significantly above the norm for rape and family trauma.

38 **"...infertility now affects 25% of couples in developing countries"** –Maya N et al, "National, Regional, and Global Trends in Infertility Prevalence Since 1990: A Systematic Analysis of 277 Health Surveys." *World Health Organization Human Reproductive Program*, www.who.int/reproductivehealth/topics/infertility December 18, 2012.

38 **"For those with normal fertility levels, the maximum conception rate each month is between 20 and 25%."** – Racowsky C: "High rates of embryonic loss, yet high incidence of multiple births in human ART: is this paradoxical?" *Theriogenology*, 1; 57(1):87-96, 2002.
"Humans have low natural fecundity, as the probability of establishing a viable conception in any one menstrual cycle is 20-25% for a healthy, fertile couple."

38 **"After two years of failing to conceive, approximately 5% of couples will have virtually no chance of becoming pregnant..."** – Freundl G et al: "Definition and prevalence of subfertility and infertility." *Human Reproduction*, 20(5):1144-1147, 2005.
"Most of the pregnancies occur in the first six cycles with intercourse in the fertile phase (80%). After that, serious subfertility must be assumed in every second couple (10%) although – after 12 unsuccessful cycles – untreated livebirth rates among them will reach nearly 55% in the next 36 months. Thereafter (48 months), approximately 5% of the couples are definitively infertile with a nearly zero chance of becoming spontaneously pregnant in the future."

38 **"On average, only half of all embryos are chromosomally normal."** – Clark DA: "Is there any evidence for immunologically mediated or immunologically modifiable early pregnancy failure?" *Journal of Assisted Reproduction & Genetics*, Vol. 20, No.2 Feb 2003.
"In the study of unfertilized oocytes, 47% were abnormal and 53% were normal. Applying this estimate to the data of *Pieters et al.*, there would be 398 normal oocytes; if 56% fertilized, 23 did not divide and 200 did, then 200/402 (50%) of dividing embryos would have been abnormal and 50% normal."

38 **"It is likely that of the remaining 50% of good quality embryos, many are being wasted on failed cycles, caused by the same immune mechanisms that cause recurrent losses."** – Birkenfeld A et al: "Incidence of autoimmune antibodies in failed embryo transfer cycles." *American Journal of Reproductive Immunology*, Mar-Apr; 31 (2-3):65-8, 1994.
The authors speculate that patients who carry viable embryos, fail to demonstrate a positive pregnancy test due to implantation failure or a very early post-implantation loss, possibly caused by autoimmune antibodies. They conclude: "Very early miscarriage or implantation failure may be related to the same pathophysiological mechanism that causes recurrent miscarriages and is diagnosed incorrectly as infertility."

NOTES

Vaquero E et al, "Diagnostic evaluation of women experiencing repeated in vitro fertilization failure." *European Journal of Obstetrics and Gynecology*, March 1, Volume 125, Issue 1, Pages 79–84, 2006.
"Our data provide two important results: thyroid abnormalities, aPL and increased NK levels are more prevalent in women experiencing IVF failure."

Zhon Y et al, "Relationship between Antithyroid Antibody and Pregnancy Outcome following in Vitro Fertilization and Embryo Transfer." *International Journal of Medical Science*, 9(2):121-125, 2012.
"Patients with antithyroid antibody showed significantly lower fertilization rate, implantation rate and pregnancy rate and higher risk for abortion following IVF-ET when compared with those without antithyroid antibody."

38 **"...women incorrectly diagnosed with unexplained infertility before their first IVF attempt have a high incidence of immune problems..."** – Putowski L et al: "The immunological profile of infertile women after repeated IVF failure (preliminary study)." *European Journal of Obstetrics, Gynecology & Reproductive Biology*, Feb 10; 112(2): 192-6, 2004.
17 women with repeated IVF failures and 10 non-pregnant women with a history of successful IVF pregnancies were included in this study. In the IVF failure group, the percentage of CD19+5+ lymphocytes was significantly higher than that of the control group. 82% of patients failing IVF had at least one abnormal result on autoimmune testing. The authors concluded: "There is a need for immunological diagnostics in the group of patients with unexplained infertility." *See also*:

Coulam C and Roussev R: "Increasing circulating T cell activation markers are linked to subsequent implantation failure after transfer of in vitro fertilized embryos." *American Journal of Reproductive Immunology*, Oct; 50(4):340-5, 2003.
Blood from 22 women undergoing IVF was analyzed for circulating T-cells expressing CD69+ and HLA-DR+. The study concluded: "T-cell activation markers CD69+ and HLA-DR+ are associated with increased implantation failure after IVF/embryo transfer."

Schmutzler A et al: "High prevalence of markers for immunological disorders in IVF patients." *International Journal of Gynecology & Obstetrics*, July; 86(1):59-60, 2004.

Recurrent Miscarriage

39 **"As much as 40% of unexplained infertility may be the result of immune problems, as are as many as 80% of 'unexplained' pregnancy losses."** – Coulam C and Hemenway N: "Immunology May Be Key to Pregnancy Loss." 2004. See:
http://www.inciid.org/article.php?cat=immunology&id=374&pagenumber=1

39 **"...approximately 1 in 25 couples fitting this category."** – *Textbook of Gynecology*, 2nd edition, edited by Copeland L and Jarrell J. Published by W.B. Saunders Company in 1999. ISBN: 0721655521.

- 312 -

NOTES

40 **"The American College of Obstetricians and Gynecologists (ACOG) claims in its May 2016 patient guide..."** – www.acog.org/Patients/FAQs/Repeated-Miscarriages?
"About 65% of women with unexplained recurrent pregnancy loss have a successful next pregnancy."

40 **"...the likelihood that the fetuses being lost are chromosomally normal increases with the number of miscarriages the woman experiences."** – Ogasawara M et al: "Embryonic karyotype of abortuses in relation to the number of previous miscarriages." *Fertility & Sterility*, 300-304, 2000.
"The frequency of normal embryonic karyotypes significantly increases with the number of previous abortions, and a normal karyotype in a previous pregnancy is a predictor of subsequent miscarriage."

40 **"...the risk of miscarriage in a first pregnancy is 11 to 13%...but the risk to a third pregnancy after two successive losses nearly triples to 38%."** – Coulam et al: "Immunotherapy for recurrent pregnancy loss: analysis of results of clinical trials." *American Journal of Reproductive Biology*, 35; 352-359, 1996.

40 **"...in a subset of recurrent miscarriage patients it is possible the risk is nearer 100%."** – Clark DA: "Unexplained sporadic and recurrent miscarriage." *Human Reproduction Update*, Vol. 7, No 5, 501-511, 2001.
"Although repeated attempts at conception should eventually lead to a normal embryo...it is possible that some [couples] have a low risk of recurrence and others a risk near 100%."

40 **"...one study found that just 3.6% of 500 couples with recurrent miscarriage had such problems."** – Regan L et al: "An informative protocol for the investigation of recurrent miscarriage: preliminary experience of 500 consecutive cases." *Human Reproduction*, July; 9(7): 1328-32, 1994.

40 **"...miscarriage is not just a benign process; it may indicate an underlying health condition and even lead to autoimmune disease."** – Chong J et al: "Immunology of recurrent spontaneous abortion." *The Female Patient*, Vol. 20, Feb 1995.
See: http://www.rialab.com/pdf/irsa.pdf
This review concludes that failure of the protective maternal response and autoantibodies production can result in repetitive pregnancy loss.

Kwak-Kim J, "Immunology and Pregnancy Losses: HLA, Autoantibodies and Cellular Immunity." *Madame Curie Bioscience Database*, 2013.
"It is clear that local and systemic immunological differences can be found in these women (with recurrent loss) compared to women with normal pregnancies."

40 **"...the chance of carrying a baby to term without immunotherapy after three miscarriages is 30%, after four miscarriages 25%, and after five miscarriages 5%."** – Matzner W: "Miscarriages Can Be Prevented."
See: http://www.americanfertility.com/pdfs/miscarriages.pdf

40 **"...the baby is automatically at greater risk of premature birth or other potentially fatal pregnancy complications."** – Sheiner E et al: "Pregnancy

NOTES

outcome following recurrent spontaneous abortions." *Euro-pean Journal of Obstetrics, Gynecology & Reproductive Biology*, Jan; 118(1):61-5, 2005.

Between 1988 and 2002, 4.9% of 154,294 births were to women with a history of recurrent consecutive miscarriage. The study concludes: "A significant association exists between consecutive recurrent abortions and pregnancy complications such as placental abruption, hypertensive disorders and Cesarean section."

Stillbirth

41 **"...the incidence of stillbirth is estimated to affect 1% of pregnancies in the US..."** – Macdorman M, Gregory E: "Fetal and perinatal mortality, United States, 2013." *National Vital Statistics Reports*; Vol 64 no 8. Hyattsville, MD: National Center for Health Statistics. 2015.

41 **"A baby born via IVF is also around twice as likely to be stillborn..."**: Davies J et al: "Perinatal Outcomes by Mode of Assisted Conception and Sub-Fertility in an Australian Data Linkage Cohort," *PLOS One*, Published: January 8, 2014.

42 **"It is estimated that 14% of deaths occurring during labor and delivery and 86% before labor begins."**
Say L et al: "The prevalence of stillbirths: a systematic review." *Reproductive Health*, 3: 1. 2006.

42 **"Chromosomal disorders are present in approximately 25% of stillbirths."** – Silver R et al, "Work up of stillbirth: A review of the evidence." *American Journal of Obstetrics and Gynecology*, May; 196(5): 433–444, 2007.
"Approximately 25% of stillbirths have been attributed to cytogenetic, mendelian or biochemical causes."

42 **"Between 10 and 25% of stillbirths are caused by an infection..."** – Goldenberg RL and Thompson C: "The infectious origins of stillbirth." *American Journal of Obstetrics & Gynecology*, Sep; 189(3):861-73, 2003.

4. THE IMMUNE SYSTEM

52 **"These surface markers, known as clusters of differentiation (CD), define the cell's function."** – See: http://www.pathologyoutlines.com

53 **"...the Th1/Th2 relationship is the focus of most medical efforts when treating...infertility, pregnancy complications and miscarriage."** – Beer AE et al: "Increased T helper 1 cytokine responses by circulating T-cells are present in women with recurrent pregnancy losses and in infertile women with multiple implantation failures after IVF." *Human Reproduction*, Apr; 18(4):767-73, 2003.
"The prevalence of dominant Th1 immune responses in peripheral blood lymphocytes may reflect the systemic contribution of Th1 cytokines to recurrent spontaneous abortion or multiple implantation failures in IVF cycles." *See also*:

Beer AE et al: "Expression of intracellular Th1 and Th2 cytokines in women with recurrent spontaneous abortion, implantation failures after IVF/embryo transfer or normal pregnancy." *American Journal of Reproductive Immunology*, Aug; 48(2):77-86, 2002.

"In women with implantation failures, absolute cell counts of TNF-alpha expressing CD3+/4- cells reflects the presence of dominant Th1 immune response. A significantly increased Th1 cytokine expression may be the underlying immune etiology for reproductive failures."

Kwak-Kim J et al, "Elevated Th1/Th2 Cell Ratios in a Pregnant Woman with a History of RSA, Secondary Sjogrens Syndrome and Rheumatoid Arthritis Complicated with One Fetal Demise of Twin Pregnancy." *American Journal of Reproductive Immunology*, 58(4):325-9, Nov 2007

"Elevated Th1/Th2 cytokine producing CD3(+)/CD4(+) cell ratios were reported in women with a history of recurrent spontaneous abortion (RSA) and multiple implantation failures."

Makhseed M et al: "Pro-inflammatory maternal cytokine profile in preterm delivery" *American Journal of Reproductive Immunology*, Vol. 49, Issue 5:p.308, 2003.

Blood samples were taken from 54 women with a history of successful pregnancy, and 30 women undergoing preterm delivery. Significantly higher levels of the type 1 cytokines, interferon-gamma and interleukin-2, were produced by the group with preterm delivery than by the normal pregnancy group.

Mosmann T et al: "Bidirectional cytokine interactions in the maternal-fetal relationship: is successful pregnancy a Th2 phenomenon?" *Immunology Today*, 14:353–356, 1993.

In this review, the authors hypothesize that Th2 cytokines inhibit Th1 responses, thereby improving fetal survival, but impairing responses against some pathogens.

Raghupathy R: "Th1-type immunity is incompatible with successful pregnancy." *Immunology Today*, 18:478-482, 1997.

"Here, evidence from murine and human pregnancy is presented to show that, since Th1-type cytokines mediate pregnancy loss, a shift towards Th1-type immunity may help resolve 'unexplained' pregnancy failure."

Raghupathy R et al: "Cytokine production by maternal lymphocytes during normal human pregnancy and in unexplained recurrent spontaneous abortion." *Human Reproduction*, 15:713-718, 2000.

23 women with a history of unexplained recurrent abortion had significantly higher concentrations of Th1 cytokines than the control group.

Rezaei A and Dabbagh A: "T-helper (1) cytokines increase during early pregnancy in women with a history of recurrent spontaneous abortion." *Medical Science Monitor*, Aug; 8(8):CR607-10, 2002.

Blood samples of a control group of 40 women with no history of pregnancy loss and 92 women with at least 3 pregnancy losses were compared. Blood from women with recurrent losses had a higher concentration of TNF-alpha, TNF beta, and IL-2 compared with that of normal pregnant women. Tissue cultures from women with recurrent abortion also showed higher concentrations of TNF-alpha, IFN-gamma, TNF beta and IL-2 than the control group.

NOTES

Saito S and Sakai M: "Th1/Th2 balance in preeclampsia." *Journal of Reproductive Immunology*, Vol. 59, No.2, pp.161-173, Aug 2003.
"In this review, we discuss that Th1 predominant immunity is closely related to inflammation, endothelial dysfunction and poor placentation."

55 **"One of the factors that make some people more likely to develop autoimmunity is genetic..."** – Jawaheer D et al: "A genomewide screen in multiplex rheumatoid arthritis families suggests genetic overlap with other autoimmune diseases." *American Journal of Human Genetics,* Apr; 68(4):927-36, 2001. *See also*:

The Wellcome Trust Case Control Consortium: "Genome-wide association study of 14,000 cases of seven common diseases and 3,000 shared controls" *Nature*, Jun 7; 447(7145): 661–678, 2007.
"Approximately 2,000 British individuals were assessed for each of 7 major diseases. "Case-control comparisons identified 24 independent association signals in bipolar disorder, 1 in coronary artery disease, 9 in Crohn's disease, 3 in rheumatoid arthritis, 7 in type 1 diabetes and 3 in type 2 diabetes. On the basis of prior findings and replication studies thus far completed, almost all of these signals reflect genuine susceptibility effects."

56 **"[Autoimmune diseases] are also more prevalent in women..."**– Faustman DL: "Autoimmunity – disease of women: Genes and sex." 56th Annual Meeting of the American Society for Reproductive Medicine, San Diego, California, U.S.A., 2000.

56 **"One in 12 women and one in 20 men in the U.S. will develop some sort of autoimmune disease in their lifetime"** – Crowson C. et al: "The Lifetime Risk of Adult-Onset Rheumatoid Arthritis and Other Inflammatory Autoimmune Rheumatic Diseases," *Arthritis and Rheumatism*, March 2011; 63 (3): 633-639.

Selected Bibliography:

How the Immune System Works, by Sompayrac L, Published by Blackwell Publishing in 2003. ISBN: 063204702X

Immunobiology – The Immune System in Health and Disease, 6th Edition, by Janeway C. Published in 2005. ISBN: 0815320442

The Baby Resistant Body

57 **"In a normal pregnancy, a woman's body accommodates... a foreign body that should be destroyed by the immune system."** – Beer AE and Kwak JYH: "Immunology of normal pregnancy." *Immunology and Allergy Clinics of North America*, May 1998.

58 **"When TNF-alpha cytokine ratios are too high, they can stop the placental cells from dividing."** – Beer AE et al: "Increased T helper 1 cytokine responses by circulating T-cells are present in women with recurrent pregnancy losses and in infertile women with multiple implantation failures after IVF." *Human Reproduction*, Apr; 18(4):767-73, 2003.
The proportions of TNF-alpha producing CD3+/CD8- cells and the Th1/Th2 ratios of TNF-alpha/IL-4 and TNF-alpha/IL-10 in CD3+/CD8- cells were

NOTES

significantly higher in women with multiple IVF failures compared with those of controls.

58 **"Dr Beer has treated thousands of women whose levels of circulating NK cells and/or TNF-alpha cytokines are extremely high..."** – Beer AE et al: "Status of peripheral blood natural killer cells in women with recurrent spontaneous abortions and infertility of unknown etiology." *Human Reproduction,* May; 16(5):855-61, 2001. *See also*:

Beer AE et al: "Up-regulated expression of CD56+, CD56+/CD16+, and CD19+ cells in peripheral blood lymphocytes in pregnant women with recurrent pregnancy losses." *American Journal of Reproductive Immunology,* Aug; 34(2):93-9, 1995.

58 **"...in preeclampsia a strong maternal inflammatory response against the pregnancy tissue causes inflammation and damage to the placenta and to the mother's blood vessels."** – Jacek R et al: "Lymphocyte subset distribution and cytokine secretion in third trimester decidua in normal pregnancy and preeclampsia." *European Journal of Obstetrics & Gynecology and Reproductive Biology,* pp.8-15, Vol. 109, Issue 1, 1 Jul 2003.
"Preeclamptic patients were characterized with an increased percentage of the CD3-/CD56+CD16+, CD8+/CD28+ and decreased percentage of CD3+, CD19+, CD4+/CD45RA+ lymphocytes. The profile of secreted cytokines shifts in favor of Th1 activity..." *See also:*

Ness R: "The consequences for human reproduction of a robust inflammatory response." *Quarterly Review Biology,* Dec; 79(4):383-93, 2004.
Several studies are reviewed that show how an over-aggressive inflammatory reaction relates to adverse reproductive outcomes, including the fallopian tube damage and preeclampsia. There is also an association between immune hyper-responsiveness and premature delivery.

Harmon A et al: " The role of inflammation in the pathology of preeclampsia." *Clinical Science,* March; 130(6): 409–419 2016
"Women with PE exhibit chronic inflammation characterized by oxidative stress, pro-inflammatory cytokines, and auto antibodies. Studies... show that restoring the balance of the immune system... reduces the blood pressure and pathophysiology associated with placental ischemia."

59 **"...there is a direct link between subclinical autoimmune dysfunction and reproductive failure."** – Beer AE et al: "Expression of intracellular Th1 and Th2 cytokines in women with recurrent spontaneous abortion, implantation failures after IVF/ET or normal pregnancy." *American Journal of Reproductive Immunology,* Aug; 48(2):77-86, 2002.
Cell counts and percentages of CD3+, CD3+/CD4+, and CD3+/CD8+ T-cell populations were studied in 15 recurrent spontaneous abortion and 13 implantation failure patients. "In women with implantation failures, absolute cell counts of TNF-alpha expressing CD3+/4- cells reflect the presence of dominant Th1 immune response. A significantly increased Th1 cytokine expression may be the underlying immune etiology for reproductive failures." *See also:*

- 317 -

NOTES

Beer AE et al: "Immunophenotypic profiles of peripheral blood lymphocytes in women with recurrent pregnancy losses and in infertile women with multiple failed in vitro fertilization cycles." *American Journal of Reproductive Immunology*, Apr; 35(4):376-82, 1996.
"Non pregnant women with recurrent spontaneous abortions (RSA) of unknown etiology have higher levels of CD56+ lymphocytes compared to normal controls…Infertile and RSA women who fail alloimmune and autoimmune therapy have significant alterations in cellular and humoral immunity involving NK cells and CD19+/CD5+ B cells."

Birkenfeld A et al: "Incidence of autoimmune antibodies in failed embryo transfer cycles." *American Journal of Reproductive Immunology*, Mar-Apr; 31(2-3):65-8, 1994.
The presence of antiphospholipid antibodies and antinuclear antibodies was tested in 56 IVF-failure patients and 14 successful IVF patients. 32.1% IVF-failure patients tested positive for one or more of the autoimmune antibodies. None of the 14 successful IVF patients tested positive for any. The report concludes that in women who produce viable embryos, "…periimplantation events may be affected by autoimmune antibodies. Very early miscarriage or implantation failure may be related to the same pathophysiological mechanism that causes recurrent miscarriages and is diagnosed incorrectly as infertility."

Shoenfeld Y et al: "Autoantibodies and prediction of reproductive failure." *American Journal of Reproductive Immunology*, Nov-Dec; 56(5-6):337-44, 2006.
269 patients with autoimmune disease and/or reproductive failure were analyzed for anti-phospholipid, anti-annexin-V, anti-lactoferrin, anti-thyroglobulin, anti-thyroid peroxidase, anti-prothrombin, anti-nuclear, and anti-saccharomycetes cerevisiae antibodies. The prevalence of anti-prothrombin, anti-annexin, anti-phospholipid and anti-nuclear anti-bodies was significantly higher than in the control group.

Geva E et al: "Autoimmunity and reproduction." *Fertility & Sterility*, Apr; 67(4):599-611, 1997.
Over 300 original and review articles were evaluated, after which it was concluded: "When abnormal autoantibody levels are present in women with reproductive failure, the reproductive failure alone should be considered as one of the possible clinical expressions of autoimmune disorders."

Gleicher N et al: "What do we really know about autoantibody abnormalities and reproductive failure: a critical review." *Autoimmunity*, 16, 115-140, 1993.
Over 200 published papers referring to autoantibody-associated forms of reproductive failure were evaluated in this review. The authors concluded: "Autoantibody associated reproductive failure, characterized by a decrease in fecundity and an increase in the risk of pregnancy loss, appears established…The evaluation of autoantibody abnormalities in all cases of suspected autoimmune-associated reproductive failure is valuable and will improve clinical care of affected patients."

Maier D et al: "Subclinical autoimmunity in recurrent aborters." *Fertility & Sterility*, Feb; 51(2):280-5, 1989.
34 women with recurrent miscarriage were evaluated for the presence of lupus-associated autoantibodies, antisperm antibodies, and evidence of complement

NOTES

abnormalities. Multiple autoimmune abnormalities were found in women with unexplained losses. "This study suggests that recurrent pregnancy loss may be a marker for subclinical autoimmune disease."

Pandey MK et al: "An update in recurrent spontaneous abortion." *Archives of Gynecology & Obstetrics*, May 19 2005.
In this review, the authors state that the majority of cases of recurrent spontaneous abortion are associated with autoimmune and alloimmune antibodies. It is concluded that alterations in the expression of the Th1 pattern of cytokines and natural killer cell activity may induce abortion. Immunotherapy is suggested as an effective method of treatment.

5. BEING TOO GENTICALLY SIMILAR

61 **"It is thought that the preference for couples who are genetically incompatible, to mate successfully..."** – Apanius V et al: "The nature of selection on the major histocompatibility complex." *Critical Reviews in Immunology,* 17(2):179-224, 1997.
The authors state that MHC diversity probably functions to both avoid genome-wide inbreeding and to produce MHC-heterozygous offspring with increased immune responsiveness. *See also*:

Penn D et al: "MHC heterozygosity confers a selective advantage against multiple-strain infections." *Procedures of the National Academy of Science U.S.A.*, Aug; 20:99(17):11260-4, 2002.

61 **"...there is a significant increase in genetic compatibility between couples with unexplained infertility and recurrent miscarriage."** – Beer AE et al: "Pregnancy outcome in human couples with recurrent spontaneous abortions: HLA antigen profiles; HLA antigen sharing; female serum MLR blocking factors; and paternal leukocyte immunization." *Experimental & Clinical Immunogenetics*, Vol. 2(3):137-53, 1985.
11 women who aborted after immunization with paternal leukocytes were compared with 14 women who delivered infants at term post-immunization. Those who aborted shared more HLA antigens with their spouses than did controls. *See also*:

Creus M et al: "Parental human leukocyte antigens and implantation failure after in vitro fertilization." *Human Reproduction,* Jan; 13(1):39-43, 1998.
In 50 couples with prior primary infertility who had not achieved a pregnancy after three or more IVF cycles, there was a statistically significant excess of HLA sharing between partners.

Gerencer M: "HLA antigen studies in women with recurrent gestational disorders." *Fertility & Sterility,* Apr; 31(4):401-4, 1979.
In this study, a greater degree of HLA compatibility was found between women with unexplained recurrent spontaneous abortions and their partners.

Ober C et al: "Human leukocyte antigen matching and fetal loss: results of a 10-year prospective study." *Human Reproduction*, Jan 13(1):33-8, 1998.
In a 10-year prospective study of 251 pregnancies among 111 Hutterite couples, significantly increased fetal losses were observed among couples who were matched for HLA.

NOTES

Thomas M et al: "HLA sharing and spontaneous abortion in humans." *American Journal of Obstetrics & Gynecology,* Apr 15; 151(8):1053-8, 1985.

21 couples with two or more unexplained fetal losses were HLA typed. "...there was a strong indication that aborting couples shared a greater portion of the chromosome that contains the major histocompatibility complex (MHC) than would be expected in random matings."

62   **"Lack of recognition can lead to 'unexplained' IVF failure and miscarriage."** – Beer AE: "Immunopathologic factors contributing to recurrent spontaneous abortions in humans." *American Journal of Reproductive Immunology,* 4:182-184, 1983. *See also*:

Faulk W and McIntyre J: "Immunological studies of human trophoblast: markers, subsets and functions." *Immunological Review,* 75:139-75, 1983.

"...components of trophoblast membranes are capable of serving as immunogens to stimulate the mother to mount immune recognition of her blastocyst. Indeed, it is presently our interpretation that successful nidation depends upon maternal recognition of the blastocyst, and that a lack of recognition results in spontaneous abortion, sometimes occurring so early that the mother is not aware that she was pregnant."

62   **"The placenta contains paternal proteins, and paternal genes play a part in governing its invasion and growth..."** – Surani M: "Evidence and consequences of differences between maternal and paternal genomes during embryogenesis in the mouse." Source: *Experimental Approaches to Mammalian Embryonic Development,* edited by Rossant J and Pederson R. Published 1988. ISBN-13: 9780521368919. See also:

Wang Xu et al: "Paternally expressed genes predominate in the placenta." *Proceedings of the National Academy of Sciences of the United States of America,* June 25, 2013.

62   **"...there are many similarities between the behaviors of invasive placental cells and invasive cancer cells."** – Harandi A et al: "Immunoplacental therapy, a potential multi-epitope cancer vaccine." *Medical Hypotheses,* 66(6):1182-1187, 2006.

"The goal of cancer immunotherapy...is to view the fetal allograft as an 'impregnating tumor' and create an immunological state in the oncological patient analogous to a spontaneous abortion in a pregnant woman. The placenta shares identical growth mechanisms, antigenic determinants, and immune-escape properties with cancer cells..." *See also*:

Ferretti C et al: "Molecular circuits shared by placental and cancer cells, and their implications in the proliferative, invasive and migratory capacities of trophoblasts." *Human Reproduction,* Update, Volume 13, Issue 2, 1 March 2007, Pages 121–141, October 2006.

Shernan G et al: "Cancer and Pregnancy: Parallels in Growth, Invasion, and Immune Modulation and Implications for Cancer Therapeutic Agents," *Mayo Clinic Proceedings,* Nov; 84(11): 985–1000, 2009.

NOTES

62 **"...'non-classical' HLA-G molecules are expressed which work to help turn off the aggressive immune response..."** – Hunt J et al: "HLA-G and immune tolerance in pregnancy." *The FASEB Journal*, 19:681-693, 2005.
"The idea that placental HLA-G proteins facilitate semiallogeneic pregnancy by inhibiting maternal immune responses to foreign (paternal) antigens via these actions on immune cells is now well established..." *See also*:

Hunt S et al: "The role of HLA-G in human pregnancy." *Reproductive Biology and Endocrinology*, 4 (Suppl 1): S10, 2006.

Kanai T et al: "Human leukocyte antigen-G-expressing cells differently modulate the release of cytokines from mononuclear cells present in the decidua versus peripheral blood." *American Journal of Reproductive Immunology*, Vol. 45, No.2, pp.94-99(6), Feb 2001.
"Upon contact with HLA-G, decidual mononuclear cells, and peripheral blood mononuclear cells modulate their ability to release cytokines in a way that may shift the Th1/Th2 balance towards relative Th2 dominance, suggesting a role for HLA-G in maintaining pregnancy."

62 **"...HLA-G molecules are able to make activated CD8 cells self-destruct..."** – Fournel S et al: "Cutting edge: soluble HLA-G1 triggers CD95 CD95/CD95 ligand-mediated apoptosis in activated CD8+ cells by interacting with CD8." *Journal of Immunology*, Jun; 164, pp.6100-6104, 2000.

62 **"HLA-G molecules...switch natural killer cell receptors from 'on' to 'off'..."** – Menier C et al: "HLA-G truncated isoforms can substitute for HLA-G1 in fetal survival." *Human Immunology,* Nov; 61(11):1118-25, 2000.
"Our results show that not only HLA-G1, but also the other HLA-G truncated isoforms, can inhibit NK cytolysis and therefore contribute to immune privilege for the fetus." See also:

Le Rond S et al: "Indoleamine 2, 3 dioxygenase and human leukocyte antigen-G inhibit the T-cell alloproliferative response through two independent pathways." *Immunology,* Nov; 116(3):297-307, 2005.
"...HLA-G is thus complementary for inducing and maintaining immune tolerance in physiological (pregnancy) and pathological (tumor and allograft) situations."

Rajagopalan S: "HLA-G-mediated NK cell senescence promotes vascular remodeling: implications for reproduction." *Cellular and Molecular Immunology*, Sep; 11(5): 460–466, 2014.

62 **"HLA G molecules...stimulate the macrophages to produce Th2 protective cytokines..."** – Blaschitz A et al: "HLA Class I protein expression in the human placenta." *Early Pregnancy*, 5(1):67-9, 2001.
"HLA class I molecules HLA-G and HLA-E are thought to be involved in the induction of immune tolerance by acting as ligands for inhibitory receptors present on NK cells and macrophages."

62 **"HLA-G molecules...encourage the production of T regulatory cells."** – Clark DA: "Tolerance signaling molecules." *Chemical Immunology & Allergy*, 89:36-48, 2005.

- 321 -

NOTES

This article states that as well as several other mechanisms to explain maternal tolerance of the fetus, "CD4+ CD25+ T regulatory cells (Treg) cells and gammadelta T-cell receptor-positive regulatory cells appear to play key roles in responding to and in generating signals." *See also*:

Ristich V et al: "Tolerization of dendritic cells by HLA-G." *European Journal of Immunology,* Apr; 35(4):1133-42, 2005.
"Dendritic cells play a critical role in the control of innate and adaptive immune responses…HLA-G is an important tolerogenic molecule on dendritic cells for the acceptance of a semiallogeneic fetus and trans-planted tissue/organ."

Zenclussen A et al: "Abnormal T-cell reactivity against paternal antigens in spontaneous abortion: adoptive transfer of pregnancy-induced CD4+ CD25+ T regulatory cells prevents fetal rejection in a murine abortion model." *American Journal of Pathology,* Mar; 166(3): 811-22, 2005.

62   **"Without HLA-G… the placenta may not develop…"** – Noci I et al: "Embryonic soluble HLA-G as marker of developmental potential in embryos." *Human Reproduction*, 20(1):138-146, 2005.
In 26 out of 66 patients, none of the obtained embryos showed any detectable HLA-G molecules and no pregnancies occurred. From these results, it was observed that HLA-G is a potential marker of embryo development. *See also*:

Sher G et al: "Influence of early ICSI-derived embryo sHLA-G expression on pregnancy and implantation rates: a prospective study." *Human Reproduction*, 20(5):1359-1363, 2005.
The media surrounding embryos derived from oocytes from 482 women less than 43 years of age were tested for HLA-G expression. Significantly improved IVF results followed the transfer of good quality embryos if at least one expressed HLA-G.

Fuzzi B et al: "HLA-G expression in early embryos is a fundamental prerequisite for the obtainment of pregnancy." *European Journal of Immunology,* Feb; 32(2):311-5, 2002.
In 101 IVF procedures, embryo implantations occurred only in women where HLA-G molecules were present in their culture samples.

63   **"If the mother and baby share a genetic DQ alpha match, the mother's immune system may be aggravated…"** – Ober C, Beer AE et al: "MHC class II compatibility in aborted fetuses and term infants of couples with recurrent spontaneous abortion." *Journal of Reproductive Immunology*, Dec; 25 (3):195-207, 1993.
In 68 couples with a history of unexplained recurrent spontaneous abortion, significantly more couples shared two HLA-DQA1 alleles as compared with fertile control couples. "HLA-DQA1 compatible fetuses may be aborted early in pregnancy, prior to the time when fetal tissue can be recovered for genetic studies." *See also:*

Pandey M et al: "Characterization of mixed lymphocyte reaction blocking antibodies (MLR-Bf) in human pregnancy." *BMC Pregnancy & Childbirth*, 3:2, 2003.
Blood samples were taken from women at different stages of pregnancy and from women with recurrent spontaneous abortion, before and after immune

NOTES

therapy. The authors state that inhibition of T-cell activation is caused by antibodies against her partner's lymphocytes. These antibodies develop during pregnancy and are associated with increased pregnancy success rates.

63 **"...there is a 10 to 15% chance that the mother will also develop new antibodies to the fatty molecules on the cells of the baby that miscarried."** – Beer AE and Kwak J: "What is the evidence for immunologic pregnancy loss? Lymphocyte immunization the supportive view." In *Molecular and Cellular Biology of the Maternal-Fetal Relationship* by Mowbray J and Chaoaut G, Paris: Inserm Libbey, 285-295, 1991.

63 **"If her blocking antibody levels are low then the couple is at higher risk of producing a pregnancy that induces an inadequate HLA-G signaling response."** – Adachi H et al: "Results of immunotherapy for patients with unexplained secondary recurrent abortions." *Clinical Immunology*, Mar; 106(3):175-80, 2003.
26 women experiencing unexplained secondary recurrent miscarriage underwent LIT. In all 26 patients, MLR-BAbs developed after vaccination. Of those who were negative for MLR-BAbs and had become pregnant without immunotherapy, pregnancy continued in only 2 cases (18.2%). Of 22 newly pregnant patients after vaccinations, pregnancy successfully continued in 20; thus, the success rate of the therapy was 90.9%.

63 **"LIT can encourage a proper blocking antibody and suppressive response..."** – Beer AE et al: "Pregnancy outcome in human couples with recurrent spontaneous abortions: HLA antigen profiles; HLA antigen sharing; female serum MLR blocking factors; and paternal leukocyte immunization." *Experimental & Clinical Immunogenetics*, 2(3): 137-53, 1985. *See also*:

Pandey MK et al: "Prevalence of MLR blocking antibodies before and after immunotherapy." *Journal of Hematotherapy & Stem Cell Research*, April Vol. 9, No.2:257-262, 2000.
Lymphocyte immunotherapy was performed on 28 recurrent aborters. Levels of blocking antibodies increased in 23 patients. The difference in the level of blocking antibodies in the pre-immunotherapy and post-immunotherapy groups was statistically significant and was associated with successful pregnancy outcome in 82.15% of cases.

64 **"For certain recurrent miscarriage patient groups with chromosomally normal embryos, the use of LIT alone has been shown to increase the livebirth rate to between 75% and nearly 100%."** – Daya S and Gunby J: "The effectiveness of allogeneic leukocyte immunization in unexplained primary recurrent spontaneous abortion." *American Journal of Reproductive Immunology*, 32:294-302, 1994.
In this review, the data from randomized controlled trials in eight centers were analyzed. It was concluded that immunotherapy significantly improved the livebirth rate in selected patient groups with recurrent miscarriage, and the effectiveness of LIT was close to 100% for those with normal karyotype embryos. *See also*:

Beer AE, Kwak J et al: "Reproductive outcome in women with recurrent spontaneous abortions of alloimmune and autoimmune causes: preconception

- 323 -

versus post-conception treatment." *American Journal of Obstetrics & Gynecology*, Jun; 166(6 Pt 1):1787-95, 1992.

94 women with recurrent spontaneous abortion were studied. Group I began autoimmune therapy 48 hours after ovulation. Group 2 started the same medication after a positive pregnancy test. Group 3 received no medication. (Controls were 19 women with no autoimmune abnormalities.) The percentages of liveborn children in groups 1, 2, and 3 were 74%, 44% and 11%, respectively. *See also*:

Pandey M et al: "Induction of MLR-Bf and protection of fetal loss: a current double-blind randomized trial of paternal lymphocyte immunization for women with recurrent spontaneous abortion." *Molecular Medicine Program, International Immunopharmacology*, Feb; 4(2): 289-98, 2004.

124 women with unknown causes of abortions received immunotherapy in this double-blind randomized trial. Women who received therapy had a pregnancy success rate of 84% compared with 30 to 44% in those who received other therapies or a placebo.

64 **"...preliminary data indicate that a combination of both LIT and intravenous immunoglobulin G (IVIG) therapy is most effective." –**
Winger E, Reed J, Stricker R: *American Journal of Reproductive Immunology*, 58: 181-237, 2007. 115 pregnancies in women with primary RSA were retrospectively evaluated. The live birth rates among primary RSA patients were: using heparin alone, 8% (1/12); using heparin + IVIG, 56% (15/27); and using heparin + IVIG + LIT, 79% (11/14). The addition of IVIG or IVIG + LIT to the heparin regimen resulted in significant improvement in the pregnancy success rate compared to heparin alone.

6. BLOOD CLOTTING DISORDERS

65 **"Pregnancy is a time when the blood is hypercoagulable..."** – Kutteh WH and Triplett DA: "Thrombophilias and recurrent pregnancy loss." *Seminars in Reproductive Medicine,* Feb; 24(1):54-66, 2006.
"Pregnancy is a hypercoagulable state, and thromboembolism is the leading cause of antepartum and postpartum maternal mortality."

66 **"Blood flow, or principally the lack of it, is one of the most important issues associated with...implantation failure, early pregnancy loss and recurrent miscarriage."** – Edi-Osagie E et al: "Characterizing the endometrium in unexplained and tubal factor infertility: a multiparametric investigation." *Fertility & Sterility*, Nov; 82(5):1379-89, 2004.
In a study of 42 women with unexplained or tubal factor infertility, "there was significantly reduced uterine artery flow velocity in all phases." *See also*:

66 **"...thrombophilia is found in approximately two thirds of women with unexplained pregnancy loss."** – Sarig G et al: "Thrombophilia is common in women with idiopathic pregnancy loss and is associated with late pregnancy wastage." *Fertility & Sterility*, Feb; 77 (2):342-7, 2002.
Of 145 patients with repeated pregnancy loss, 66% demonstrated at least one thrombophilic defect. "Thrombophilia was found in the majority (66%) of women with idiopathic pregnancy loss."

NOTES

Habara T et al: "Elevated blood flow resistance in uterine arteries of women with unexplained recurrent pregnancy loss." *Human Reproduction & Embryology*, Vol.17, No.1, pp.190-194, Jan 2002.

66   **"Thrombophilia, both inherited and acquired, is very common... and is associated with the following conditions..."** – Arkel YS and Ku DH: "Thrombophilia and pregnancy: review of the literature and some original data." *Clinical & Applied Thrombosis/ Hemostasis,* 2001 Oct; 7(4):259-68, 2001.
"... thrombophilia is responsible for a large number of the serious complications of pregnancy such as venous thrombosis, pulmonary embolism, fetal loss, pregnancy loss, intrauterine fetal demise, and preeclampsia. The inherited thrombophilia abnormalities: factor V Leiden mutation, prothrombin gene mutation 20210A, and antithrombin III, protein C, and protein S deficiency, and the acquired disorders: the anticardiolipin syndrome and lupus inhibitor, are responsible for a large share of the incidences of premature termination of pregnancy and many of the above complications." *See also*:

Kutteh WH and Triplett DA: "Thrombophilias and recurrent pregnancy loss." *Seminars in Reproductive Medicine,* Feb; 24(1):54-66, 2006.
"... multiple inherited thrombophilic defects associated with secondary hypercoagulable states, have a particularly strong association with adverse pregnancy outcome."

Cyle S et al: "Which Thrombophilic Gene Mutations are Risk Factors for Recurrent Pregnancy Loss?" *American Journal of Reproductive Immunology;* Vol.56 Issue 4, Oct 2006.
A total of 550 women with a history of recurrent pregnancy loss were tested for gene mutations for thrombophilia. It was concluded that their presence corresponded with recurrent pregnancy loss and such testing identifies individuals at risk.

66   **"Thrombophilia, both inherited and acquired, is very common and is associated with...subchorionic hemorrhages or hematomas."** – Heller DS et al: "Subchorionic hematoma associated with thrombophilia: report of three cases.*" Pediatric and Developmental Pathology*, May-Jun; 6 (3):261-4, 2003.
"...the underlying etiology of SCH may be related to hypercoagulability in the maternal circulation... it is suggested that these women should undergo a thrombophilia work-up."

Phospholipids: Building the Baby's Life Support System

67   **"The phospholipid ethanolamine also acts like 'glue' on the sperm enabling it to attach to the egg..."**   Martínez P and Morros A. "Membrane lipid dynamics during human sperm capacitation." *Frontiers in Bioscience 1*, 103-117, July 1, 1996.

67   **"When these cell membrane molecules are targeted, the chances of a successful pregnancy may stand at less than 10%."** – Rai R et al: "High prospective fetal loss rate in untreated pregnancies of women with recurrent miscarriage and antiphospholipid antibodies." *Human Reproduction*, 10:3301-4, 1995.

- 325 -

NOTES

Of 20 pregnancies in women with APAs and history of recurrent miscarriage who declined pharmacological treatment in their next pregnancy, 18 (90%) miscarried compared with 34 of 100 women (34%) without APAs.

67 **"Anticoagulant medication can increase the livebirth rate to approximately 70%."** – Heilmann L et al: "Antiphospholipid syndrome in obstetrics." *Clinical Application of Thrombosis/ Hemostasis,* Apr; 9(2):143-50, 2003.
"The general failure rate of heparin/aspirin treatment is approximately 30%. In such cases, intravenous immunoglobulin in combination with heparin and aspirin has been used to treat Antiphospholipid Syndrome."

Empson, M., M. Lassere, J. Craig, and J. Scott, "Prevention of recurrent miscarriage for women with antiphospholipid antibody or lupus anticoagulant." *Cochrane Database of Systemic Reviews,* 2005.

The Antibodies that can Switch the Baby's Life Support System Off

68 **"Antibodies to phospholipid molecules prevent the structural transformations that are vital for implantation from taking place."** – Matsubayashi H et al: "Different antiphospholipid antibody specificities are found in association with early repeated pregnancy loss versus recurrent IVF failure patients." *American Journal of Reproductive Immunology*, Nov; 46(5): 323-9, 2001.

68 **"They can also trigger an immune reaction that damages the inside of the blood vessel walls."** – Robertson DL: "Antiphospholipid antibody thrombosis; another source of chronic wounds." *Journal of Wound Ostomy Continence Nursing,* Jan-Feb; 31(1):18-22, 2004.
"Several theories exist speculating on the mechanism of thrombosis involving antiphospholipid antibodies, and each focuses on changes at the interface between the vessel, cell wall membrane, and its interaction with circulating antibodies."

69 **"Approximately 70% of people diagnosed with antiphospholipid syndrome are female."** – Bertolaccini ML et al, "Report on antiphospholipid syndrome laboratory diagnostics and trends." *Autoimmune Review*, 2014, Sep;13(9): 917-30.doi: 10.1016/ j.autrev. 2014. 05.001. Epub 2014 May 10

69 **"Up to 30% of women who repeatedly miscarry, or are infertile, test positive for antiphospholipid antibodies."** – Stojanovic L: "Role of antiphospholipid antibodies in human reproduction." *Vojnosanit Pregl*, Mar-Apr; 55(2 Suppl.):35-40, 1998.
In a group of 931 women with a history of unexplained recurrent miscarriage, 254 (27%) tested positive for APAs. *See also*:

Kaider BD et al: "Antiphospholipid antibody prevalence in patients with IVF failure." *American Journal of Reproductive Immunology,* Apr; 35(4):388-93, 1996.
In 42 women with IVF failure and 42 women who successfully conceived after IVF treatment, the presence of APAs was 26.2% and 4.8% respectively. *See also*:

NOTES

Coulam C et al: "Antiphospholipid antibodies associated with implantation failure after IVF/ET." *Journal of Assisted Reproduction & Genetics,* Nov; 14(10):603-8, 1997.
The prevalence of APAs among 312 women with implantation failure was compared with that of 100 fertile control women. Positive APAs were detected in 69 (22%) of the 312 women with implantation failure compared with 5 (5%) of the 100 control women.

Birkenfeld A et al: "Incidence of autoimmune antibodies in failed embryo transfer cycles." *American Journal of Reproductive Immunology*, 31:65-68, 1994.
In women undergoing IVF embryo transfer 18 (32%) of 56 patients who had a failed IVF cycle were positive for one or both lupus anticoagulant and anticardiolipin antibodies, compared with none of 14 women with successful implantation.

da Silva Santos T et al: "Antiphospholipid syndrome and recurrent miscarriage: A systematic review and meta-analysis." *Journal of Reproductive Immunology*, Volume 123, September 2017.

69 **"...with every IVF failure or miscarriage, there is a 10% chance that the woman will develop an antibody to a phospholipid molecule."** – Fisch B et al: "The relationship between IVF and naturally occurring antibodies: evidence for the increased production of antiphospholipid antibodies." *Fertility & Sterility*, 56:718-24, 1991.
35 patients who had undergone at least one previous IVF attempt and 36 age- and sex-matched controls were analyzed. "Serum levels of antiphospholipid (but not antinuclear) autoantibodies increase after IVF treatment."

69 **Implantation failure in IVF can occur when the first pregnancy tissue to be formed, the trophoblast, is destroyed by APAs..."** – McIntyre J: "Antiphospholipid antibodies in implantation failures" *American Journal of Reproductive Immunology*, Vol. 49, p.221, April 2003.
"The trophoblast is targeted by antiphospholipid antibodies...Cardiolipin is not present in the trophoblast plasma membrane, nonetheless, anticardiolipin (aCL) has been implicated in trophoblast pathology... recent reports from several independent laboratories document that aPE are associated significantly with very early (embryonic) recurrent pregnancy loss."

69 **"The majority of losses of chromosomally normal fetuses among women with high levels of APAs occur within the first 12 weeks."** – Rai R et al: "High prospective fetal loss rate in untreated pregnancies of women with recurrent miscarriage and antiphospholipid antibodies." *Human Reproduction,* Dec; 10(12):3301-4, 1995.
Of 20 pregnancies in women with APA and a history of recurrent miscarriage 18 (90%) miscarried in their next pregnancy. The majority of the miscarriages (94%) occurred in the first trimester.

70 **"A large review was carried out by the American Society for Reproductive Immunology (ASRI)..."** – American Society for Reproductive Immunology Antiphospholipid Antibody Committee, "A rational basis for antiphospholipid antibody testing and selective immunotherapy in assisted reproduction: a

NOTES

rebuttal to the American Society for Reproductive Medicine Practice opinion." *Fertility & Sterility*, Oct; 74(4):631-4, 2000.

70 **"Around 15% of people with systemic lupus erythematosus have antiphospholipid syndrome."** – Bertero M et al: "Antiphospholipid syndrome in northwest Italy (APS Piedmont Cohort) : demographic features, risk factors, clinical and laboratory profile." *Lupus,* 2012 Jun;21(7):806-9. doi: 10.1177/0961203312446974.

70 **"...APAs are just one among several markers that point to an activated immune system."** – Berman J et al: "TNF-alpha is a critical effector and a target for therapy in antiphospholipid antibody-induced pregnancy loss." *Journal of Immunology*, Jan 1; 174(1):485-90, 2005. *See also*:

Sher G et al: "Antibodies to phosphatidylethanolamine and phosphatidylserine are associated with increased natural killer cell activity in non-male factor infertility patients." *Human Reproduction*, Sep; 15(9): 1932-6, 2000.
In this double-blind study, antibodies to serine and ethanolamine were measured in 197 IVF candidates. 45% were APA positive; of these 57% tested positive for antibodies to serine and ethanolamine. 78% of those with antibodies to serine and/or ethanolamine had elevated NK cell levels. In those without APAs, the rate was just 8%. The study concludes: "It is possible that APAs do not directly cause reproductive failure but rather function as markers or intermediaries for an under-lying abnormal activation of cellular immunity."

Beer AE et al: "Up-regulated expression of CD56+, CD56+/CD16+, and CD19+ cells in peripheral blood lymphocytes in pregnant women with recurrent pregnancy losses." *American Journal of Reproductive Immunology*, Aug; 34(2):93- 9, 1995.
"Women with recurrent spontaneous abortion and antiphospholipid antibodies showed significantly elevated NK cells when compared with women without antiphospholipid antibodies."

Salmon J and Girardi G: "Antiphospholipid antibodies and pregnancy loss: a disorder of inflammation." *Journal of Reproductive Immunology*, Jan;77(1):51-6, 2008.
Conventional treatment for APS patients is heparin throughout pregnancy. In our experimental model of APS... anticoagulation in and of itself is not sufficient to prevent pregnancy complications.

More on the Sticky Subject of the Antiphospholipid Syndrome

71 **"...this immune mediated blood clotting syndrome was linked to autoimmune disease, fetal loss and other thrombotic events."** – Hanly JG: "Antiphospholipid syndrome: an overview." *Canadian Medical Association Journal*, Jun 24; 168 (13), 2003. *See also:*

Asherson RA and Cervera R: "Unusual manifestations of the antiphospholipid syndrome." *Clinical Reviews in Allergy & Immunology*, Aug; 25(1):61-78, 2003.

McIntyre JA et al: "Antiphospholipid antibodies: discovery, definitions, detection and disease." *Progressive Lipid Research*, May; 42(3):176-237, 2003.

NOTES

"The persistent finding of aPL in patients in association with abnormal blood clotting and a myriad of neurological, obstetrical and rheumatic disorders often compounded by autoimmune diseases has led to an established clinical diagnosis termed antiphospholipid syndrome (APS)."

71   **"In a study of those who tested positive for APAs, many relatives were found to have other autoimmune diseases."** – Goldberg SN et al: "Antibody associated with autoimmune disorders found to cluster in families." *American Journal of Medicine*, 99(5):473-9, Nov 1995. *See also*:
Diogenes MJ et al: "Cutaneous manifestations associated with antiphospholipid antibodies." International Journal of Dermatology, Sep; 43(9): 632-7, 2004.
60 patients with APS were screened. 40% of the patients had a cutaneous acrocyanosis (13), urticaria (9), diffuse alopecia (9), livedo reticularis (7), Raynaud's phenomenon (3), purpura (2), ulcers and necrosis (4), nodules (4), pterygium ungueum (1) and subungual hemorrhage (1).

Corinne Richard-Miceli C and Lindsey A Criswell L: "Emerging patterns of genetic overlap across autoimmune disorders." *Genome Medicine*, 4:6, 2012.

71   **"Many women with endometriosis will also test positive for antiphospholipid antibodies."** – Ulcova-Gallova Z et al: "Endometriosis in reproductive immunology." *American Journal of Reproductive Immunology*, May; 47 (5):269-74, 2002.
The researchers observed that patients with lesions of endometriosis stage I-II had more autoantibodies than those with stage III-IV and were immunologically more active.

72   **"...women in their 20s and 30s are four to five times more likely to develop deep vein thrombosis or pulmonary embolism...if they are pregnant, undergoing IVF, or taking contraceptive pills..."** – Martinelli I et al: "Interaction between the G20210A mutation of the prothrombin gene and oral contraceptive use in deep vein thrombosis." *Arteriosclerosis, Thrombosis & Vascular Biology,* 19:700-3, 1999. *See also*:

Bloemenkamp KW et al: "Higher risk of venous thrombosis during early use of oral contraceptives in women with inherited clotting defects." *Archives of Internal Medicine*, 160:49-52, 2000.

73   **"...the immune system dysfunctions that cause these events are ultimately extremely damaging to the woman's own health."** – Bick R and Hoppensteadt D: "Recurrent miscarriage syndrome and infertility due to blood coagulation protein/platelet defects: a review and update." *Clinical Application of Thrombosis/ Hemostasis*, Jan; 11 (1):1-13. 2005.
351 women with recurrent miscarriages were assessed. 60% had antiphospholipid syndrome. The report concludes: "...thrombophilia is a common cause of recurrent miscarriage and all patients with no anatomical, hormonal or chromosomal defect should be evaluated for thrombophilia or a bleeding disorder." *See also*:

Quenby S et al: "Recurrent miscarriage and long-term thrombosis risk: a case-control study." *Journal of Human Reproduction*, Jun; 20(6): 1729-32, 2005.

- 329 -

NOTES

141 women with recurrent miscarriage were studied over a number of years. The report concludes that both unexplained and APS-associated recurrent miscarriages carry a long-term risk of thrombosis.

Inherited Thrombophilia

74 **"...these conditions affect about 15% of people in the United States and kill more Americans than breast cancer, AIDS, and car accidents combined." –** *Redbook Magazine*, June 2004 article by Tamara Eberlein (referring to a March of Dimes report).

74 **"Indeed, thrombosis is one of the most common cause of death worldwide."** – Kutteh WH and Triplett DA: "Thrombophilias and recurrent pregnancy loss." *Seminars in Reproductive Medicine,* Feb; 24 (1):54-66, 2006.

74 **"...particularly affects those who carry genes for more than one condition."** – Regan L et al: "Genetic thrombophilic mutations among couples with recurrent miscarriage." *Human Reproduction,* May; 21 (5):1161-1165, 2006. "In couples with recurrent miscarriage, multiple genetic thrombophilic mutations in either partner significantly increase the risk of miscarriage in a subsequent pregnancy." *See also*:

Kutteh WH and Triplett DA: "Thrombophilias and recurrent pregnancy loss." *Seminars in Reproductive Medicine,* Feb; 24(1):54-66, 2006. "Current understanding indicates that a combination of risk factors, including multiple inherited thrombophilic defects associated with secondary hypercoagulable states, have a particularly strong association with adverse pregnancy outcome."

74 **"...laboratory-based testing has made it possible to identify a genetic cause in up to half of patients with venous thromboembolism."** – Laffan M et al: "Science, medicine, and the future: assessing thrombotic risk." *British Medical Journal*, 317(7157):520-3, 1998. "In most cases thrombosis arises from a combination of external circumstances and the inherited and acquired predisposition to thrombosis of an individual. Only 30-40% of cases seem to be completely spontaneous....We can now identify a genetic contribution to thrombosis in roughly half of patients presenting with a first thrombotic episode..." *See also*:

Paschoa AF and Guillaumon AT: "Impact of screening on thrombophilia for patients with venous thrombosis." *International Angiology*, Mar; 25(1):52-9, 2006. In 84 patients with venous thrombosis, a genetic cause was found in 32.12% (27/84).

Factor V Leiden

74 **"In white Europeans and North Americans, this mutation is present in approximately 4 to 7% of the general population..."** – Rees DC et al: "World distribution of factor V Leiden." *Lancet*, 346: 11.33-34, 1995. 3,380 chromosomes from 24 populations were analyzed for the presence of factor V Leiden. The allele frequency in 618 Europeans was 4.4%, with the highest prevalence among Greeks, at 7.0%. Factor V Leiden was not found in

- 330 -

NOTES

any of 1,600 chromosomes from Africa, Southeast Asia, Australasia and the Americas.

74 **"The highest rate is found in Europe, with a prevalence of 10 to 15% in southern Sweden."** – Kujovich JL: "Hereditary resistance to activated protein C, factor V Leiden mutation." *Gene Reviews*, updated May 2004. See: http://www.geneclinics.org/profiles/factor-v-leiden/details.html

75 **"In women with recurrent miscarriage, a rate of 20 to 27% has been reported."** – Santoro R et al: "Prothrombotic gene mutations in women with recurrent abortions and intrauterine fetal death." *Minerva Ginecologie*. Aug; 57(4):447-50, 2005.
150 women with a history of unexplained recurrent pregnancy loss were studied for hereditary thrombophilia. The factor V Leiden mutation was significantly more prevalent in women with fetal death (19.6%). *See also:*

Mahjoub T et al: "Association between adverse pregnancy outcomes and maternal factor V G1691A (Leiden) and prothrombin G20210A genotypes in women with a history of recurrent idiopathic miscarriages." *American Journal of Hematology*, Sep; 80(1):12-9, 2005.
Of 200 women with 3 or more consecutive early or late recurrent pregnancy losses, the factor V Leiden mutation was seen in 27% of patients compared with 11.5% of controls.

Mtiraoui N et al: "Prevalence of antiphospholipid antibodies, factor V G1691A (Leiden) and prothrombin G20210A mutations in early and late recurrent pregnancy loss." *European Journal of Obstetrics, Gynecology & Reproductive Biology*. Apr 1; 119(2):164-70, 2005.
Of 146 patients with 3 or more consecutive early or late recurrent pregnancy losses, 20.5% carried the factor V Leiden mutation compared with 6.06% of controls.

Sarig G et al: "Thrombophilia is common in women with idiopathic pregnancy loss and is associated with late pregnancy wastage." *Fertility & Sterility*, Feb; 77(2):342-7, 2002.
In 145 patients with repeated pregnancy loss and 145 matched controls, the prevalence of factor V Leiden was 25% and 7.6% respectively.

75 **"If both genes are affected, the clotting risk during pregnancy is 34 times greater..."** – Wu O et al: "Screening for thrombophilia in high-risk situations: systematic review and cost-effectiveness analysis. The Thrombosis: Risk and Economic Assessment of Thrombophilia Screening (TREATS) study." *Health Technology Assessment Reports*, Apr; 10(11):1-110, 2006.

75 **"...without ongoing therapy, the chance of experiencing a thrombotic event over a lifetime is virtually 100%."** – Rosendaal F: "High risk of thrombosis in patients homozygous for factor V Leiden (activated protein C resistance)." *Blood*, Mar; 15; 85(6):1504-8, 1995.

75 **"Studies have also shown that women with a history of recurrent miscarriage...have a livebirth rate of less than 40%...when this clotting disorder is left untreated."** – Regan L et al: "Factor V Leiden and recurrent

miscarriage – prospective outcome of untreated pregnancies." *Human Reproduction*, 17, pp.442-445, 2002.

In 25 women heterozygous for the factor V Leiden with a history of recurrent early miscarriage, the livebirth rate for their next pregnancy was 37.5% (6/16). *See also*:

Reznikoff-Etievan M et al: *British Journal of Obstetrics & Gynaecology*, Dec; 108(12):1251-4, 2001.

260 women with early, unexplained recurrent miscarriage and a control group of 240 healthy women were screened for protein C, factor V Leiden and the prothrombin G20210A mutation. The study found that early recurrent miscarriage was significantly associated with Factor V Leiden or prothrombin G20210A mutations.

Protein C and Protein S Deficiencies

75 **"The incidence of protein C deficiency in women with two or more consecutive pregnancy losses ranges from 20% to 40%."** – Coumans AB et al: "Haemostatic and metabolic abnormalities in women with unexplained recurrent abortion." *Human Reproduction*, 14(1):211-4, 1999. *See also*:

Rawan Nahas, MD et al: "The Prevalence of Thrombophilia in Women with Recurrent Fetal Loss and Outcome of Anticoagulation Therapy for the Prevention of Miscarriages." *Clinical and Applied Thrombosis/ Hemostasis*, Vol. 24(1) 122-128, 2018.

"490 pregnant women with recurrent miscarriage were referred for thrombophilia screening. The most common thrombophilia in our study group was factor V Leiden mutation with a prevalence of 20.9% followed by protein S deficiency with a prevalence of 19%."

Younis JS et al: "Activated protein C resistance and factor V Leiden mutation can be associated with first as well as second-trimester recurrent pregnancy loss." *American Journal of Reproductive Immunology*, 43; pp.31-35, 2000.

In 78 women with two or more unexplained post-embryonic recurrent pregnancy losses, the incidence of activated protein C resistance was 38% (30/78) and the incidence of the factor V Leiden mutation was (15/78).

Sarig G et al: "Thrombophilia is common in women with idiopathic pregnancy loss and is associated with late pregnancy wastage." *Fertility & Sterility*, Feb; 77(2):342-7, 2002.

Of 145 patients with repeated pregnancy loss, activated protein C resistance was documented in 39% of women with pregnancy loss compared with 3% of the control patients.

Prothrombin 20210 Mutation

76 **"This gene mutation...can activate the clotting process and lead to pregnancy loss."** Reznikoff-Etievan MF et al: "Factor V Leiden and G20210A prothrombin mutations are risk factors for very early recurrent miscarriage." *British Journal of Obstetrics & Gynaecology*, 108: 1251-1254, 2001. *See also*:

NOTES

Pihusch R et al: "Thrombophilic gene mutations and recurrent spontaneous abortion: prothrombin mutation increases the risk in the first trimester." *American Journal of Reproductive Immunology*, Aug; 46(2): 124-31, 2001.

76   **"...the incidence of thrombosis is five times greater than in unaffected people."** – Amy P et al: "Evaluation of the hypercoagulable state, whom to screen, how to test and treat." *Postgraduate Medicine*, Vol. 108:4 Sept 15, 2000.

MTHFR Mutation (Leading to Hyperhomocysteinemia)

77   **"Those with the defective MTHFR gene are unable to process folate properly, so homocysteine concentrations build up, increasing their risk of arterial and venous thrombosis."** – Loralie J et al: "Hyperhomocysteinemia and the increased risk of venous thromboembolism." *Archives of Internal Medicine*, 160:961-964, 2000. *See also*:

Arrula V et al: "The mutation Ala677-Val in the methylene tetrahydro-folate reductase gene: a risk factor for arterial disease and venous thrombosis." *Thrombosis Haemostasis*, 77:818-821, 1997.

77   **"High concentrations are also found in approximately 30% of women with recurrent pregnancy loss"** – Raziel et al: "Hypercoagulable thrombophilic defects and hyperhomocysteinemia in patients with recurrent pregnancy loss." *American Journal of Reproductive Immunology*, Feb; Vol. 45 no.2 pp.65-71, 2001.
The prevalence of heritable thrombophilic defects was evaluated in 36 non-pregnant recurrent aborters and 40 normal controls. "Hyperhomocysteinemia was found in 31% of those experiencing recurrent miscarriage." *See also:*

Couto E et al: "Association of anticardiolipin antibody and C677T in methylenetetrahydrofolate reductase mutation in women with recurrent spontaneous abortions: a new path to thrombophilia?" *Sao Paulo Medical Journal*, Vol.123 no.1 São Paulo, Jan 2005.

77   **"Low levels of folic acid and vitamin B12 are also associated with the MTHFR genetic mutation, which increases the risk of neural tube defects in the baby..."** – Xiao S et al: "Maternal folate deficiency results in selective up-regulation of folate receptors and heterogeneous nuclear ribonucleoprotein-E1 associated with multiple subtle aberrations in fetal tissues." *Birth Defects Research Part A. Clinical & Molecular Teratology*, Jan; 73(1):6-28, 2005. *See also*:

Grandone E et al: "Homocysteine metabolism in families from southern Italy with neural tube defects: role of genetic and nutritional determinants." *Prenatal Diagnosis*, Jan; 26(1):1-5, 2006.
"The T677 MTHFR allele is significantly associated with the occurrence of neural tube defects (NTDs)...Homocysteine levels in children with NTDs are significantly higher than those of the paediatric population from the same geographical area."

77   **"The incidence of this genetic condition [heterozygous] in women with reproductive failure is approximately 25 to 30%."** – Data collected by Jane

- 333 -

NOTES

Reed from Yahoo Reproductive Immunology Support Group members since August 17, 2003 in an ongoing poll. Dr Beer's patients have a 29.9% (49/164) incidence of the heterozygous MTHFR mutation as of 4/11/06.

77 **"During pregnancy...psychological stress and alterations in diet and metabolism can increase homocysteine levels."** – Stoney C: "Plasma homocysteine levels increase in women during psychological stress." *Life Sciences*, 64(25): 2359 65, 1999. *See also*:

Zhang H et al: "Association of Increased Maternal Plasma Homocysteine with the Adverse Birth Outcomes Following Prenatal Psychological Stress." *International Journal of Pediatric Research*, 3:026, 2017.
"(In 60 women with Prenatal psychological stress (PPS) there was) a significant association with maternal plasma homocysteine and adverse birth outcomes and increased maternal plasma homocysteine may be related to the impacts of PPS on poor birth outcomes."

77 **"The homozygous MTHFR condition is found in approximately 19% of patients with arterial disease, 11% with venous thrombosis..."** – Arruda VR et al: "The mutation Ala677-->Val in the methylene tetrahydrofolate reductase gene: a risk factor for arterial disease and venous thrombosis." *Thrombosis and Haemostasis,* May; 77(5):818-21, 1997.
In 191 patients with arterial disease and 127 individuals with venous thrombosis, the prevalence of the homozygous MTHFR C677T mutation was 19% and 11% respectively.

77 **"The homozygous MTHFR condition is found in approximately...14% of women with recurrent miscarriage."** – Data collected by Jane Reed from Yahoo Reproductive Immunology Support Group members since August 17, 2003 in an ongoing poll. Dr Beer's patients have a 14.0% (23/164) incidence of the homozygous MTHFR mutation as of 4/11/06.

7. IMMUNITY TO PREGNANCY

79 **"[ANAs] are also found in approximately 30% of women with recurrent miscarriage and in 20% of those who are infertile."** – Xu L et al: "Antinuclear antibodies in sera of patients with recurrent preg-nancy wastage." *American Journal of Obstetrics & Gynecology*, Nov; 163(5 Pt 1):pp.1493-7, 1990.
Antinuclear antibodies were detected in 40% of 30 women with unexplained fetal losses and 53.3% of 30 women with explained fetal losses. Levels among 61 healthy pregnant women and 61 healthy non-pregnant women were 8.2% and 5.6% respectively. *See also*:

Iijima T et al: "Effects of autoantibodies on the course of pregnancy and fetal growth." *Obstetrics & Gynecology*, Sep; 90(3):364-9, 1997.
1,179 pregnant women were assessed for autoantibodies. In 228 cases (19.3%), at least one autoantibody was found. "A significantly higher rate of spontaneous abortion was observed in antibody-positive subjects, especially those with antithyroid microsomal (10.4%) or antinuclear antibodies (16.0%), compared with all antibody-negative subjects (5.5%)."

NOTES

Kaider AS et al: "Immunodiagnostic evaluation in women with reproductive failure." *American Journal of Reproductive Immunology*, Dec; 42(6):335-46, 1999.
Of all patients with reproductive failure, 75.6% had at least one abnormal test. The most frequent abnormal result was an elevation of NK (CD56+) cells (37%), followed by ANA (34%).

Cubillos J et al: "Incidence of autoantibodies in the infertile population." *Early Pregnancy*, Jun; 3(2):119-24, 1997.
In 43 women with primary infertility, the incidence of antinuclear antibodies was 37.2%. In a group of patients with a history of miscarriage, 31.8% were positive for ANAs. In the control group, the incidence of ANA was 5.7%.

Stern C et al: "Antibodies to beta2 glycoprotein I are associated with in vitro fertilization implantation failure as well as recurrent miscarriage: results of a prevalence study." *Fertility & Sterility*, Jul; 72(1):187-8, 1999.
In a trial involving women with recurrent first trimester miscarriages and those undergoing IVF, 23% of the 360 samples tested were positive for at least one autoantibody.

79 **"...the 'Reproductive Autoimmune Failure Syndrome.'"** – Gleicher N and el-Roeiy A: "The reproductive autoimmune failure syndrome." *American Journal of Obstetrics & Gynecology,* Jul; 1;59 1:223-7, 1988.
"...abnormal autoimmune function may lead to reproductive failure at different stages of the reproductive process, depending on the quality and possibly quantity of the abnormal autoimmune response."

80 **"ANAs are often associated with hyperactivated NK cells..."** – Geva E et al: "Circulating autoimmune antibodies may be responsible for implantation failure in in vitro fertilization." *Fertility & Sterility*, Oct; 62 (4):802-6, 1994. *See also*:

Taniguchi F: "Results of prednisolone given to improve the outcome of in vitro fertilization-embryo transfer in women with antinuclear antibodies." *Journal of Reproductive Medicine*, Jun; 50(6):383-8, 2005.
In 120 women aged 22-42 years old, ANA positivity was noted in 20.0% of patients (24/120) and 25.1% of IVF cycles (56/223). Implantation and clinical pregnancy rates in the prednisolone non-treated ANA-positive group were 0% (0/41 transplanted embryos) and 0% (0/15 cycles).

80 **"...the miscarriage rate for women with SLE is much higher than that of the general population."** – Hochberg M: "Epidemiology of rheumatic disease: systemic lupus erythematosus." *Rheumatic Disease Clinics of North America*, 16(3):617-637, 1990.
In this study of 45 women diagnosed with SLE, 39 of them had experienced a miscarriage.

Singh A and Chowdhary V: "Pregnancy-related issues in women with systemic lupus erythematosus." *International Journal of Rheumatic Diseases*, Feb;18(2):172-81, 2015.
"Established risk factors for adverse pregnancy outcomes include active disease within 6 months prior to conception and during pregnancy, active nephritis, maternal hypertension, antiphospholipid antibodies and hypocomplementemia."

NOTES

80 **"...when ANA damage is seen in the placenta..."** – Guzman L et al: "Placental abnormalities in systemic lupus erythematosus: in situ deposition of anti-antinuclear antibodies." *Journal of Rheumatology,* Oct; 14(5):924-9, 1987. Five placentas from patients with SLE were examined. ANAs were deposited along the villi, trophoblast and amnion.

80 **"Some medications can also cause 'drug-induced lupus.'"** – Rubin R: "Drug-induced lupus." *Toxicology*, Apr 15; 209(2):135-47, 2005.

81 **"[ANAs] affect approximately 80% of patients with Sjögren's syndrome..."** – Nardi N et al: "Circulating autoantibodies against nuclear and non-nuclear antigens in primary Sjögren's syndrome: Prevalence and clinical significance in 335 patients." *Clinical Rheumatology*, May; 25(3):341-6, 2006. Of 335 patients diagnosed with primary SS, ANA were detected in 278 (83%) patients.

81 **"...up to 95% of patients with scleroderma have ANAs."** – Barnett A and McNeilage N: "Antinuclear antibodies in patients with scleroderma (systemic sclerosis) and in their blood relatives and spouses." *Annals of the Rheumatic Diseases*, Vol. 52, pp.365-368, 1993. Of 58 patients with scleroderma 55 (95%) tested positive for ANAs. *See also*:

Jacobsen S et al: "Clinical features and serum antinuclear antibodies in 230 Danish patients with systemic sclerosis." *British Journal of Rheumatology,* Jan; 37(1):39-45, 1998. Sera from 230 patients with systemic sclerosis were tested for the presence of ANAs; 82% of the patients were women. ANAs were found in 86% of the patients.

81 **"Approximately 50% of those with alopecia areata...are ANA- positive."** – Seyrafi H et al: "Evaluation of the profile of alopecia areata and the prevalence of thyroid function test abnormalities and serum autoantibodies in Iranian patients." *BMC Dermatology,* Oct 31; 5:11, 2005. Positive autoimmune antibodies were found in 51.4% of 123 patients with alopecia areata.

81 **"Their development can also be accelerated by viral or bacterial infection and environmental factors."** – von Herrath M: "A viral epitope that mimics a self antigen can accelerate but not initiate autoimmune diabetes." *Journal of Clinical Investigation*, Nov 114 (9): 1290 -8, 2004. *See also*:

Nicolson G: "Autoimmune illnesses and degenerative diseases." See: http://www.immed.org/illness/autoimmune_illness_research.html

81 **"In a 2005 study, ANAs were detected in women with high blood levels of a chemical called bisphenol A..."** – Sugiura-Ogasawara M et al: "Exposure to Bisphenol A is associated with recurrent miscarriage." *Human Reproduction*, Jun 9, 2005. Bisphenol A levels were tested in 45 patients with a history of three or more consecutive first trimester miscarriages. Blood levels of Bisphenol A in miscarriage patients were significantly higher than in the control group. *See also*:

Shen Y et al: "Higher Urinary Bisphenol A Concentration Is Associated with Unexplained Recurrent Miscarriage Risk: Evidence from a Case-Control Study in Eastern China." *Public Library of Science*, 10(5); 2015.
"A higher level of urinary BPA was significantly associated with an increased risk of recurrent miscarriage."

81 **"A higher than average incidence of ANAs has been detected in mercury sensitive individuals."** – Bartova J et al: "Dental amalgam as one of the risk factors in autoimmune diseases." *Neuroendocrinology Letters,* Feb-Apr; 24(1-2):65-7, 2003.
Blood samples were obtained from patients with autoimmune thyroiditis and increased response to mercury in vitro, and tested for ANAs. "...in some patients with thyroiditis, mercury from dental amalgam can stimulate the production of antinuclear antibodies. Dental amalgam may be a risk factor in some patients with autoimmune disease."

8. ANTIBODIES TO SPERM

83 **"Approximately 7% of women who are unable to conceive normally have produced antibodies to sperm."** – Busacca M et al: "Evaluation of antisperm antibodies in infertile couples with immunobead test: prevalence and prognostic value." *ACTA Europaea Fertilitatis*, Mar-Apr; 20(2):77-82, 1989.
"We studied the prevalence of the immune response against spermatozoa in infertile couples using immunobead test. 16.2% of the men were autoimmune and 7.3% of the women isoimmune." See also:

83 **"Over 50% of men with low sperm motility and 66% of men with no live sperm have been found to carry these antibodies."** – Madar J et al: "Immunologically conditioned fertility disorders in men – experience of the immunobiological department of the Institute for Maternal and Child Care" – *Ceska Gynekologie*, Dec; 69 Supplement 1:15-20, 2004.
The semen from 1,680 men was analyzed. Increased cell-mediated immunity was identified in 10.2% of fertile men, in 18.5% of men with a low sperm count and in 66.3% men with no live sperm. In those with a severe lack of motile sperm, cell-mediated immunity against spermatozoa was identified in over 50% of cases.

83 **"There is an even higher incidence in those who have undergone a vasectomy or vasectomy reversal, where up to to 74% of men can be affected."** – Jarow J et al: "Relationship between antisperm antibodies and testicular histologic changes in humans after vasectomy." *Urology*, Apr; 43 (4):521-4, 1994.
Antisperm antibody status was determined in 19 vasectomized men and 21 fertile control subjects. Antisperm activity was present in 74% of the vasectomized men but in none of the control subjects.

Reza Nowroozi M et al: "Antisperm Antibody Formation Following Vasectomy." www.researchgate.net/publication/228655654
"This case series was performed on 80 healthy men at Imam Khomeini hospital. Blood antisperm antibody was checked at the time of vasectomy and 3 months later, when they came to assure vasectomy results... Only 2 patients had antisperm antibody before surgery. Three months after vasectomy 56.49% of the patients had antisperm antibody."

NOTES

83 **"Studies have shown that antibodies that attach to the head of the sperm stop it from binding to the egg, while those that attach to the tail affect motility."** – Bronson R et al: "Sperm-specific isoantibodies and autoantibodies inhibit the binding of human sperm to the human zona pellucida." *Fertility & Sterility,* Dec; 38(6):724-9, 1982. *See also*:

Bronson R: "Correlation between regional specificity of antisperm antibodies to the spermatozoan surface and complement-mediated sperm immobilization." *American Journal of Reproductive Immunology,* Aug; 2(4):222-4, 1982.
"A high degree of immobilization was found only when IgG binding occurred on the distal two-fifths to three-fifths of the principal piece of the tail or when IgM bound to the sperm tail end piece."

Tripti N et al: "Evaluation of Serum Antisperm Antibodies in Infertility." The *Journal of Obstetrics and Gynecology of India*, May / June 2011.
"Antibodies against sperm prevent their motility through the female reproductive tract and hamper the process of fertilization."

84 **"The woman can also develop reproductive problems by being exposed to this antibody coated sperm..."** – Witkin SS and Chaudhry A: "Association between recurrent spontaneous abortions and circulating IgG antibodies to sperm tails in women." *Journal of Reproductive Immunology,* May; 15(2):151-8, 1989.
This study concludes: "Antisperm antibodies may be a marker for defective immunosuppression in women with recurrent miscarriages. Alternatively, exposure of sperm-sensitized pregnant women to sperm may activate the maternal immune system to respond to paternal antigens present on the embryo." *See also*:

Witkin SS and David SS: "Effect of sperm antibodies on pregnancy outcome in a subfertile population." *American Journal of Obstetrics and Gynecology*, Jan; 158(1):59-62, 1998.
Of 109 infertile couples, conception occurred in 33 couples over an 18-month period. Of these, 16 women suffered a spontaneous miscarriage during the first trimester. Antisperm antibodies were present in 2 of 17 women with successful pregnancies, 7 of 16 women who miscarried, and 29 of 76 who did not conceive.

84 **"...antisperm antibody levels of 109 prostitutes were measured and compared to those of 40 age-matched women..."** – Bahraminejad R al: "Reproductive failure and antisperm-antibody production among prostitutes." *Acta Obstetrica et Gynecologica Scan-dinavica*, 70(6): 483-5, 1991.

85 **"Immunotherapy is an effective way of preventing these problems"**– Beer AE et al: "Circulating antisperm antibodies in recurrently aborting women." *Fertility & Sterility*, Feb; 45(2):209-15, 1986.
173 women with a history of three or more recurrent consecutive abortions were analyzed for circulating antisperm antibodies. There were no full-term pregnancies in women who were antisperm antibody positive unless they were inoculated with their partner's leukocytes as treatment for an immune basis (not related to antisperm antibodies) for their recurrent abortions. *See also*:

NOTES

Sugi T et al: "Influence of immunotherapy on antisperm antibody titer in unexplained recurrent aborters." *American Journal of Reproductive Immunology*, Mar; 29(2):95, 1993.
This study concludes: "The data of the present study suggest that antisperm antibodies have potential for use as a marker for a deficiency in maternal genital tract immunosuppressor mechanisms and that immunotherapy could be an effective treatment for women with antisperm antibodies who have unexplained recurrent abortions."

Tripti N et al: "Evaluation of Serum Antisperm Antibodies in Infertility." *The Journal of Obstetrics and Gynecology of India*, May / June 2011.
"Low-dose prednisolone was useful in infertility associated with ASA by improving sperm quality and giving rise to pregnancies."

9.   HIGH NATURAL KILLER CELL LEVELS

87   **"For many years, scientists considered natural killer cells to be the 'blunt instrument' of the body's immune system."** – School of Life Sciences, University of Science and Technology of China, Hefei, Anhui 230027, China.

88   **"Pregnant women with a history of recurrent pregnancy loss have significantly higher circulating NK cell levels…"** – Beer AE et al: "Up-regulated expression of CD56+, CD56+/CD16+, and CD19+ cells in peripheral blood lymphocytes in pregnant women with recurrent pregnancy losses." *American Journal of Reproductive Immunology*, August; 34(2):93-9, 1995. *See also*:

Beer AE et al: "Status of peripheral blood natural killer cells in women with recurrent spontaneous abortions and infertility of unknown etiology." *Human Reproduction,* May; 16(5):855-61, 2001.
NK cell levels of 40 women with unexplained infertility or recurrent miscarriage and 13 normal healthy controls were compared. "A significant increase in CD69 expression on CD56+ NK cells was demonstrated in women with recurrent abortion and infertility compared with that of normal controls."

Coulam C et al: "Systemic CD56+ cells can predict pregnancy outcome." *American Journal of Reproductive Immunology*, 33:40-46, 1995.
114 pregnant women were studied prospectively. 70 women had a history of infertility and 44 had two or more previous spontaneous abortions. CD56+ cells were significantly elevated in women treated for infertility.

Coulam C and Roussev R: "Correlation of NK cell activation and inhibition markers with NK cytoxicity among women experiencing immunologic implantation failure after in vitro fertilization and embryo transfer." *Journal of Assisted Reproduction &Genetics*, Feb; 20(2):58-62, 2003.
Blood samples from 22 infertile women undergoing IVF were compared with those from 26 fertile control women. Infertile women had a significantly higher expression of NK cell activation markers than those who were fertile. None of the successfully pregnant women had elevated levels of NK cytotoxicity, but 50% of those experiencing a chemical pregnancy loss and those not becoming pregnant had elevated levels of NK cytotoxicity.

NOTES

Emmer P et al: "Peripheral natural killer cytotoxicity and CD56+ CD16+ cells increase during early pregnancy in women with a history of recurrent spontaneous abortion." *Human Reproduction,* 15:1163-1169, 2000.
43 women with subsequent pregnancy, 37 healthy controls and 39 women who had undergone a successful IVF procedure were included in the study. "...NK cell numbers below 12% were strongly associated with a subsequent pregnancy carried to term...the analysis of peripheral NK cell characteristics appears a suitable diagnostic tool in recurrent spontaneous abortion."

Yamada H et al: "High NK cell activity in early pregnancy correlates with subsequent abortion with normal chromosomes in women with recurrent abortion." *American Journal of Reproductive Immunology,* Aug; 46(2):132-6, 2001.

Seshadri S and Sunkara S: "Natural killer cells in female infertility and recurrent miscarriage: a systematic review and meta-analysis." *Human Reproduction Update*, May-Jun;20(3):429-38 2014.
"Meta-analysis of studies that evaluated peripheral NK cell percentages in women with recurrent miscarriage versus controls showed significantly higher NK cell percentages in women with recurrent miscarriage."

Ramos-Medina R et al: "New decision-tree model for defining the risk of recurrent reproductive failure." *Human Reproduction*, 28:144– 145, 2013.
By multivariate analysis, blood NK cells expansion was an independent risk factor for recurrent miscarriages and implantation failures. Women with age above 35 years and with 13% or above $CD56^+$ $CD16^+$ NK cells showed the highest risk of further pregnancy loss (100%).

Sacks G: "Enough! Stop the arguments and get on with the science of natural killer cell testing." *Human Reproduction* 30(7) · May 2015

88 **"...uterine NK cells (uNKs) make up the majority of the white blood cell population in the uterus..."** – Chao K et al: "The expression of killer cell inhibitory receptors on natural killer cells and activation status of CD4+ and CD8+ T-cells in the decidua of normal and abnormal early pregnancies." *Human Immunology,* Sep; 60(9):791-7, 1999.
"The establishment of the human placenta in early pregnancy is characterized by the presence of large numbers of natural killer cells within the maternal decidua. These NK cells have an unusual phenotype, CD3- CD16- CD56 (bright), distinguishing them from peripheral blood NK cells."

89 **"...uNKs make structural changes that increase the capacity of the blood supply channels leading to the placenta/fetus..."** – Croy B and Xie X: "In vivo models for studying homing and function of murine uterine natural killer cells." *Methods in Molecular Medicine,* 122:77-92, 2006,
"uNK cells are central to initiation of spiral arterial modification (i.e., structural changes that increase capacity of the blood supply channels leading to the placenta)."

89 **"...uNKs release a spectrum of cytokines that enable them to influence the implantation process."** – Saito S et al: "Cytokine production by CD16- CD56+ natural killer cells in the human early pregnancy decidua." *International Immunology*, Vol.5, 605-613, 1993.

NOTES

89 **"Although they [uNKs] have considerable destructive potential..."** – King A et al: "Expression of perforin, granzyme A and TIA-1 by human uterine CD56+ cells implies they are activated and capable of effector functions." *Human Reproduction*, Vol.8, pp.2061-2067, 1993.

89 **"...uNKs deliver just 15% of the killing power of the NK cells that circulate in the blood."** – Kopcow H et al: "Human decidual NK cells form immature activating synapses and are not cytotoxic." *Proceedings of the National Academy of Sciences of the United States of America,* Oct 25; 102(43):15563-8, 2005.
"Even though they are granular and express the essential molecules required for lysis, fresh decidual NK displayed very reduced lytic activity on classical MHC I negative targets K562 and 721.221, approximately 15% of that of peripheral NK cells."

89 **"After this, they undergo a slow form of cell death..."** – Zhang J et al: "Uterine natural killer cells: their choices, their missions." *Cellular and Molecular Immunology*, Vol.2, No.2 Apr 2005.
"Uterine NK cells progressively increased in number, with the peak at gestation day 10-12...After gestation day 12, uNK cells undergo a slow form of cell death and disappear from implantation sites...the cells are absent from term decidua of normal pregnancy."

89 **"...and by week 20 have virtually disappeared."** – King A et al: "Human uterine lymphocytes." *Human Reproduction Update*, Vol.4, No.5, pp.480-485, 1998.
"The presence of NK cells in the uterine mucosa is a feature only of early pregnancy as they become less conspicuous after approximately 20 weeks' gestation."

89 **"...CD56+/CD16+ NK cells...higher rates of recurrent pregnancy loss, IVF failure and pregnancy complications (e.g., preeclampsia and low birth weight)."** – Beer AE et al: "Increased T-helper 1 cytokine responses by circulating T-cells are present in women with recurrent pregnancy losses and in infertile women with multiple implantation failures after IVF." *Human Reproduction*, Apr; 18(4):767-73, 2003. *See also*:

Beer AE et al: "Expression of intracellular Th1 and Th2 cytokines in women with recurrent spontaneous abortion, implantation failures after IVF/ET or normal pregnancy." *American Journal of Reproductive Immunology,* Aug; 48(2):77-86, 2002.
"In women with implantation failures, absolute cell counts of TNF-alpha expressing CD3+/ 4- cells reflects the presence of dominant Th1 immune response. A significantly increased Th1 cytokine expression may be the underlying immune etiology for reproductive failures."

Daher S et al: "Cytokines in recurrent pregnancy loss." *Journal of Reproductive Immunology*, Vol.62, Issues 1-2 June 2001.
Blood samples from 29 recurrent miscarriers and 27 women with a history of successful pregnancies were compared. Significantly higher levels of IFN-gamma and a trend toward increased TNF-alpha production were seen in women with recurrent miscarriage.

Darmochwal-Kolarz D et al: "The expressions of intracellular cytokines in the lymphocytes of preeclamptic patients." *American Journal of Reproductive Immunology*, 48:381-386, 2002.
Blood samples were taken from 20 patients with preeclampsia and 16 healthy pregnant women. In patients with preeclampsia, the expressions of Il-2 were significantly higher compared with women with uncomplicated pregnancy. "These results suggest that in patients with preeclampsia there is Th1/Th2 imbalance, with predominant Th1 immunity."

Dong R et al: "Influences of active immunotherapy on T helper cell type 1 and 2 cytokines in women with unexplained habitual abortion." *Zhonghua Fu Chan Ke Za Zhi*, June; 38(6):362-5, 2003.
55 patients with unexplained recurrent miscarriage were found to "...have Th1 type immunity to trophoblast and produce high-level Th1 type cytokines which probably result in pregnancy loss."

Figueroa R et al: "Evaluation of amniotic fluid cytokines in preterm labor and intact membranes." *Journal of Maternal & Fetal Neonatal Medicine,* Oct; 18 (4): 241-7, 2005.
52 women with preterm labor and intact membranes between 21 and 35 weeks of gestation were included in the study. 62% of women delivered within 7 days and 38% delivered after 7 days of amniocentesis. The amniotic fluid concentrations of pro-inflammatory cytokines were significantly higher in women who delivered within 7 days.

Jacek R et al: "Lymphocyte subset distribution and cytokine secretion in third trimester decidua in normal pregnancy and preeclampsia." *European Journal of Obstetrics & Gynecology & Reproductive Biology*, Vol.109, Issue 1: pp.8-15, July 2003.
In this study, 21 preeclamptic patients were characterized by an increased percentage of the CD3−/CD56+CD16+, CD8+/CD28+ lymphocytes. "The profile of secreted cytokines shifts in favor of Th1 activity..."

Makhseed M et al: "Pro-inflammatory maternal cytokine profile in preterm delivery." *American Journal of Reproductive Immunology*, Vol.49, No.5 p.308, May 2003.
Blood samples from 54 women with a history of successful pregnancy and 30 women undergoing preterm delivery were compared. "Significantly higher levels of the type 1 cytokines, interferon-gamma and interleukin 2, were produced by the preterm delivery group than by the normal pregnancy group..."

El-Shazly S: "Increased expression of pro-inflammatory cytokines in placentas of women undergoing spontaneous preterm delivery or premature rupture of membranes." *American Journal of Reproductive Immunology*, Vol.52, Issue 1, p.45, July 2004.

Reed J and Winger E: "IVIg therapy increases delivery birthweight in babies born to women with elevated preconception proportion of peripheral blood (CD56+/CD3-) natural killer cells." *Clinical Experimental Obstetrics and Gynecology."* 44(3):384-391, 2017
"In women with elevated preconception peripheral NK cells, mean birthweight at delivery is low without IVIg but significantly improved with IVIg Precon-

eption immune testing may be a tool for determining which patients are at risk for low birthweight and may benefit from immunotherapy."

89 **"In women with reproductive failure... NK cells that are usually situated in the bloodstream are associated with higher rates of recurrent pregnancy loss, IVF failure and pregnancy complications..."** – Beer AE et al: "Immunopathology of the implantation site utilizing monoclonal antibodies to natural killer cells in women with recurrent pregnancy losses." *American Journal of Reproductive Immunology*, Jan; 41(1):91-8, 1999.
Placental tissue blocks from prior pregnancy losses of 71 women were obtained, re-cut and analyzed. "Some women with recurrent spontaneous abortions demonstrate abnormal placental lesions at the implantation site." *See also*:

Chao K et al: "Decidual natural killer cytotoxicity decreased in normal pregnancy but not in anembryonic pregnancy and recurrent spontaneous abortion." *American Journal of Reproductive Immunology*, 34:274, 1995.
The researchers examined the immune cell subpopulations in those with pregnancy failure or spontaneous abortion. They concluded: "...decidual NK activity was higher in anembryonic pregnancies and in recurrent spontaneous abortions than it was in normal pregnancies."

Lachapelle M et al: "Endometrial T, B and NK cells in patients with recurrent abortion: altered profile and pregnancy outcome." *Journal of Immunology*, May; 15:156(10):4027-34, 1996.
"...endometrial lymphocytes of recurrent spontaneous aborters harbor a distinct immunophenotypic profile that antedates implantation and suggests that endometrial immunologic conditions are intrinsically altered in recurrent aborters...a role for NK cells in the abortion process is suggested by their altered subsets in all repetitive aborters."

Fukui A et al: "Natural killer cell subpopulations and cytotoxicity for infertile patients undergoing in vitro fertilization." *American Journal of Reproductive Immunology*, 41:413-22, 1999.
In this study involving women undergoing IVF, on the day of embryo transfer, the percentages of CD56+ cells and CD16+/CD56+ cells in the peripheral blood were significantly higher in the failed group than in the group with successfully implanting embryos. In the endometrial tissue, the decrease in the percentage of CD56+/CD16- cells in the failed group was also significant when compared with those of the successful group.

Emmer P et al: "Peripheral natural killer cytotoxicity and CD56 (pos) CD16 (pos) cells increase during early pregnancy in women with a history of recurrent spontaneous abortion." *Human Reproduction,* 2000 May; 15(5):1163-9, 2000.

89 **"Culture studies have shown that TNF-alpha disrupts cellular mitosis."** – Di Pietro R et al: "Effects of TNF-alpha/colchicine combined treatment on Burkitt lymphoma cells: molecular and ultra-structural changes." *Cytokine*, Feb; 11(2):144-50, 1999.
"Tumour necrosis factor alpha (TNF-alpha) kills Daudi cells (Human Burkitt Lymphoma), inducing either necrosis or apoptosis without DNA fragmentation." *See also*:

NOTES

Vieira K et al: "Tumor necrosis factor alpha interferes with the cell cycle of normal and papillomavirus-immortalized human keratin-ocytes." *Cancer Research*, May 15; 56(10):2452-7, 1996.
"In this report, we investigated the expression of mitotic regulatory proteins, such as cyclin A, cyclin B, and p34cdc2. After exposure to TNF-alpha, normal and HPV-16-immortalized cells exhibited a dramatic decrease in the expression of these proteins."

89   **"...high concentrations of these cytokines in the endometrium are associated with delayed embryonic development and implantation failure."** – Lalitkumar P et al: "Endometrial tumor necrosis factor is a likely mediator of early luteal phase mifepristone-mediated negative effector action on the preimplantation embryo." *Reproduction*, 129, pp.323-335, 2005.
The study concludes: *"...increased levels of TNF-alpha in endometrial and luminal compartments around the time of uterine receptivity adversely affect the growth and viability of preimplantation stage embryos." See also*:

Ledee-Bataille N et al: "Role of the endometrial tripod interleukin-18, -15, and -12 in inadequate uterine receptivity in patients with a history of repeated in vitro fertilization-embryo transfer failure." *Fertility & Sterility,* Mar; 83(3):598-605, 2005.
Blood samples from women who failed to become pregnant after repeated IVF embryo transfer and fertile control subjects were compared. "...IL-18 and IL-15 seems to be involved in the local recruitment and the activation of uterine natural killer (uNK) cells. IL-18 was itself correlated with IL-15 and IL-12, suggesting a local control of uNK cells activation."

Stewart-Akers A et al: "Endometrial leukocytes are altered numerically and functionally in women with implantation defects." *American Journal of Reproductive Immunology,* 39:1-11, 1998.
Endometrial leukocyte populations in women with autoimmune thyroid disease were measured. "A significant increase in the endometrial T-cell population was observed in women with autoimmune thyroid disease compared with controls. Both the leukocyte numbers and cytokine expression profile were altered significantly in a well-defined group of women with implantation defects."

Inagaki N et al: "Analysis of intrauterine cytokine concentration and matrix-metalloproteinase activity in women with recurrent failed embryo transfer." *Human Reproduction,* Mar; 18(3):608-15, 2003.

Spandorfer S et al: "Maternal serum levels of interferon-gamma and interleukin-2 soluble receptor-alpha predict the outcome of early IVF pregnancies." *Human Reproduction*, Jun; 19(6):1357-63, 2004.

90   **"High TNF-alpha concentrations can even activate the coagulation system..."** – Esmon C: "The impact of the inflammatory response on coagulation." *Thrombosis Research*, 114(5-6):321-7, 2004.
"Inflammatory mediators like endotoxin and tumor necrosis factor alpha (TNF-alpha) elicit the expression of tissue factor on blood cells ...Natural anticoagulant mechanisms limit the thrombotic response, but these pathways are depressed by inflammatory mediators...antiphospholipid antibodies severely impair the protein C pathway ...Inflammatory mediators like interleukin 6 can increase both platelet count and their responsiveness to agonists like thrombin.

- 344 -

NOTES

All of these events tend to shift the hemostatic balance in favor of clot formation." *See also:*

Pircher J et al: "Prothrombotic effects of tumor necrosis factor alpha in vivo are amplified by the absence of TNF-alpha receptor subtype 1 and require TNF-alpha receptor subtype 2." *Arthritis Research Therapy*, Oct 18;14(5): 2012.
"TNF-a accelerates thrombus formation in an in vivo model of arteriolar thrombosis."

90 **"Subchorionic hematomas can be associated with autoimmune activity that kills the cells of adjacent tissue."** – Baxi L and Pearlstone M: "Subchorionic hematomas and the presence of autoantibodies." *American Journal of Obstetrics & Gynecology*, Nov; 165(5 Pt 1):1423-4, 1991.
"Five cases of subchorionic hematoma detected by ultrasonography in patients with threatened abortion are presented. Three of these subjects had antinuclear antibodies, and the remaining two subjects had anticardiolipin antibodies."

90 **"...the stimulation protocol in IVF can make the situation even worse..."** – Carruba G et al: "Estrogen regulates cytokine production and apoptosis in PMA-differentiated, macrophage-like U937 cells." *Journal of Cellular Biochemistry*, Sep 1; 90(1):187-96, 2003. *See also*:

Hunt J et al: "Female steroid hormones regulate production of pro-inflammatory molecules in uterine leukocytes." *Journal of Reproductive Immunology*, Nov 15; 35(2):87-99, 1997.
"In uterine mast cells TNF-alpha is promoted by E2..."

90 **"For women with a history of infertility who are undergoing IVF there may be problems with egg quality and embryonic cell division."** – Soto P et al: "Actions of tumor necrosis factor-A on oocyte maturation and embryonic development in cattle." *American Journal of Reproductive Immunology*, Vol. 50, No.5 p.380, Nov 2003.
"TNF-alpha can have deleterious actions on oocyte maturation that compromise development of the resultant embryo."

91 **"...when peripheral blood concentrations of NK cells exceed 18%, there is a strong likelihood that the pregnancy will not succeed."** – Beer AE et al: "Immunophenotypic profiles of peripheral blood lymphocytes in women with recurrent pregnancy losses and in infertile women with multiple failed in vitro fertilization cycles." Apr; 35(4):376 -82, 1996.
"Elevations of CD56+ lymphocytes to over 18% during a pregnancy are a good prognostic indicator of impending pregnancy loss. We have not seen a liveborn infant in women with levels of 18% or higher without IVIG therapy..."

91 **"When appropriate treatment is provided, up to 85% of these women are able to deliver a healthy baby within three natural or IVF cycles."** – Beer AE et al: "Elevated peripheral blood natural killer cells are effectively down-regulated by immunoglobulin G infusion in women with recurrent spontaneous abortions." *American Journal of Reproductive Immunology*, Apr; 35(4):363-9, 1996.
73 women with recurrent miscarriage and elevated NK cells received IVIG therapy and anticoagulation treatment. 86% had a successful outcome in their next pregnancy when their NK cells were significantly suppressed.

NOTES

Thyroid Disease

92 **"Approximately 30% of women experiencing repeated spontaneous abortions test positive for one or both antibodies..."** – Dendrinos et al: "Thyroid autoimmunity in patients with recurrent spontaneous miscarriages." *Gynecological Endocrinology*, Aug; 14(4):270-4, 2000.
30 women with recurrent miscarriages, aged 25 to 37, were tested for thyroid antibodies and compared with 15 matched controls. The frequency of those with ATAs was 37% versus 13%. "This may represent an additional marker for impaired regulation of the maternal immune system." *See also*:

Poppe K et al: "Assisted reproduction and thyroid autoimmunity: an unfortunate combination?" *Journal of Clinical Endocrinology & Metabolism*, Vol.88, No.9, 4149-4152, 2003.
234 women were screened for thyroid peroxidase antibodies, among others, before their first ART cycle. 14% tested positive. The miscarriage rate in this group was 53% compared with 23% of women without thyroid antibodies. The researchers state, "We conclude that women who test positive for antithyroid peroxidase antibodies before the first ART cycle have a significantly increased risk for miscarriage."

Toulis K: "Risk of spontaneous miscarriage in euthyroid women with thyroid autoimmunity undergoing IVF: a meta-analysis." *European Journal of Endocrinology*, Apr;162(4):643-52, 2010.
"Four prospective studies that reported data on 1098 subfertile women undergoing IVF (141 with thyroid autoimmunity and 957 controls) were included in the meta-analysis. Women with thyroid autoimmunity undergoing IVF demonstrated significantly higher risk for miscarriage compared with controls."

92 **"They are also associated with reproductive failure in general."** – Zhong Y et al: "Relationship between Antithyroid Antibody and Pregnancy Outcome following in Vitro Fertilization and Embryo Transfer." International Journal of Medical Sciences, 9(2): 121–125, 2012.
"Patients with antithyroid antibody showed significantly lower fertilization rate, implantation rate and pregnancy rate and higher risk for abortion following IVF-ET when compared with those without antithyroid antibody."

92 **"Women with antithyroid antibodies (ATAs) may also have elevated levels of CD56+ NK cells, CD19+/5+ cells and activated T-cells..."** – Hidaka Y: "Increase in peripheral natural killer cell activity in patients with autoimmune thyroid disease." *Autoimmunity*, 11(4): 239-6, 1992. *See also:*
In this study involving 43 subjects, the researchers conclude: "...an increase of NK activity is associated with exacerbation of autoimmune thyroid disease both in Hashimoto's thyroiditis and in Graves' disease and suggests that NK cells might have an important role for the control of disease activity in autoimmune thyroid disease."

Stewart-Akers A et al: "Endometrial leukocytes are altered numerically and functionally in women with implantation defects." *American Journal of Reproductive Immunology,* Jan; 39(1):1-11, 1998.
This study involving a large number of women concluded that both the leukocyte numbers and cytokine expression profile were altered significantly in

NOTES

women with implantation defects who suffered from autoimmune thyroid disease.

92 **"That is why these antibodies are considered markers for at risk pregnancies."** – Stagnaro-Green A et al: "Detection of at risk pregnancy by means of highly sensitive assays for thyroid antibodies." *Journal of the American Medical Association*, 264, 1422-1425, 1990.
The report concludes: "...thyroid autoantibodies are an independent marker of an at-risk pregnancy." *See also*:

Rodien P et al: "Thyroid dysfunction and pregnancy." *Revue du Prat*, Jan; 31:55(2):174-9, 2005.
"Thyroid autoimmunity is associated with hypofertility, particularly with spontaneous abortion. Screening for thyroid dysfunction during pregnancy, although not systematic, should have broad indications."

Prummel M and Wiersinga W: "Thyroid autoimmunity and miscarriage." *European Journal of Endocrinology*, Jun; 150(6):751-5, 2004.
This meta-analysis of both case-controlled and longitudinal studies performed since 1990 shows a clear association between the presence of thyroid antibodies and miscarriage. "This association may be explained by a heightened autoimmune state affecting the fetal allograft, of which thyroid antibodies are just a marker."

93 **"ATAs can be elevated in those with systemic lupus erythematosus..."** – Park D et al: "Thyroid disorders in Korean patients with systemic lupus erythematosus." *Scandinavian Journal of Rheumatology,* 24(1):13-7, 1995.
In 63 SLE patients, the prevalence of antithyroid autoantibodies was 27.0%. "Antithyroid autoantibodies may be good predictors for the detection of Hashimoto's thyroiditis developing in SLE." *See also*:

Pyne D and Isenberg D: "Autoimmune thyroid disease in systemic lupus erythematosus." *Annals of Rheumatic Disorders,* Jan; 61(1):70-2, 2002.
In 300 patients with SLE, the prevalence of hypothyroidism was higher than in the normal population. 14% had thyroid antibodies, rising to 68% in the subgroup who also had thyroid disease.

93 **"... some studies have found a higher prevalence of thyroid antibodies in women suffering from clinical depression."** – Hage M and Azar S: "The Link between Thyroid Function and Depression." *Journal of Thyroid Research,* 590648, 2012.
"Today, it is well recognized that disturbances in thyroid function may significantly affect mental status including emotion and cognition Subclinical hypothyroidism occurs in up to 40% of these patients with depression. Furthermore, thyroid hormones are reported by many authors to be an effective adjunct treatment for depression."

93 **"Some doctors have also suggested that this test should be performed before a woman with infertility embarks on an IVF program."** – Pratt D et al: "Antithyroid antibodies and the association with non-organic-specific antibodies in recurrent pregnancy loss." *American Journal of Obstetrics & Gynecology*, Mar; 168(3 Pt 1):837-41, 1993.

NOTES

"...we may conclude that thyroid hormones and thyroid antibodies could be assessed in infertile women before ART, to delineate women at risk for clinical miscarriage."

93   **"Graves' disease is stimulated by a particular virus that can activate the disease process."** – Jaspan J et al: "Evidence for a retroviral trigger in Graves' disease." *Autoimmunity,* 20(2):135-42, 1995.

In 40 patients with Graves' disease, 87.5% showed a positive reaction against several HIAP-1-associated proteins. Only 2% (2/105) of normal controls showed positive reactivity.

93   **"Antibodies to this virus have also been found in a high percentage of people with SLE and other autoimmune conditions."** – Sander D et al: "Involvement of human intracisternal A-type retroviral particles in autoimmunity." *Microscopy Research and Technique,* Nov; 68 (3-4):222-34, 2005.

"A substantial majority of patients with systemic sclerosis (SS) or systemic lupus erythematosus (SLE) have serum antibodies to the proteins of this human retrovirus (HIAP-I)." Additional studies suggest that HIAP or related viruses may be involved in SLE and other autoimmune conditions. *See also*:

Jaspan J et al: "The interaction of a type A retroviral particle and class II human leukocyte antigen susceptibility genes in the pathogenesis of Graves' disease." *Journal of Clinical Endocrinology & Metabolism,* Jun; 81(6):2271-9, 1996.

35 members of 3 families were selected because of a high family prevalence of Graves' disease. The results showed that retroviral exposure together with genetic HLA susceptibility were the two major predisposing factors underlying the pathogenesis of the disease.

94   **"As a result of increased NK cell activity, women with thyroid damage often display a Th1-dominant autoimmune profile."** – Colin I et al: "Functional lymphocyte subset assessment of the Th1/Th2 profile in patients with autoimmune thyroiditis by flow-cytometric analysis of peripheral lymphocytes." *Journal of Biological Regulators and Homeostatic Agents (Milano)*, Jan-Mar; 18(1):72-6, 2004.

The white blood cell levels of 23 consecutive patients with Hashimoto's thyroiditis were compared with 17 healthy control subjects. The Th1: Th2 ratio measured on CD3 T cells was significantly increased in patients with Hashimoto's thyroiditis compared with controls.

94   **"In addition, the baby's neural growth may be affected..."** – Rodien P et al: "Thyroid dysfunction and pregnancy," *Revue du Prat,* Jan 31; 55(2):174-9, 2005.

In this review, hyperthyroidism is described as being associated with maternal, fetal and neonatal complications. "Untreated or inappropriately treated maternal hypothyroidism can lead to...poorer performances of offspring in intelligence tests."

Endometriosis

95   **"Endometriosis is a leading cause of reproductive failure and is undiagnosed in many cases of "unexplained" infertility."** – Gleicher N and

NOTES

Pratt D: "Abnormal (auto) immunity and endometriosis." *International Journal of Gynecology and Obstetrics*, 40: Supplement S21-7, 1993.
"Many cases of unexplained infertility may represent undiagnosed endometriosis. This is supported by the observation that immunologic profiles in endometriosis and unexplained infertility are very similar." *See also*:

Dmowski W: "Immunological aspects of endometriosis." *International Journal of Gynecology & Obstetrics*, 50: Supplement 1:S3-10, 1995.
"Studies from our laboratories support the theory that endometrial cells misplaced during menses can implant in ectopic locations only in women with genetically or environmentally altered cell-mediated immune function...We recently observed that the presence of autoantibodies in endometriosis was associated with significantly lower in vitro fertilization/embryo transfer pregnancy rates. Interestingly, in about 30% of women with unexplained infertility, immune changes characteristic of endometriosis were also present, suggesting a sub-clinical form of this disease." *See also:*

http://www.endo.org.uk:
"As recently as March 2006, it was reported that 68% of British sufferers were misdiagnosed with conditions such as irritable bowel syndrome and depression and that after their first visit to a doctor it took on average, eight years to be given a correct diagnosis."

95 **"...this condition is often associated with high levels of autoantibodies, and dysfunctional immune activity."** – Ulcova-Gallova Z et al: "Endometriosis in reproductive immunology." *American Journal of Reproductive Immunology*, May; 47(5):269-74, 2002.
The immune responses of over 300 women with endometriosis were compared with those of 101 healthy women. All were tested for seven antiphospholipid antibodies plus anti-zona pellucida antibodies (aZPA). Those with stage I-II endometriosis had higher levels of APAs and 40% were positive for aZPA. Women with stage I-II endometriosis had more autoantibodies than those with stage III-IV, and may be immunologically more active. "This result may be significant for future treatments such as in vitro fertilization and embryo transfer." *See also*:

Gazvani R and Templeton A: "Peritoneal environment, cytokines and angio-genesis in the pathophysiology of endometriosis." *Reproduction*, Feb; 123(2):217-26, 2002.
"In women with endometriosis, there appears to be an alteration in the function of peritoneal macrophages, natural killer cells and lymphocytes. Furthermore, growth factors and inflammatory mediators in the peritoneal fluid, produced mainly by peritoneal macrophages, are altered in endometriosis, indicating a role for these immune cells and mediators in the pathogenesis of this disease."

Seery J: "Endometriosis associated with defective handling of apoptotic cells in the female genital tract is a major cause of autoimmune disease in women." *Medical Hypotheses*, 66(5):945-9, 2006.
"Endometriosis is characterized by defective clearance of apoptotic endometrial cells in a pro-oxidant inflammatory environment. It is proposed that this combination of abnormalities triggers autoantibody production in women affected by endometriosis...The hypothesis is supported by epidemiological

studies which show a strong association between endometriosis and female-predominant autoimmune disorders."

95　**"In endometriosis, an abnormal decrease in NK cell cytotoxicity means the tissue from the lining of the uterus is not destroyed so it continues to grow elsewhere."** – Berkkanoglu M and Arici A: "Immunology and endometriosis." *American Journal of Reproductive Immunology*, Jul; 50(1):48-59, 2003.
"There is substantial evidence that immunologic factors play a role in the pathogenesis of endometriosis...Decreased natural killer cell cytotoxicity leads to an increased likelihood of implantation of endometriotic tissue. In addition, macrophages and a complex network of locally produced cytokines modulate the growth and inflammatory behavior of ectopic endometrial implants."

96　**"Its cytotoxic activity can also compromise egg development, fertilization and implantation."** – Dmowski W et al: "The effect of endometriosis, its stage and activity and of autoantibodies on in vitro fertilization and embryo transfer success rates." *Fertility & Sterility*, Mar; 63(3):555-62, 1995.
In an analysis of 237 consecutive IVF cycles, 119 in women with and 118 without endometriosis, the study concludes that women with endometriosis have autoantibodies that "may affect adversely implantation of embryos." *See also*:

Bullimore DW: "Endometriosis is sustained by tumor necrosis factor-alpha." *Medical Hypotheses*, Jan; 60(1):84-8, 2003.
"...abnormal production of tumor necrosis factor-alpha is required for the establishment and maintenance of endometriosis and also is responsible for the associated infertility through its effect on sperm motility and function and oocyte development."

Pellicer A: "Exploring the mechanism(s) of endometriosis-related infertility: an analysis of embryo development and implantation in assisted reproduction." *Human Reproduction*, Supplement 2:91-7, Dec 1995.
The outcome of 96 IVF cycles in 78 patients with tubal infertility was compared with that of 96 cycles in 59 women with endometriosis. Endometriosis patients had a poor IVF outcome in terms of a reduced pregnancy rate per cycle, a reduced pregnancy rate per transfer, and a reduced implantation rate per embryo replaced. The same poor results were also seen with donor eggs. Furthermore, in embryos created by women with endometriosis, significantly more failed to develop, compared with controls.

96　**"Despite the fact that their TNF-alpha levels are high, women with endometriosis usually have normal or even low levels of circulating NK cells in their bloodstream."** – Hua L et al: "The measurement of natural killer cell activity in peripheral blood and peritoneal fluid of patients with endometriosis." *Zhonghua Fu Chan Ke Za Zhi,* Oct; 31(10):586-9, 1996.
NK cell activity in peripheral blood and peritoneal fluid of 72 patients with endometriosis was lower than that of infertile and fertile controls and decreased as the stage of endometriosis progressed. *See also:*

Somigliana E et al: "Endometriosis and unexplained recurrent spontaneous abortion: pathological states resulting from aberrant modulation of natural killer cell function?" *Human Reproduction Update*, Jan-Feb; 5(1):40-51, 1999.

NOTES

"The observation that natural killer cell activity is abnormally low in endometriosis patients and abnormally high in women with otherwise unexplained recurrent spontaneous abortion represents, at present, an intriguing curiosity. There is evidence suggesting that these conditions are associated with an opposite regulation of NK cell behavior."

96 **"A study of over 3,500 women found that women with endometriosis were far more likely to suffer from additional autoimmunities..."** – Sinaii N et al: "High rates of autoimmune and endocrine disorders, fibromyalgia, chronic fatigue syndrome and atopic diseases among women with endometriosis: a survey analysis." *Human Reproduction*, Oct; 17(10):2715-2724, 2002.
In a survey of 3,680 members of the Endometriosis Association, 90% of women of reproductive age had clinically diagnosed endometriosis. 20% had more than one other disease, up to 31% of those with co-existing diseases had fibromyalgia or chronic fatigue syndrome, and some of these had another autoimmune or endocrine disease. Chronic fatigue syndrome was more than 100 times more common than in the female U.S. population. Hypothyroidism was 7 times more common, and fibromyalgia was twice as common. SLE, Sjögren's syndrome, rheumatoid arthritis and multiple sclerosis also occurred more frequently. 61% of endometriosis sufferers had allergies, compared with 18% of the U.S. general population, and 12% had asthma compared with 5%. Two thirds reported that relatives also had either diagnosed or suspected endometriosis.

96 **"Many women with endometriosis also manufacture antiphospholipid antibodies..."** – Lucena E and Cubillos J: "Immune abnormalities in endometriosis compromising fertility in IVF-ET patients." *Journal of Reproductive Medicine*, May; 44(5):458-64, 1999.
This study analyzed the incidence of alloantibodies and autoantibodies in 100 women with endometriosis and 62 patients with unexplained infertility without endometriosis. 27% of the group of patients with endometriosis tested positive for antinuclear antibodies. Of these, 30% (15/50) had primary infertility and 24% (12/50), secondary infertility. 48% of the infertile patients had antiphospholipid antibodies, which was significantly higher than in controls. *See also*:

Ulcova-Gallova Z et al: "Endometriosis in reproductive immunology." *American Journal of Reproductive Immunology*, May 47(5):269-74, 2002.
Over 320 women with endometriosis were assessed for the prevalence of antibodies. Those with stages 1 and 2 of the disease were found to have significantly higher serum levels of antiphospholipid antibodies and anti-zona pellucida antibodies than controls.

97 **"...removing the adhesions does not reduce the immune activity..."** – Gleicher N and Pratt D: "Abnormal (auto)immunity and endometriosis." *International Journal of Gynecology and Obstetrics*, 40: Supplement S pp. 21 7, 1993.
"Currently available medical and surgical techniques are effective in relieving symptomatology associated with endometriosis, although this is often temporary. A new clinical approach is needed that considers systemic presentation and likely immunologic pathophysiology."

NOTES

97 **"Dr Beer's anti-TNF-alpha treatment for patients with endometriosis... 73% ongoing pregnancy success rate."** – This data was presented at a medical conference in San Jose for Santa Clara county physicians, Feb 9, 2006. Results incorporated in paper by Winger E and Reed J: "Treatment with tumor necrosis factor inhibitors improves live birth rates in women with recurrent spontaneous abortion." *American Journal of Reproductive Immunology* 60:9-16, 2008.

Pelvic Inflammatory Disease and Tubal Blockages

97 **"The incidence of ectopic pregnancy is continuing to rise..."** – Tay J et al: "Ectopic pregnancy." *British Medical Journal,* 320:916-919, 2000.
"Ectopic pregnancy...incidence is increasing worldwide. In northern Europe between 1976 and 1993 the incidence increased from 11.2 to 18.8 per 1000 pregnancies and in 1989 in the United States admissions to hospital for ectopic pregnancy increased from 17,800 in 1970 to 88,400."

97 **"Sexually transmitted infections...are responsible for many premature and low weight births."** – Locksmith G and Duff P: "Infection, antibiotics, and preterm delivery." *Seminars in Perinatology*, Oct; 25 (5):295-309, 2001.
"The relationship between genital tract infection and preterm delivery has been established on the basis of biochemical, microbiological, and clinical evidence." *See also:*

Hillier S et al: "Association between bacterial vaginosis and preterm delivery of a low birthweight infant." *New England Journal of Medicine*, 333:1737-1742, 1995.
Bacterial vaginosis was detected in 16% of 10,397 pregnant women. "Bacterial vaginosis was associated with the preterm delivery of low birthweight infants independently of other recognized risk factors."

98 **"...pro-inflammatory cytokines are secreted...which damage the lining of the uterus and create a hostile environment for the developing embryo."** – Spandorfer S et al: "Relationship of abnormal vaginal flora, pro-inflammatory cytokines and idiopathic infertility in women undergoing IVF." *Journal of Reproductive Medicine*, Sep; 46 (9):806-10, 2001.
331 IVF patients were evaluated for bacterial vaginosis and cervical cytokine production. The study concludes: "Abnormal vaginal flora, including that causing bacterial vaginosis, is associated with elevated cervical levels of IL-1 beta and IL-8. The induction of proinflammatory cytokines by an altered vaginal ecosystem may be a previously unrecognized cause of idiopathic infertility." *See also:*

Suzuki Y et al: "Evaluation levels of cytokines in amniotic fluid of women with intrauterine infection in the early second trimester." *Fetal Diagnosis & Therapy,* 21(1):45-50, 2006.
Amniotic fluid from 180 patients at 16-22 weeks of gestation was tested for cytokines. In all cases of abortion and preterm labor, levels of IL-6 and IL-8 were significantly elevated.

98 **"Many common autoimmune diseases (e.g., inflammatory bowel disease, Sjögren's, Hashimoto's, Graves', Reiter's and Crohn's disease) have been linked to chronic bacterial infections..."** – Haier J et al: "Detection of

- 352 -

NOTES

mycoplasmal infections in blood of patients with rheumatoid arthritis." *British Journal of Rheumatology*, 38:504-509, 1999.
This report concludes: "...results suggest that a high percentage of rheumatoid arthritis patients have systemic mycoplasmal infections." *See also*:

Nicolson G et al: "High prevalence of mycoplasma infections among European chronic fatigue syndrome patients." *FEMS Immunology & Medical Microbiology*, 34:209-214, 2002.

Chlamydia

98 **"Statistics show that chlamydia remains the most common type of sexually transmitted bacterial infection in England"** – See:
http://www.hpa.org.uk/infections/topics_az/hiv_and_sti/stichlamydia/chlamydia.htm

98 **"(Chlamydia) is the most common notifiable disease in the U.S."**
CDC Sexually Transmitted Disease Surveillance 2017.

99 **"Chlamydia can directly activate the NK cells, which then produce high levels of TNF-alpha and INF-gamma."** – Hook C: "Effects of Chlamydia trachomatis infection on the expression of natural killer (NK) cell ligands and susceptibility to NK cell lysis." *Clinical & Experimental Immunology*, Oct; 138(1):54-60, 2004.
In this study, the investigators discovered that recognition of Chlamydia trachomatis organisms activates the NK cells to produce cytokines including IFN-gamma. In addition, infection of cells with Chlamydia trachomatis renders them susceptible to destruction by NK cells. *See also*:

Reddy B et al: "Cytokine expression pattern in the genital tract of Chlamydia trachomatis positive infertile women: implication for T-cell responses." *Clinical & Experimental Immunology*, Sep; 137(3):552-8, 2004.
"Flow cytometric analysis of cervical secretions in chlamydia positive women revealed recruitment of both CD4 and CD8 lymphocytes to the genital tract was up-regulated...IFN-gamma, TNF-alpha, IL-10 and IL-12 were up-regulated."

Severin J and Ossewaarde J: "Innate immunity in defense against Chlamydia trachomatis infections." *Drugs Today*, (Barc). Mar; 42 Suppl. A:75-81, 2006.

Gonorrhea

99 **"...gonorrhea, which can infect the cervix, uterus and fallopian tubes, and cause an increase in NK cell activity and TNF-alpha cytokine production."**
– Gregg C et al: "Gonococcal infection of human fallopian tube mucosa in organ culture: relationship of mucosal tissue TNF-alpha concentration to sloughing of ciliated cells." *Sexually Transmitted Diseases*, Mar, 26(3). 160-5, 1999.
"Gonococcal infection of fallopian tube mucosa in organ culture also results in the production of easily quantified tumor necrosis factor-alpha (TNF-alpha) by the mucosa...TNF-alpha is a mediator of the mucosal damage that attends gonococcal infection." The researchers conclude that tissue concentrations of TNF-alpha can be used to predict the extent of mucosal damage. The results also indicate that TNF-alpha may mediate infertility and ectopic pregnancy.

NOTES

Candida

99 **"The accompanying symptoms of itching and burning...caused by the candida IgA antibodies."** – Pivarcsi A et al: "Microbial compounds induce the expression of pro-inflammatory cytokines, chemokines and human beta defensin-2 in vaginal epithelial cells." *Microbes & Infection*, Apr 19, 2005.

100 **"IL-1, IL-6, TNF-alpha and more IgA antibodies are rapidly fired out..."** – Schaller M et al: "Candida albicans-secreted aspartic proteinases modify the epithelial cytokine response in an in vitro model of vaginal candidiasis." *Infection & Immunity*, May; 73(5): 2758-65, 2005.
"Vaginal infection with the Candida albicans wild-type strain induced strong interleukin 1 alpha (IL-1alpha), IL-1beta, IL-6, IL-8, IL-10, granulocyte-macrophage colony-stimulating factor, gamma interferon, and tumor necrosis factor alpha responses..."

100 **"This immunological onslaught can soon far exceed the actual degree of threat."** – Yordanov M: "Candida albicans cell-wall fraction exacerbates collagen-induced arthritis in mice." *Scandinavian Journal of Immunology*, Apr; 61(4): 301-8, 2005.
Candida albicans was shown to exacerbate inflammation and T-helper 1 cytokine production in mice with collagen type II-induced arthritis. "Commensal micro-organisms can express molecular structures that mimic self-epitopes. During acute infection, such pathogens may activate self-reactive T-cell clones, promoting autoimmunity."

Herpes

100 **"Women with herpes often have elevated and cytotoxic NK cells in their blood and in their tissues."** – Ellermann-Eriksen S: "Macrophages and cytokines in the early defence against herpes simplex virus." *Virology Journal*, Aug 3; 2:59, 2005.
"In a first wave of responses, cytokines, primarily type I interferons (IFN) and tumor necrosis factor are produced and exert a direct antiviral effect and activate the macrophages themselves. In the next wave, interleukin (IL)-12 together with the above and other cytokines induce production of IFN-gamma in mainly NK cells...This results in the generation of an alliance against the viral enemy."

101 **"Approximately 12% of the US population tests positive for herpes virus HSV-2,"**– From the October 2002 edition of *Sexually Transmitted Diseases Journal*: "Infection with HSV-2, the virus that commonly causes genital herpes, currently affects approximately 22% of the US population..." Research suggests that the incidence of HSV-2 infection among those aged 15 to 39 years will rise to 51 million infected individuals in the U.S. by the year 2025 compared with 28 million in 2000.

101 **"In a 2004 study of infertile women, the herpes virus was detected in 64% of the 42 women who were examined."** – Dimitrios T et al: "The effect of valacyclovir treatment on natural killer cells of infertile women." *American Journal of Reproductive Immunology*, Vol. 51, Issue 3, p.248, Mar; 2004.
"Herpes virus DNA was detected in 64.3% of the 42 women examined. Prior to valacyclovir treatment mean NK cell concentration in herpes-negative group

NOTES

was statistically higher from control group but lower from herpes positive group."

Dysplasia (Genital Warts)

101   **"HPV infection can create immunologic dysfunction that has been linked to miscarriage and infertility."** – Hermonat P et al: "Human papillomavirus is more prevalent in first trimester spontaneously aborted products of conception compared with elective specimens." *Virus Genes*, 14(1):13-7, 1997.
The researchers found that human papillomavirus (HPV) infection is three times more prevalent in tissue samples from spontaneous abortions. *See also*:

Pretet J et al: "Immunohistochemical analysis of CD4+ and CD8+ T-cell subsets in high risk human papillomavirus-associated pre-malignant and malignant lesions of the uterine cervix." *Gynecologic Oncology*, Jan 19, 2006.
"Humoral and cellular immune responses are likely to play a key role for the clearance or persistence and progression of high risk (HR) HPV-associated cervical lesions."

Sasagawa T et al: "Increased secretion patterns of interleukin-10 and tumor necrosis factor-alpha in cervical squamous intraepithelial lesions." *Human Pathology*, Nov; 35(11):1376-84, 2004.
"Cytokines are released in response to infection of the uterine cervix by high-risk HPV."

Allergies

103   **"...the onset of hives is a symptom that Dr Beer has observed in women with hypersensitivity to hormones, particularly progesterone."** – Baptist A: "Autoimmune progesterone dermatitis in a patient with endometriosis: case report and review of the literature." *Clinical & Molecular Allergy*, 2:10, 2004.
"Autoimmune progesterone dermatitis (APD) is a condition in which the menstrual cycle is associated with a number of skin findings such as urticaria, eczema, angioedema, and others. In affected women, it occurs three to ten days prior to the onset of menstrual flow, and resolves two days into menses."

Irritable Bowel Syndrome and Crohn's Disease

103   **"Irritable bowel syndrome (IBS) affects approximately 7% of people in the U.S."** – Andrews E: "Prevalence and demographics of irritable bowel syndrome: results from a large web-based survey." *Alimentary Pharmacology & Therapeutics*, (22):935-942, 2005.
31,829 individuals were randomly selected and sent screening question-naires to evaluate irritable bowel syndrome symptoms. Irritable bowel syndrome prevalence was 7%. Prevalence was higher in women vs. men and unmarried individuals vs. married individuals.

104   **"In Crohn's disease...there is a shift towards a Th1-mediated response and the NK cells secrete TNF-alpha..."** – Wang J: "Tumor necrosis factor family members and inflammatory bowel disease." *Immunological Review*, Apr; 204:144-55, 2005.
"Tumor necrosis factor is one of the most potent effector cytokines in the pathogenesis of inflammatory bowel disease."

- 355 -

NOTES

104 **"...women with IBD who have an inherited or acquired blood clotting disorder combined with excessive TNF-alpha output, are at greater risk of experiencing increased rates of implantation failure and miscarriage."** – Koutroubakis I: "Role of thrombotic vascular risk factors in inflammatory bowel disease." *Digestive Diseases*, 18(3): 161-7, 2000.

"It is recognized that a hypercoagulable state exists in IBD which involves all components of the clotting system...Recent studies have shown that genetic defects such as factor V Leiden mutation and C677T methylenetetrahydrofolate reductase polymorphism associated with hyperhomocysteinemia seem to interfere in the thrombotic manifestations of IBD. Acquired factors such as antiphospholipid antibodies could also participate in the development of the thrombotic process."

104 **"If IBD is active and untreated during pregnancy, the risks of spontaneous abortion, premature delivery and stillbirth are significantly increased."** – Burakoff R and Opper F: "Pregnancy and nursing." *Gastroenterology Clinics of North America*, Sep; 24(3):689-98, 1995.

"Active IBD during pregnancy is associated with increased stillbirths and spontaneous abortions..." *See also*:

Elbaz G et al: "Inflammatory bowel disease and preterm delivery." *International Journal of Gynaecology & Obstetrics*, Sep; 90(3):193-7, 2005.

In 48 deliveries to patients with Crohn's disease and 79 deliveries to patients with ulcerative colitis, higher rates of preterm delivery were found among patients with IBD compared with the controls. In addition, these patients had higher rates of fertility treatments.

Stress

105 **"Autoimmune women tend to have higher levels of CD8+ T-cells, higher levels of toxic TNF-alpha, higher autoimmune inducing Th1: Th2 ratios, and lower serotonin levels – the same markers that are seen in women with stress triggered miscarriages."** – Arck P et al: "Stress and immune mediators in miscarriage." *Human Reproduction*, Jul; 16(7):1505-11, 2001.

94 women who had suffered a first trimester abortion completed a questionnaire to measure their own perceived stress level. Uterine tissue samples were analyzed to detect the presence of NK cells, CD8+, CD3+ T-cells, mast cells and TNF-alpha. Women with high stress scores had significantly higher numbers of mast cells, CD8+ cells and TNF-alpha. "Stress-triggered abortion in humans, identified by a questionnaire, can be linked to immunological imbalances." *See also:*

Clark DA et al: "Th1 cytokines and the prothrombinase fgl2 in stress-triggered and inflammatory abortion." *– American Journal of Reproductive Immunology*, Apr; 49(4):210-20, 2003.

In stressed mice there were two distinct cytokine patterns leading to similar abortion rates: an increase in TNF-alpha and an IL-12-triggered cascade characterized by the up-regulation of TNF-alpha and IFN-gamma.

105 **"This is why patients with illnesses characterized by a hyperactive immune system often suffer from stress and depression."** – Vuitton D et al: "Psychoimmunology: a questionable model?" *Revue de Medecine Interne*, Oct; 20(10):934-46, 1999.

NOTES

"In autoimmune diseases, a high prevalence of depression, as well as a particular sensitivity to stressful events seems to modify the course of conditions such as systemic lupus erythematosus, rheumatoid arthritis or Sjögren's disease."

105 **"Chronic stress can, in turn, reduce the immune system's ability to respond to anti-inflammatory signals..."** – Miller G et al: "Chronic psychological stress and the regulation of pro-inflammatory cytokines: a glucocorticoid-resistance model." *Health Psychology*, Nov; 21(6): 531-41, 2002.
50 adults were studied; half were parents of cancer patients, and half were parents of healthy children. Parents of cancer patients reported higher levels of psychological distress. There was evidence that chronic stress impaired the immune system's response to anti-inflammatory signals. The capacity of corticosteroids to suppress pro-inflammatory cytokine production was diminished among parents of cancer patients. "Findings suggest a novel pathway by which chronic stress might alter the course of inflammatory disease." *See also*:

Elenkov I et al: "Cytokine dysregulation, inflammation and well-being." *Neuroimmunomodulation*, 12(5):255-69, 2005.
"Under certain conditions...stress hormones may actually facilitate inflammation through induction of interleukin (IL)-1, IL-6, IL-8, IL-18, tumor necrosis factor-alpha and C-reactive protein production...Thus, a dysfunctional neuroendocrine-immune interface associated with abnormalities of the 'systemic anti-inflammatory feedback' and/or 'hyperactivity' of the local pro-inflammatory factors may play a role in the pathogenesis of atopic/allergic and autoimmune diseases, obesity, depression, and atherosclerosis."

Raison C and Miller A: "The neuroimmunology of stress and depression." *Seminars in Clinical Neuropsychiatry,* Oct; 6(4):277-94, 2001.
In this review of the literature, the authors report that immune system activation is associated with the development of behavioral symptoms similar to those of chronic stress or major depression.

106 **"Those who were suffering prolonged grief had 53.4% more inflammation in their bodies than those who were not."**
Fagundes C et al: "Spousal bereavement is associated with more pronounced ex vivo cytokine production and lower heart rate variability: Mechanisms underlying cardiovascular risk?" *Psychoneuroendocrinology*, Volume 93, July 2018, Pages 65-71.
This study by Chris Fagundes builds on previous research confirming the link between chronic stress and markers for inflammation such as pro-inflammatory cytokines.

106 **"...evidence of a specific immune profile that involves genes for stress activated and inflammatory responses."** – Sternberg W and Liebeskind J. "The analgesic response to stress: genetic and gender considerations." *European Journal of Anaesthesiology Supplement,* May; 10:14-7, 1995.
"Mice can be bred for a high or low analgesic response to stress and there is evidence that this is determined by a single gene."

106 **"Such abortions can largely be prevented with immunotherapy."** – Clark DA et al: "Stress-induced murine abortion associated with substance P-

- 357 -

NOTES

dependent alteration in cytokines in maternal uterine decidua." *Biology of Reproduction*, Vol.53, 814-819, 1995.

This study demonstrates that stress associated with recurrent spontaneous abortion is associated with the production of Th1 cytokines such as TNF-alpha by NK cells. Immunotherapy may protect against stress-triggered spontaneous abortion. *See also*:

Clark DA et al: "Stress-triggered abortion in mice prevented by alloimmunization." *American Journal of Reproductive Immunology,* Apr; 29 (3):141-7, 1993.

When mice were subjected to high levels of stress, the abortion rate of those that had been treated with immunotherapy prior to conception was significantly less than that of untreated mice.

106 **"A common human genetic variant...is another key factor in explaining the body's hyper reactivity to stress and excessive Th1 cytokine production."** – Williams R et al: "Central nervous system serotonin function and cardiovascular responses to stress." *Psychosomatic Medicine,* Mar-Apr; 63(2):300-5, 2001.

The researchers discovered that people with a common variant of a specific gene reacted negatively to mental stress and were at a much greater risk of suffering adverse cardiovascular responses. The genetic profile responsible for causing a deficiency of serotonin was particularly prevalent among African Americans, who have higher rates of hypertension and stress than white Europeans.

106 **"...chronic stress (including social isolation stress) can have the opposite effect in some women, temporarily depressing the immune system..."** – Segerstrom S et al: "Psychological Stress and the Human Immune System: A Meta-Analytic Study of 30 Years of Inquiry." *Psychological Bulletin,* Vol. 130, No. 4. 2004.

This meta-analysis of 293 independent studies found that chronic stressors (where undesirable situations seem endless and beyond control) were associated with the most suppression of immunity. *See also*:

Wu W et al: "Social isolation stress enhanced liver metastasis of murine colon 26-L5 carcinoma cells by suppressing immune responses in mice." *Life Sciences,* Mar 31; 66(19):1827-38, 2000.

Increased cancer proliferation was seen in mice that were socially isolated, compared with the group-housed mice. Suppressed NK cell activity and decreased macrophage-mediated cytotoxicity were also observed.

Elenkov I and Chrousos G: "Stress, cytokine patterns and susceptibility to disease." *Baillieres Best Practice & Research: Clinical Endocrinology & Metabolism,* Dec; 13(4):583-95, 1999.

"...systemically, stress might induce a Th2 shift, while, locally, under certain conditions, it might induce pro-inflammatory activities...stress may influence the onset and/or course of infectious, autoimmune/ inflammatory, allergic and neoplastic diseases."

NOTES

10. ANTIBODIES TO HORMONES AND NEUROTRANSMITTERS

107 **"...endocrinal disorders can indicate immune activity that is associated with infertility and pregnancy loss."** – Erlebacher A et al: "Ovarian insufficiency and early pregnancy loss induced by activation of the innate immune system." *Journal of Clinical Investigation*, 114: 39-48, 2004.
The researchers demonstrate that immune activity that inhibits the reproductive endocrine system can lead to pregnancy failure.

107 **"Infertile women and women experiencing recurrent miscarriage, often have significantly higher levels of NK cells and CD19+/5+ B cells."** – Beer AE et al: "Immunophenotypic profiles of peripheral blood lymphocytes in women with recurrent pregnancy losses and in in-fertile women with multiple failed in vitro fertilization cycles." *American Journal of Reproductive Immunology*, Apr; 35(4):376-82, 1996.
"Infertile and RSA women who fail alloimmune and autoimmune therapy have significant alterations in cellular and humoral immunity involving NK cells and CD19+/CD5+ B cells." *See also*:

Chernyshov V et al: "Immune disorders in women with premature ovarian failure in initial period." *American Journal of Reproductive Immunology*, Sep; 46(3):220-5, 2001.
This report concluded: "An increase of autoantibody producing B cells (CD19+5+)...suggested a primary autoimmune process in the initial period of premature ovarian failure."

Darmochwal-Kolarz D et al: "The immunophenotype of patients with recurrent pregnancy loss." *European Journal of Obstetrics, Gynecology & Reproductive Biology*, Jun 10; 103(1):53-7, 2002.
In this study, the percentage of CD19+5+ cells was significantly higher in women with unexplained habitual miscarriages in comparison with healthy women.

107 **"...elevated numbers of circulating CD19+/5+ cells correlate with high levels of antiphospholipid antibodies in some APS patients..."** – Youinou P and Renaudineau Y: "The antiphospholipid syndrome as a model for B cell-induced autoimmune diseases." *Thrombosis Research*, 114(5-6):363-9, 2004.
"Raised numbers of circulating CD19+5+ B cells correlate with high levels of antiphospholipid antibodies in some APS patients, and participate in altered immunity of women with recurrent spontaneous abortion...Various B cell receptor-associated transmembrane glycol-proteins are also involved in the behavior of the cells. These include CD19 which amplifies the message." *See also:*

Sato S et al: "Quantitative genetic variation in CD19 expression correlates with autoimmunity." *The Journal of Immunology*, 165.6635-6643, 2000.
"...modest changes in the expression or function of regulatory molecules such as CD19 may shift the balance between tolerance and immunity to autoimmunity."

- 359 -

NOTES

Antibodies to Hormones

108 **"High FSH and estradiol levels three days after the first day of menstruation are signs that antibodies to hormones could be at work." –** Cameron I et al: "Occult ovarian failure: a syndrome of infertility, regular menses, and elevated follicle-stimulating hormone concentrations." *Journal of Clinical Endocrinology & Metabolism*, 67: p.1190-1194, 1988.
Of 10 women with infertility and failed IVF cycles, antibodies to the adrenal or thyroid glands were present in 50% of women and antiovarian antibodies were present in 40%. *See also*:

Kauffman P: "Premature ovarian failure associated with autoimmune polyglandular syndrome: Pathophysiological mechanisms and future fertility." *Journal of Women's Health*, Jun; Vol.12, No.5:513-520, 2003.
The author states: "An autoimmune response to steroidogenic enzymes and ovarian steroid cells appears to mediate destruction of ovarian function."

108 **"...in... women undergoing IVF, 92% of low responders had antibodies to follicle-stimulating hormones..."** – Meyer W et al: "Evidence of gonadal and gonadotropin antibodies in women with a suboptimal ovarian response to exogenous gonadotropin." *Obstetrics & Gynecology*, 77:795-799, 1990.
Sera from 26 women identified as "low responders" were assessed for specific antibodies to human ovary and gonadotropins. 92% of low responders had antibodies to FSH and 65% had antibodies to LH.

Antibodies to Estrogen

109"Too little estradiol can restrict the development of the uterine lining..." – Hillard T et al: "Differential effects of transdermal estradiol and sequential progesterones on impedance to flow within the uterine arteries of postmenopausal women." *Fertility & Sterility*, 58; 959-963, 1992.
In 12 postmenopausal women, treatment with estradiol and progestin improved blood flow in the uterine arteries. The report concludes: "Gonadal hormones have a profound effect on arterial tone in post-menopausal women; this action may help explain some of the beneficial effects of estrogen on arterial disease risk." *See also*:

de Ziegler D et al: "Vascular resistance of uterine arteries: physiological effects of estradiol and progesterone." *Fertility & Sterility*, 55,775-779, 1991.
After receiving estradiol and progesterone, there was a significant decrease in vascular resistance in the uterine arteries of six women with non-functioning ovaries.

109 **"Because estrogen receptors are found on the surfaces of all the cells in the body, this hormone can...exacerbate autoimmune disease."** – Kanda N et al: "Estrogen enhancement of anti-double-stranded DNA antibody and immunoglobulin G production in peripheral blood mononuclear cells from patients with systemic lupus erythematosus." *Arthritis & Rheumatology*, Feb; 42(2):328-37, 1999. *See also*:

Delpy L et al: "Estrogen enhances susceptibility to experimental autoimmune myasthenia gravis by promoting type 1-polarized immune responses." *Journal of Immunology*, Oct 15; 175(8):5050-7, 2005.

NOTES

Antibodies to Progesterone

110 **"[Progesterone] acts on the uterus to stimulate and maintain uterine functions that encourage embryonic growth, implantation and the formation of the placenta."** – Rider V: "Progesterone and the control of uterine cell proliferation and differentiation." *Frontiers in Bioscience*, Jun 1; 7:1545-55, 2002.
"Progesterone is the only steroid hormone that is essential for the establishment and maintenance of pregnancy in all mammalian species that have been studied."

110 **"...progesterone inhibits T-cell activity by working as an immuno-suppressant."** – Stites D and Siiteri P: "Steroids as immunosuppressants in pregnancy." *Immunological Review*, 75:117-138, 1983.
"Specific functions of human T-lymphocytes and macrophages are inhibited by concentrations of progesterone known to occur in the placenta." *See also*:

Szekeres-Bartho J and Wegmann T: "A progesterone-dependent immuno-modulatory protein alters the Th1:Th2 balance." *Journal of Reproductive Immunology*, Vol.31, Issues 1-2, Aug 1996.
"In the presence of progesterone, lymphocytes from pregnant females produce an immunomodulatory protein known as progesterone induced blocking factor." In experiments on mice, it was shown that this blocking factor affected the Th1:Th2 ratio and contributed to decreased cell-mediated immune responses during pregnancy.

110 **"A small number of women were also experiencing skin reactions..."** – Baptist A: "Autoimmune progesterone dermatitis in a patient with endo-metriosis: case report and review of the literature." *Clinical & Molecular Allergy*, Aug 2; 2(1):10, 2004.

110 **"...a state of estrogen dominance that can add yet more fuel to the inflammatory process."** – Grimaldi C et al: "Estrogen alters thresholds for B cell apoptosis and activation." *Journal of Clinical Investigation*, Jun 15; 109(12):1625–1633, 2002.
This study found that estrogen increased antibody expression levels by between 15 and 27%. "...estrogen induces a genetic program that alters survival and activation of B cells in a B cell-autonomous fashion and thus skews the naive immune system toward autoreactivity."

110 **"...levels of pro-inflammatory estrogens, particularly estradiol, are often significantly elevated in those with rheumatoid arthritis or SLE."** – Cutolo M et al: "Sex hormones influence on the immune system: basic and clinical aspects in autoimmunity." *Lupus*, 2004; 13 (9):635-8.
The review states that levels of pro-inflammatory estrogens, particularly estradiol, are significantly elevated in rheumatoid arthritis and SLE patients. "...locally increased estrogens might exert activating effects on cell proliferation, including macrophages and fibroblasts, suggesting new roles for estrogens in autoimmunity."

- 361 -

NOTES

Antibodies to HCG

111 **"Antibodies to HCG are found in the blood of some women with infertility."** – Amato F et al: "Infertility caused by hCG autoantibody." *The Journal of Clinical Endocrinology & Metabolism*, Vol. 87, No.3, pp.993-997, 2002.
"An anti-hCG autoantibody was found in a patient with a 9-yr history of secondary infertility. Although the patient had regular menstrual cycles, had conceived spontaneously, and had good hormonal and follicular responses to gonadotropic stimulation regimens during the in vitro fertilization work-up, she presented with apparent recurrent pregnancy loss...We suggest that the persisting titer of the antibody is responsible for the patient's infertility." *See also*:

Wang L et al: "Analysis on the treatment of 1,020 patients with immunologic infertility." *Zhonghua Fu Chan Ke Za Zhi*, Apr; 34(4):234-6, 1999.
In 1,020 women with primary or secondary infertility, antibodies to HCG were found in 23.61% of patients.

111 **"...these antibodies have even been developed for use as a contraceptive vaccine."** – Talwar G et al: "The HSD- hCG Vaccine Prevents Pregnancy in Women: Feasibility Study of a Reversible Safe Contraceptive Vaccine." *American Journal of Reproductive Immunology*, 06 September 2011.
"Reversible fertility control is feasible with the HSD- hCG vaccine without impairment of ovulation or disturbance of menstrual regularity."

111 **"A reaction to LH suppressors could therefore potentially stimulate an antibody reaction to HCG."** – Pala A et al: "Immunochemical and biological characteristics of a human autoantibody to human chorionic gonadotropin and luteinizing hormone." *Journal of Clinical Endocrinology & Metabolism*, Vol. 67; pp.1317-1321, 1988.
"Immunoglobulins isolated from a pool of serum obtained during the post-abortion period neutralized the activity of both hCG and LH in an in vivo bioassay, and the binding affinity of the antibodies toward both hormones was high."

Premature Ovarian Failure

112 **"Approximately one in a hundred women is affected by premature ovarian failure..."** Haller-Kikkatalo K et al, "The prevalence and phenotypic characteristics of spontaneous premature ovarian failure: a general population registry-based study." *Human Reproduction,* 2015 May; 30(5):1229-38

112 **"...their presence is often a marker for premature ovarian failure."** – Luborsky J et al: "Ovarian antibodies, FSH and inhibin B: independent markers associated with unexplained infertility." *Human Reproduction*, May; 15(5):1046-51, 2000. *See also*:

Luborsky J et al: "Ovarian antibodies detected by immobilized antigen immunoassay in patients with premature ovarian failure." *Journal of Clinical Endocrinology & Metabolism*, Jan; 70(1):69-75, 1990.

- 362 -

NOTES

69% of 45 patients with premature ovarian failure tested positive for either ovarian or oocyte antibodies. "This supports the concept that some forms of premature ovarian failure are associated with an autoimmune process."

112 **"Studies have shown that in many cases of premature ovarian failure the woman will have an additional autoimmune disorder, the most common being hypothyroidism."** – Belvisi L et al: "Organ-specific autoimmunity in patients with premature ovarian failure." *Journal of Endocrinological Investigation,* 16, 889-892, 1993.
Sera from 45 women with premature ovarian failure and a control group of 28 women were compared. 18 patients with premature ovarian failure (40%) were positive for at least one autoantibody. In the control group, only one woman (3.6%) showed autoimmunity. Antithyroid was the most common autoimmunity (20%). *See also*:

Ishizuka B et al: "Antinuclear antibodies in patients with premature ovarian failure." *Human Reproduction*, Vol.14, No.1, 70-75, Jan 1999.
The prevalence of antinuclear antibodies was assessed in 32 consecutive patients with premature ovarian failure. "ANA were found in 77% (10/13) of premature ovarian failure patients with normal karyotypes who developed amenorrhea at or under the age of 30."

112 **"Women with elevated antiovarian antibody levels are often poor responders to ovulation induction..."** – Meyer W et al: "Evidence of gonadal and gonadotropin antibodies in women with a suboptimal ovarian response to exogenous gonadotropin." *Obstetrician Gynecologist*, 75:795-799, 1990.
In sera from 26 women identified as "low responders" during the IVF ovarian stimulation protocol, 77% had ovarian antibodies. None of the "good responders" had antibodies to gonadotropins or to ovarian tissue.

112 **"Those with elevated antiovarian antibody levels...have lower pregnancy success rates."** – Geva E et al: "The possible role of anti-ovary antibodies in repeated in vitro fertilization failures." *American Journal of Reproductive Immunology*, Nov; 42(5):292-6, 1999.
In 80 IVF patients with five or more failed treatment cycles, ovarian antibodies were found in 10 patients compared with none in the control groups. 9 of the patients were treated with corticosteroids in their following cycle. A statistically significant improvement in embryo grading was noted. 3 patients conceived after treatment, with a take-home baby rate of 22%, compared with only 8.6% among the untreated group.

112 **"In one study, 58% of women with failed IVF cycles had antiovarian antibodies compared with 25% of those who were successful."** – Luborsky J et al: "Pregnancy outcome and ovarian antibodies in infertility patients undergoing controlled ovarian hyperstimulation." *American Journal of Reproductive Immunology*, 44(5):261-265, 2000.
"Women who became pregnant had a lower frequency of ovarian antibodies than women who did not become pregnant: 25.0% versus 58.1% respectively."

NOTES

How Autoimmunity, Obesity and Infertility Can Interrelate

113 **"More than 60% of American women are now obese or overweight..."** – Institute for Health Metrics and Evaluation reported in 2018 that "an estimated 160 million Americans are either obese or overweight. Nearly three-quarters of American men and more than 60% of women are obese or overweight. These are also major challenges for America's children, nearly 30% of boys and girls under age 20 are either obese or overweight, up from 19% in 1980."

113 **"This is also an extremely serious threat to health, as the percent-ages of instances where obesity is linked to disease show."** – Data compiled from research and information from the National Institute of Diabetes & Digestive & Kidney Diseases (NIDDK). See:
www.webmd.com/

114 **"As fatty tissue expands, it creates inflammation..."** – Trayhurn P: "Endocrine and signaling role of adipose tissue: new perspectives on fat." *Acta Physiologica Scandinavia*, Aug; 184(4):285-93, 2005.
"Obesity is characterized by a state of mild inflammation and the expression and release of inflammation related adipokines generally rises as adipose tissue expands...increased circulating levels of inflammatory markers reflecting spill-over from an 'inflamed' tissue, leading to the obesity associated pathologies of type 2 diabetes and the metabolic syndrome." *See also*:

Das U: "Is obesity an inflammatory condition?" *Nutrition*, Nov-Dec; 17 (11-12):953-66, 2001.
"Overweight and obese children and adults have elevated serum levels of C-reactive protein, interleukin-6, tumor necrosis factor-alpha, and leptin, which are known markers of inflammation..."

Calabro P: "Release of C-reactive protein in response to inflammatory cytokines by human adipocytes: Linking obesity to vascular inflammation." *Journal of the American College of Cardiology,* Sep 20, Vol. 46: pp.1112-1113, 2005.

114 **"Due to this increased inflammatory activity, obesity also carries more risks for women who are pregnant, with a greater incidence of miscarriage, preeclampsia, hyperinsulinemia (high blood sugar) and gestational diabetes."** – Baeten JM et al: "Pregnancy complications and outcomes among overweight and obese nulliparous women." *American Journal of Public Health*, Mar; 91(3):436-40, 2001.
96,801 women were categorized by body mass index. "Compared with lean women, both overweight and obese women had a significantly increased risk for gestational diabetes, preeclampsia, eclampsia, Cesarean delivery, and delivery of a macrosomic (large) infant." *See also*:

Lashen H et al: "Obesity is associated with increased risk of first trimester and recurrent miscarriage: matched case-control study." *Human Reproduction*, Vol. 19, No. 7, 1644-1646, Jul 2004.
Using a population sourced from a maternity database, 1,644 obese women were compared with 3,288 normal weight, age-matched controls. The risks of early miscarriage and recurrent early miscarriage were significantly higher among the obese patients.

NOTES

Linné Y: "Effects of obesity on women's reproduction and complications during pregnancy." *Obesity Reviews*, Vol. 5, Issue 3, p.137, Aug 2004.
It was observed that obese women have a higher risk of complications during pregnancy such as hypertensive diagnoses and gestational diabetes. They also have higher rates of Caesarean sections and prolonged deliveries.

Ramsay J: "Maternal obesity is associated with dysregulation of metabolic, vascular, and inflammatory pathways." *The Journal of Clinical Endocrinology & Metabolism*, Vol.87, No.9, 4231-4237, 2002.
This report concludes: "...obesity in pregnancy is associated not only with marked hyperinsulinemia (without necessarily glucose dysregulation) and dyslipidemia, but also impaired endothelial function, higher blood pressure, and inflammatory up-regulation."

Melczer R: "Role of tumor necrosis factor in insulin resistance during normal pregnancy." *European Journal of Obstetrics, Gynecology & Reproductive Biology*, Vol.105, Issue 1, pp.7-10, Oct 2002.
This study involving 40 patients concludes: "TNF-alpha may contribute to the insulin resistance during the course of normal pregnancy."

114 **"...biochemical changes associated with obesity, and things can become very difficult for these women hoping to become pregnant..."** – Ferlitsch K et al: "Body mass index, follicle-stimulating hormone and their predictive value in in vitro fertilization." *Journal of Assisted Reproduction & Genetics*, Dec; 21(12):431-6, 2004.
This study involving 171 women concludes: "...obesity and hormonal function may be independent risk factors for failure in assisted reproduction." *See also*:

Lintsen A et al: "Effects of subfertility cause, smoking and body weight on the success rate of IVF." Human Reproduction, Jul; 20(7): 1867-75, 2005.
The success rate of IVF was examined in 8,457 women. Women with a BMI above normal had a significantly lower delivery rate, compared with normal weight women.

114 **"Specialists have recently predicted that already low fertility rates are set to plummet even further because of what it calls an 'obesity crisis.'"** –
"Infertility to rise as obesity crisis widens." Environmental Health News report in *The Age*, July 5, 2004.

Type 2 Diabetes – Both the Result and Possible Cause of Autoimmunity

116 **"According to the U.S. Center for Disease Control, as of 2015 almost one in 10 US adults has diabetes and more than a third has prediabetes."**
www.cdc.gov/diabetes/data/statistics-report

116 **"This excess of 'free-insulin' acts as a toxin within the body. It speeds up cell production on the artery walls, creating conditions for abdominal obesity, hypertension and ultimately, heart disease."** – Hurst R and Lee R: "Increased incidence of coronary atherosclerosis in type 2 diabetes mellitus: mechanisms and management." *Annals of Internal Medicine*, Nov 18; 139(10):824-34, 2003. *See also*:

NOTES

Hollmann M et al: "Impact of waist-hip-ratio and body mass index on hormonal and metabolic parameters in young, obese women." *International Journal of Obesity Related Metabolic Disorders*, 21:476-483, 1997.
Blood analysis of a group of 58 obese women found that the rate of obesity was associated with increased levels of plasma triglycerides, cholesterol, insulin resistance and blood pressure. "Women with android obesity (central obesity or 'apple shape') seemed to be more prone to developing menstrual irregularity and infertility. The hyperinsulinaemia may be the pathway."

116 **"Increased levels of Th1 cytokines and activated CD4+ and CD8+ white blood cells are commonly found in those with type 2 diabetes."** – Stentz F and Kitabchi: A: "Activated T lymphocytes in Type 2 diabetes: implications from in vitro studies." *Current Drug Targets*, Aug; 4(6):493-5503, 2003.
The authors state: "Our studies show that patients with diabetic ketoacidosis and hyperglycemia have increased pro-inflammatory cytokines and activated CD4+ and CD8+ T lymphocytes. The diabetic state, where effective insulin concentrations are low and both glucose and free fatty acids are high, provides an environment of oxidative stress and activation of the inflammatory pathways." *See also*:

Giulietti A et al: "Monocytic expression behavior of cytokines in diabetic patients upon inflammatory stimulation." *Annals of the New York Academy of Science*, Dec; 1037:74-8, 2004.
In this study, type 2 diabetes was shown to present an inflammatory cytokine imbalance. TNF-alpha, IL-1, and IL-6 were elevated in type 2 diabetic patients compared with healthy controls, suggesting an important "pro-inflammatory milieu." *See also*:

Kalousova M: "Oxidative stress, inflammation and autoimmune reaction in type 1 and type 2 diabetes mellitus." *Prague Medical Report*, 105 (1):21-8, 2004.
Advanced oxidation protein products, C-reactive protein and anti-beta glycoprotein-2 antibodies were significantly elevated in patients with type 2 diabetes.

Pickup J: "Inflammation and activated innate immunity in the pathogenesis of type 2 diabetes." *Diabetes Care,* Mar; 27(3):813-23, 2004.
"Activated immunity may be the common antecedent of both type 2 diabetes and atherosclerosis, which probably develop in parallel."

Syed M et al: "Is type 2 diabetes a chronic inflammatory/autoimmune disease?" *Diabetes Nutrition & Metabolism*, Apr; 15(2):68-83, 2002.
Islet-cell autoimmunity, which is characteristic of type 1 diabetes, was found to be present in up to 10 to 15% of those diagnosed clinically with type 2 diabetes. The authors speculated, "If islet-cell autoimmunity is truly present in 10-15% of subjects clinically diagnosed with type 2 diabetes, up to two million Americans might have an unidentified autoimmune form of [the disease]..."

117 **"Glycodelin suppresses NK cell activity in the uterus..."** – Okamoto N et al: "Suppression by human placental protein 14 of natural killer cell activity." *American Journal of Reproductive Immunology*, Dec; 26 (4):137-42, 1991.
(Glycodelin-A is known as placental protein-14 or PP14.) Laboratory testing led to the following conclusion: "PP14 suppresses the function of NK cells, which

NOTES

might be involved in prevention of maternal immune rejection of fetus at the feto-maternal interface." *See also*:

Mishan-Eisenberg G et al: "Differential regulation of Th1/Th2 cytokine responses by placental protein 14." *Journal of Immunology*, Nov 1; 173 (9):5524-30, 2004.
The authors state: "...the T-cell inhibitor placental protein 14 (PP14; glycodelin) preferentially inhibits Th1 cytokine responses and chemokine expression when present during ex vivo priming of CD4+ T-cells... Significantly, PP14 impairs the down-regulation of GATA-3 transcriptional regulator expression that normally accompanies T-cell activation, which is a prerequisite for Th1 development. Taken together, these data document for the first time the ability of PP14 to skew Th responses."

Polycystic Ovary Syndrome – Another Disorder Weighted by Insulin-Resistance

117 **"Polycystic ovarian syndrome (PCOS) is a pre-diabetic condition that is associated with weight gain."** – Norman R et al: "Metabolic approaches to the sub-classification of polycystic ovary syndrome." *Fertility & Sterility*, 63:329-335, 1995.
In 122 patients with PCOS, five clusters were identified: a non-obese group, a moderately obese group and three very obese groups. The non-obese group exhibited the lowest level of insulin. The moderately obese group had the second lowest level of insulin, whereas the three very obese groups had significantly higher levels of insulin. *See also:*

Gonzalez F et al: "In vitro evidence that hyperglycemia stimulates tumor necrosis factor-{alpha} release in obese women with polycystic ovary syndrome." *Journal of Endocrinology*, Mar; 188(3):521-9, 2006.
"Women with polycystic ovary syndrome (PCOS) are often insulin resistant and have chronic low-level inflammation." The researchers note how an increase in TNF-alpha also corresponds to the amount of adipose fat.

117 **"The syndrome affects up to 10% of women..."** – Hart R et al: "Definitions, prevalence and symptoms of polycystic ovaries and poly-cystic ovary syndrome." *Best Practice and Research Clinical Obstetrics & Gynaecology*, Oct; 18(5):671-83, 2004.
"Polycystic ovary syndrome (PCOS) is a common and perplexing endocrine disorder of women in their reproductive years, with a prevalence of up to 10%."

117 **"...around 40% of the sisters and 35% of the mothers of affected women have the syndrome to varying degrees."** – Azziz R and Kashar Miller M: "Family history as a risk factor for the polycystic ovary syndrome." *Journal of Pediatric Endocrinology & Metabolism,* 13, Supplement 5:1303-6, 2000.
In the relatives of 195 PCOS patients, 35% of mothers and 40% of sisters were affected by PCOS themselves. "...the heritability of PCOS is probably more complex, similar to that of diabetes mellitus type 2 and cardiovascular disease."

117 **"PCOS is not just a reproductive problem; it is an important health concern."** – Carmina E and Lobo RA: "Polycystic ovary syndrome (PCOS): arguably the most common endocrinopathy is associated with significant morbidity in women." *Clinical Endocrinology & Metabolism*, Jun; 84(6):1897-9, 1999.

NOTES

The authors state that at the age of menopause, women with PCOS have a high prevalence of diabetes (16%) and hypertension (40%) and are at seven times greater risk of myocardial infarction. Coronary disease is more prevalent in women with PCOS and there is an increased risk of endometrial cancer due to chronic unopposed estrogen exposure in combination with obesity, hypertension and diabetes.

118 **"Elevated levels of insulin prompt the ovaries to produce testosterone..."** – Misugi T et al: "Insulin-lowering agents inhibit synthesis of testosterone in ovaries of DHEA-induced PCOS rats." *Gynecologic and Obstetric Investigation*, Feb 13; 61(4):208-215, 2006.
Testosterone deposits in ovarian tissue were reduced by feeding rats insulin-lowering agents.

118 **"Up to 75% of women with PCOS have insulin resistance."** March W et al: "The prevalence of polycystic ovary syndrome in a community sample assessed under contrasting diagnostic criteria." *Human Reproduction*, Volume 25, Issue 2, 1 February 2010

118 **"In a 2004 study, 36.8% of women with PCOS also had elevated levels of C-reactive protein..."** – Boulman N et al: "Increased C-reactive protein levels in the polycystic ovary syndrome: a marker of cardiovascular disease." *Journal of Clinical Endocrinology & Meta-bolism,* May; 89(5):2160-5, 2004.

118 **"...an excess of insulin can interfere with the normal blood clotting balance, leading to restricted uterine blood flow."** – Chekir C et al: "Impaired uterine perfusion associated with metabolic disorders in women with polycystic ovary syndrome." *Acta Obstetrica et Gyne-cologica Scandinavica,* Feb; 84(2):189-95, 2005.
25 women with PCOS and 45 control women with regular menstrual cycles were compared. Women with PCOS had a significantly higher body mass index and serum testosterone. They also showed insulin resistance, a greater incidence of reduced uterine arterial blood flow and reduced endometrial thickness during the luteal phase.

118 **"Glycodelin...inhibits NK cell and T cell activity."** – Okamoto N et al: "Suppression by human placental protein 14 of natural killer cell activity." *American Journal of Reproductive Immunology,* Dec; 26(4):137-42, 1991. *See also*:

Rachmilewitz J et al: "Placental protein 14 functions as a direct T-cell inhibitor." *Cellular Immunology,* 191:26-33, 1999.

118 **"...low levels of this key protein can increase the chance of miscarriage."** – Dalton C et al: "Endometrial protein PP14 and CA-125 in recurrent miscarriage patients; correlation with pregnancy outcome." *Human Reproduction*, Nov; 13(11):3197-202, 1998.
In this study, the concentrations of PP14 in women with recurrent miscarriage were significantly lower in those who went on to miscarry compared with those who had a livebirth after a subsequent pregnancy. *See also*:

Nestler J et al: "Reduced serum glycodelin and insulin-like growth factor-binding protein-1 in women with polycystic ovary syndrome during first

- 368 -

trimester of pregnancy." *Journal of Clinical Endocrinology & Metabolism*, Feb; 89(2):833-9 2004.

118   **"For women with untreated PCOS...increase the risk of miscarriage by between 30% and 50% during the first trimester."**– Jakubowicz D: "Effects of metformin on early pregnancy loss in the polycystic ovary syndrome." *Journal of Clinical Endocrinology & Metabolism,* Feb; 87(2):524-9, 2002.
65 women received metformin during pregnancy and 31 women did not. The early pregnancy loss rate in the metformin group was 8.8% (6 of 68 pregnancies) compared with 41.9% (13 of 31 pregnancies) in the control group. In women with a prior history of miscarriage, the early pregnancy loss rate was 11.1% (4 of 36 pregnancies) in the metformin group, compared with 58.3% (7 of 12 pregnancies) in the control group.

118   **"...several PCOS-related cellular dysfunctions are associated with autoimmunity, including higher circulating levels of inflammatory mediators such as TNF-alpha."** – Dhindsa G et al: "Insulin resistance, insulin sensitization and inflammation in polycystic ovarian syndrome."
Journal of Postgraduate Medicine, Apr-Jun; 50(2):140-4, 2004.
"Recent studies have shown that PCOS women have higher circulating levels of inflammatory mediators like C-reactive protein, tumor necrosis factor-alpha, tissue plasminogen activator and plasminogen activator inhibitor-1." *See also*:

Reimand K: "Autoantibody studies of female patients with reproductive failure." *Journal of Reproductive Immunology*, Aug; 51(2):167-76, 2001.
This study included 108 women with menstrual cycle disturbances, polycystic ovaries and polycystic ovary syndrome. The results indicated a high prevalence of autoimmune reactions in this group.

van Gelderen C and Gomes dos Santos M: "Polycystic ovarian syndrome: evidence for an autoimmune mechanism in some cases." *Journal of Reproductive Medicine,* May; 38(5):381-6, 1993.
"Antiovarian autoantibodies localized to the granulosa cells were detected in 50% of a group of eight patients diagnosed with polycystic ovarian syndrome."

Amato G et al: "Serum and follicular fluid cytokines in polycystic ovary syndrome during stimulated cycles." *Obstetrics & Gynecology* Jun; 101 (6):1177-82, 2003.
31 patients with PCOS undergoing IVF were compared with 39 age-matched controls. The patients with PCOS had higher serum and follicular fluid TNF-alpha IL-6 concentrations and lower follicular fluid estradiol levels than the control group.

Antibodies to Neurotransmitters

120   **"Women who have difficulty conceiving or suffer early pregnancy losses can have levels well above 10%."** – Beer AE et al: "Immunophenotypic profiles of peripheral blood lymphocytes in women with recurrent pregnancy losses and in infertile women with multiple failed in vitro fertilization cycles." *American Journal of Reproductive Immunology,* Apr; 35(4):376-82, 1996.
"Infertile and recurrent spontaneous abortion women who fail alloimmune and autoimmune therapy have significant alterations in cellular and humoral immunity involving NK cells and CD19+/CD5+ B cells."

NOTES

When Autoimmunity Gets Depressing

121 **"Studies have also shown that women deplete their serotonin more rapidly than men..."** – Nishizawa S et al: "Differences between males and females in rates of serotonin synthesis in human brain." *Procedures of the National Academy of Science U.S.A.*, 94(10):5308-5313, 1997.
"The mean rate of synthesis in normal males was found to be 52% higher than in normal females; this marked difference may be a factor relevant to the lower incidence of major unipolar depression in males." *See also*:

Muck-Seler D et al: "Sex differences, season of birth and platelet 5-HT levels in schizophrenic patients." *Journal of Neural Transmission,* 106 (3-4):337-347, 1999.
Platelet 5-HT concentrations in 116 control subjects were significantly higher in men than in women.

121 **"...around the middle of a normal 28-day cycle, endorphins and enkaphlins (natural opiates and pain relievers) help prepare the uterine lining..."** – Wahlstrom T et al: "Immunoreactive beta-endorphin is demonstrable in the secretory but not in the proliferative endometrium." *Life Science*, Mar 11; 36(10):987-90, 1985.
The presence of endorphins in the endometrium was studied at various stages of the menstrual cycle. Endorphins were found in the endometrium during the secretory phase of the cycle but not in the proliferative phase or during the first three postovulatory days of the cycle. *See also*:

Petraglia F: "Endogenous opioid peptides in uterine fluid." Fertility & Sterility, Aug; 46(2):247-51, 1986.
This study demonstrates that concentrations of enkephalins in the uterine fluid of fertile women are higher in the secretory than in the proliferative phase of the menstrual cycle.

121 **"Serotonin relaxes the vessels in the uterus, increasing the blood circulation so the embryo can implant successfully."** – Cohen M and Wittenauer L: "Serotonin receptor activation of phosphoinositide turnover in uterine fundal vascular and tracheal smooth muscle." *Journal of Cardiovascular Pharmacology*, 10:176-181, 1987.
This study was designed to explore the effects of serotonin to enhance phosphoinositide turnover in several smooth muscle preparations. Serotonin produced significant elevations of smooth muscle cell proliferation in the rat uterus. *See also*:

Pakala R et al: "Effect of serotonin, thromboxane A_2, and specific receptor antagonists on vascular smooth muscle cell proliferation." *Circulation,* 96:2280-2286, 1997.
"Stimulation of endothelial cells by 5-HT resulted in an increase in tritiated thymidine uptake and an increase in cell number..."

Maekawa F and Yamanouchi K: "Effect of deprivation of serotonin by pchlorophenylalanine on induction and maintenance of pseudo-pregnancy in female rats." *Brain Research Bulletin*, 39(5):317- 21, 1996.

The effect of serotonin on deciduoma formation was examined in female rats. The study showed that "some levels of serotonin are required to induce and maintain pseudopregnancy."

121 **"Serotonin may also play a role in egg maturation and the early cellular development phase of the embryo."** – Amireault P and Dube F: "Serotonin and its antidepressant sensitive transport in mouse cumulus-oocyte complexes and early embryos." *Biology of Reproduction*, April 27, 2005.
This study indicates that "5-HT may be produced locally by cumulus cells and that it can be actively taken up by mammalian oocytes and embryos as part of a likely larger serotonergic network possibly regulating various developmental processes much earlier than previously thought."

121 **"...serotonin is an important regulator of TNF-alpha production..."** – Kubera M et al: "Effects of serotonin and serotonergic agonists and antagonists on the production of tumor necrosis factor alpha and interleukin-6." *Psychiatry Research,* Apr 30; 134(3):251-8, 2005.
In this study, the researchers found 5-HT significantly decreased IL-6 and TNF-alpha production. *See also*:

Pollak Y and Yirmiya R: "Cytokine-induced changes in mood and behaviour: implications for 'depression due to a general medical condition', immunotherapy and antidepressive treatment." *Brain, Behavior & Immunity*, Oct; 16(5):544, 2002.
This report states that evidence to indicate that depression is cytokine-mediated includes: (1) Depression is highly prevalent in various medical conditions, including infectious, autoimmune and neurodegenerative diseases; (2) Experiments in humans and in animals demonstrate that exposure to cytokines induces depressive-like mood and behavioral alterations; (3) Cytokine immunotherapy in cancer and hepatitis patients elicits a major depressive episode in a large percentage of the patients; (4) Several types of depression that are not directly associated with a physical disease (e.g., major depression, melancholia, dysthymia) are also associated with cytokine hypersecretion; (5) Antidepressant drugs possess anti-inflammatory characteristics, which may partly account for their therapeutic effect.

121 **"...antidepressant medication has been shown to regulate the inflammatory immune response."** – Szuster-Ciesielska A et al: "In vitro immunoregulatory effects of antidepressants in healthy volunteers." *Polish Journal of Pharmacology*, May-Jun; 55(3):353-62, 2003.
A study of 16 healthy volunteers was carried out to observe the effect of antidepressant medication on the in vitro production of Th1-like cytokines. "The results indicate that antidepressants exert immunoregulatory effects on human leukocyte functions, especially on cytokine production." *See also*:

Kenis G and Maes M: "Effects of antidepressants on the production of cytokines." – *International Journal of Neuropsychopharmacology*, Dec; 5(4):401-12, 2002.
"There is now evidence that major depression is associated with an up-regulation of the inflammatory response system...and the hyper-production of pro-inflammatory cytokines...Current data indicate a normalization of cytokine plasma levels and cytokine production after antidepressant treatment."

NOTES

121 **"Indeed, several studies have described a link between depression and bleeding in pregnancy, preeclampsia..."** – Preti A et al: "Obstetric complications in patients with depression – a population-based case-control study." *Journal of Affective Disorders,* 61:101-6, 2000. *See also*:
Chung TK et al: "Antepartum depressive symptomatology is associated with adverse obstetric and neonatal outcomes." *Psychosomatic Medicine,* 63(5): 830-4, 2001.

Zarajskaya M et al: "Peculiarities of biogenic amines supply of placental cellular structures during chronic placental insufficiency." *Frontiers in Fetal Health,* Vol.3 May 2001.
45 placentas were taken from 30 patients with chronic placental insufficiency and 15 patients with normal pregnancy. Placental serotonin levels in the study group were significantly lower than in the control group. The greatest difference in serotonin concentrations was seen in fetal membranes.

121 **"Low levels of serotonin are also associated with increased sensitivity to the effects of stress..."** – Bethea C et al: "Sensitivity to stress-induced reproductive dysfunction linked to activity of the serotonin system." *Obstetrics Gynecology Survey,* Jul; 60(7):448-450, 2005.
"Highly stress-resistant animals have higher endogenous serotonin levels than do stress-sensitive animals in the absence of stress." *See also*:
Coplan J et al: "Plasma anti-serotonin and serotonin anti-idiotypic antibodies are elevated in panic disorder." *Neuropsychopharmacology,* 20; 386-391,10:1038, 1999.

Autoimmunity Can Be a Real Headache

122 **"[Migraine headaches] are...more prevalent in those suffering from depression."** – Gesztelyi G: "Primary headache and depression." *Orvosi Hetilap (Budapest),* Nov 28; 145(48):2419-24, 2004.
"Depression is more prevalent in headache patients than in the headache-free population. Prospective epidemiological studies suggest a common genetic, biochemical or environmental background behind primary headaches and depression. This theory is supported by the role of the same neurotransmitter systems (mostly serotonin and dopamine) in headaches as well as in depression."

122 **"The size of the cerebral arteries and blood vessels is partly regulated by serotonin..."** – Bonvento G et al: "Serotonergic innervation of the cerebral vasculature: relevance to migraine and ischaemia." *Brain Research,* Sep-Dec; 16(3):257-63, 1991.
"Multiple and complex interactions exist between the cerebral circulation and a potent vasoactive (and neurotransmitter) agent, serotonin...It appears that, by its very nature, the pattern of the serotonergic innervation is singular to blood vessels of the brain..."

123 **"High concentrations of TNF-alpha and the cells that produce it are often present in those with migraines..."** – Perini F et al: "Plasma cytokine levels in migraineurs and controls." *Headache,* Jul-Aug; 45 (7):926-31, 2005.
In 25 migraine patients, circulating levels of IL-10, TNF-alpha, and IL-1 beta during attacks were significantly higher in comparison to their levels outside attacks. *See also:*

- 372 -

NOTES

Martelletti P et al: "Pro-inflammatory pathways in cervicogenic head-ache." *Clinical & Experimental Rheumatology,* Mar-Apr; 18(2 Suppl. 19):S33-8, 2000. "Cervicogenic headache (CEH) is a relatively common form of head-ache arising from the neck structures...Higher levels of both IL-1 beta and TNF-alpha were detected in the sera of CEH patients than the levels in patients with migraine without aura and in healthy subjects."

123 **"...inflammatory cytokines and antibodies to neurotransmitters are the hallmarks of other classic manifestations of autoimmunity..."** – Pizova N: "Cerebral vascular pathology in systemic sclerosis." *Zh Nevrol Psikhiatr Im S S Korsakova,* 104(4):19-23, 2004.
In 30 patients with systemic sclerosis, 83% had hemispheric asymmetry of blood flow and difficulties with venous outflow. *See also*:

Chaudhuri A and Behan P: "The clinical spectrum, diagnosis, pathogenesis and treatment of Hashimoto's encephalopathy (recurrent acute disseminated encephalomyelitis)." *Current Medicinal Chemistry,* Oct; 10(19):1945-53, 2003. "Hashimoto's encephalopathy may present with a wide variety of different neurological symptoms and signs. These include recurrent severe migrainous headache..."

Weder-Cisneros N et al: "Prevalence and factors associated with headache in patients with systemic lupus erythematosus." *Cephalalgia,* Dec; 24(12):1031-44, 2004.
"Headache is common in systemic lupus erythematosus with reported prevalence as high as 70%...In systemic lupus erythematosus patients the risk factors associated with headaches were Raynaud's phenomenon..."

123 **"Serotonin reuptake inhibitors (antidepressants) are more effective..."** – Ferrari M et al: "Oral triptans (serotonin 5-HT agonists) in acute migraine treatment: A meta-analysis of 53 trials." *Lancet*, 358: 1668–1675, 2001.
In 53 trials involving 24,089 patients, up to 67% reported relief of headache pain, compared with 13% taking a placebo. "The triptans, selective serotonin 5-HT (1B/1D) agonists, are very effective acute migraine drugs with a well-developed scientific rationale." *See also*:

Diamond M et al: "Antidepressants suppress production of the Th1 cytokine interferon-gamma, independent of monoamine transporter blockade." *European Neuropsychopharmacology,* Dec 30, 2005.
"...our results indicate that IFN-gamma producing T-cells (Th1 cells) are the major target for the immunomodulatory actions of antidepressants..."

123 **"Migraines can also be aggravated by restricted blood flow as a result of thrombophilia."** – Kowa H et al: "The homozygous C677T mutation in the methylenetetrahydrofolate reductase gene is a genetic risk factor for migraine." *American Journal of Medical Genetics (Neuropsychiatry & Genetics)*, 96:762-764, 2000.
This study was designed to determine the prevalence of the MTHFR mutation in 74 patients with migraine and tension-type headaches. The incidence of the gene mutation in migraine sufferers (20.3%) was significantly higher than that in controls (9.6%). The incidence of MTHFR in people with migraine headaches with aura was 40.9%. *See also*:

NOTES

Wammes-van der Heijden E et al: "A thromboembolic predisposition and the effect of anticoagulants on migraine." *Headache,* May; 44(5): 399-402, 2004.
Four migraine sufferers with one or more thromboembolic risk factors were treated with anticoagulants. Two patients, both with factor V Leiden heterozygosity, experienced a clear improvement of migraine. "...migraine, as a phenotype, has different underlying mechanisms, amongst which is a thromboembolic tendency."

Raynaud's Syndrome

124   **"Women with inherited thrombophilia are particularly prone to this condition..."** – Regeczy N et al: "The Leiden mutation of coagulation factor V in Hungarian SLE patients." *Clinical & Applied Thrombosis/Hemostasis*, Jan; 6(1):41-5, 2000.
120 patients were studied. Patients with the factor V Leiden mutation had a significantly higher prevalence of fetal losses and higher prevalence of Raynaud's syndrome.

124   **"...this syndrome occurs in up to 95% of people with scleroderma (which itself is strongly associated with the over expression of autoantibody producing CD19 B cells)."** – Excerpt from "Momentum builds with key Raynaud's discovery." *Scleroderma Research Foundation*, 2000. *See also*:

Tsuchiya N et al: "Association of a functional CD19 polymorphism with susceptibility to systemic sclerosis." *Arthritis & Rheumatology*, Dec; 50 (12): 4002-7, 2004.

125   **"Immunotherapy with anti-inflammatory and antidepressant medica-tions..."** – Robertson J.: "Serotonergic type-2(5-HT2) antagonists: a novel class of cardiovascular drugs." *Journal of Cardiovascular Pharmacology,* 17 Suppl. 5:S48-53, 1991.
"Serotonin, acting via the 5-HT2 receptor, can contribute to a range of cardiovascular problems including portal hypertension, Raynaud's phenomenon... 5-HT2 antagonists have a potential therapeutic role in all these conditions." *See also*:

Buecking A et al: "Treatment of Raynaud's phenomenon with escitalopram." *International Journal of Neuropsychopharmacology,* Jun; 8(2): 307-8, 2005.
"Serotonin has been shown to play a significant role in diseases related to vascular dysregulation like Raynaud's phenomenon (Hollenberg, 1988)...In recent years, there have been several reports on the efficacy of the selective serotonin reuptake inhibitors (SSRIs) fluoxetine (Coleiro et al., 2001; Jaffe, 1995; Rey et al., 2003) and sertraline (Rey et al., 2003) in the treatment of Raynaud's phenomenon."

Coleiro B et al: "Treatment of Raynaud's phenomenon with the selective serotonin reuptake inhibitor fluoxetine." *Rheumatology (Oxford),* Sep; 40(9):1038-43, 2001.
26 patients with primary and 27 patients with secondary Raynaud's phenomenon were assigned randomly to receive 6 weeks of treatment with fluoxetine (20 mg daily) or nifedipine...A significant improvement in the thermographic response to cold challenge was also seen in female patients with primary Raynaud's phenomenon treated with fluoxetine..."

NOTES

The Wreckage That Is Left After a B-Cell Blitz – Chronic Fatigue Syndrome and Fibromyalgia

126 **"...60 to 80% of T cells are activated, compared to a healthy person where 80% are resting."** – From a lecture by Dr N. Klimas, MD of the University of Miami Medical Center. Dr Klimas spoke at the Massa-chusetts CFIDS Spring Lecture Series on April 27. Nancy Klimas is editor of the *Journal of Chronic Fatigue Syndrome* and President of the American Association of Chronic Fatigue Syndrome.

126 **"...many of the symptoms and clinical characteristics of fibromyalgia closely match those of CFS."** – Buchwald D: "Fibromyalgia and chronic fatigue syndrome: similarities and differences." *Rheumatic Disease Clinics of North America*, May; 22(2):219-43, 1996.

126 **"In both conditions, there are elevated levels of antibodies to serotonin."** – Klein R and Berg P: "High incidence of antibodies to 5-hydroxytryptamine, gangliosides and phospholipids in patients with chronic fatigue and fibromyalgia syndrome and their relatives: evidence for a clinical entity of both disorders." *European Journal of Medical Research*, Oct 16; 1(1):21-6, 1995. Autoantibodies to serotonin were previously found in 73% of 100 patients with FMS. 62% of the CFS patients had antibodies to serotonin. *See also*:

Klein R et al: "Clinical relevance of antibodies against serotonin and ganglio-sides in patients with primary fibromyalgia syndrome." *Psychoneuro-endocrinology*, 17(6):593-8, 1992.
50 fibromyalgia patients were tested for non-organ-specific and organ-specific antibodies. 74% had antibodies against serotonin.

Yamamoto S et al: "Reduction of serotonin transporters of patients with chronic fatigue syndrome." *Neuroreport,* Dec 3; 15(17):2571-4, 2004.
It was observed that the density of serotonin transporters in the brain was significantly reduced in patients with chronic fatigue syndrome. "...an alteration of serotonergic system...plays a key role in patho-physiology of chronic fatigue syndrome."

126 **"...up to two-thirds of sufferers experiencing prior or concurrent major depression."** – Manu P et al: "Food intolerance in patients with chronic fatigue." *International Journal of Eating Disorders*, 13:203-209, 1993.
In 54 patients with CFS, approximately 65% suffered from depressive disorders. *See also*:

Lane T et al: "Depression and somatization in the chronic fatigue syndrome." *American Journal of Medicine*, 91:335-344, 1991.
"Patients with CFS have a high prevalence of unrecognized, current psychiatric disorders, which often predate their fatigue syndrome."

126 **"High cytokine levels are typically associated with CFS and fibromyalgia."** – Wallace D et al: "Cytokines play an aetiopathogenetic role in fibromyalgia: a hypothesis and pilot study." *Rheumatology*, 40:743-749, 2001.
In this study, it was found that patients who were sick for over two years were more likely to have high cytokine levels, which increased with the duration of the sickness.

NOTES

126 "...triggers for all this immunological mayhem can include exposure to a viral or bacterial infection or a reaction to environmental toxins..." – Chia J: "The role of enterovirus in chronic fatigue syndrome." *Clinical Pathology,* Nov; 58(11):1126-32, 2005.
A summary of the available experimental and clinical evidence that supports the role of enterovirus in chronic fatigue syndrome. *See also*:

Knox K et al: "Persistent active human herpes virus (HHV6) infections in patients with CFS." *AACFS Proceedings: Cambridge, MA*, Oct; 10-12, 1998.

Buchwald D and Garrity D: "Comparison of patients with chronic fatigue syndrome, fibromyalgia, and multiple chemical sensitivities." *Archives of Internal Medicine*, Sep 26; 154 (18):2049-53, 1994.
"Chronic fatigue syndrome (CFS), fibromyalgia (FM), and multiple chemical sensitivities (MCS) are conditions associated with fatigue and a variety of other symptoms that appear to share many clinical and demographic features... Symptoms that are considered typical of each disorder are prevalent in the other two conditions."

126 "...antibodies to phospholipids have been detected in 90% of those with the disease and are equally prevalent among CFS sufferers." – Berg D et al: "Chronic fatigue syndrome (CFS) &/or fibromyalgia (FM) as a variation of antiphospholipid antibody syndrome (APS): An explanatory model and approach to laboratory diagnosis." *Blood Coagulation & Fibrinolysis,* 10: pp.1-4, 1999. *See also*:

Berg D et al: "Is CFS/FM due to an undefined hypercoagulable state brought on by immune activation of coagulation? Does adding anti-coagulant therapy improve CFS/FM patient symptoms?" *AACFS Proceedings: Cambridge, MA,* Oct; 10-12, p.62, 1998.
"CFS &/or FM patients who have a hereditary deficiency for thrombophilia or hypofibrinolysis may be unable to control thrombin generation properly. We have found that 3 out of 4 CFS &/or FM patients have a genetic deficiency (unpublished data)...Since this hypercoagulable state does not necessarily result in a thrombosis, but rather in fibrin deposition, we suggest that an alternative name for this antiphospholipid antibody process would be Immune System Activation of Coagulation (ISAC)." This retrospective study of 20 patients also demonstrates that a hypercoagulable state and symptoms of CFS/ fibromyalgia can be successfully treated with anticoagulant therapies.

126 "...the results of a retrospective study of over 400 chronically ill patients showed that 83% had one or more coagulation protein defects." – Berg D: Data presented at the International Society of Thrombosis and Hemostasis meeting, July 2001.

11. HOPE FOR OLDER MOTHERS TO BE

129 "What is not so well known is that the loss of chromosomally normal fetuses also increases." – Stein D et al: "Maternal age and spontaneous abortion." Source: pp.107-127, *Human Embryonic and Fetal Death* by Porter IH and Hook EB. Published by Academic Press in 1980. ISBN: 0125628609.

NOTES

129 **"...it moves away from the reproductive mode to the pathogen-defense mode of an older woman."** – Hasler P and Zouali M: "Immune receptor signaling, aging, and autoimmunity." *Cellular Immunology,* Feb; 233(2):102-8, 2005.
"With advancing age, the immune system undergoes changes that predispose to autoimmune reactivity." *See also*:

Goronzy J et al: "Telomeres, immune aging and autoimmunity." *Experimental Gerontology,* Mar; 41(3):246-51, 2006.
"...accelerated T-cell aging combined with telomeric shortening may predispose for autoimmune responses and thereby explain the increased susceptibility for chronic inflammatory diseases in the elderly."

129 **"Immunotherapy has been shown to reduce the rate of miscarriage in older women and to improve the success rates of those receiving donor eggs."** – Beer AE et al: "Impact of age on reproductive outcome in women with recurrent spontaneous abortions and infertility of immune etiology." *American Journal of Reproductive Immunology*, Apr; 35(4):408-14, 1996.
124 women with 3 or more recurrent miscarriages and 36 women with unexplained infertility were studied. The report concludes: "Age does not affect pregnancy outcome or conception rate in women with repetitive spontaneous abortion. In women with infertility of immune etiology, conception rate was significantly reduced over age 40, although pregnancy outcome was no different with advanced age."

129 **"In IVF, the ovarian response to fertility treatment can predict the likely outcome in women with both a normal and abnormal ovarian reserve."** – Yih M et al: "Egg production predicts a doubling of in vitro fertilization pregnancy rates even within defined age and ovarian reserve categories." *Fertility & Sterility,* Jan; 83(1):24-9, 2005.
"In an age-independent fashion, ovarian response is highly predictive of IVF outcome in women with normal and abnormal ovarian reserve. These findings highlight the importance of not solely relying on age when presenting and discussing IVF outcome data and are useful information when helping patients interpret their IVF cycle response."

129 **"Therefore, age is not the absolute determining factor in predicting a woman's chances of success."** – Akande V et al: "Biological versus chronological aging of oocytes distinguishable by raised FSH levels in relation to the success of IVF treatment." *Human Reproduction*, Vol.17, No.8, 2003-2008, Aug 2002.
1,019 infertile but ovulating women were studied in their first cycle of IVF treatment. The study concludes that ovarian aging could occur independently of chronological age and that serum basal FSH measurements were a valuable prognostic indicator.

130 **"If the FSH is below 12 and the estradiol 35 or below, a fertile cycle will usually follow."** – Ashrafi M et al: "Follicle-stimulating hormone as a predictor of ovarian response in women undergoing controlled ovarian hyperstimulation for IVF." *International Journal of Gynecology & Obstetrics*, Oct; 91(1):53-7, 2005.
In this study of 212 IVF cycles, the number of follicles, oocytes retrieved and embryos transferred was found to correspond with the level of luteinizing

NOTES

hormone. Higher levels were associated with a greater number of canceled cycles. The researchers concluded: "...day 3 serum FSH level was a predictor of ovarian response and IVF outcome in this study."

130 **"In a study of women aged 45 and over who had conceived spontaneously and experienced successful pregnancies, it was discovered that they possessed a distinctive genetic profile."** – Laufer et al: "Enrichment of DNA repair genes expression in women conceiving spontaneously after the age of 45." *European Society for Human Reproduction & Embryology 21st Annual Meeting*, presented June 21, 2005.
250 participants over the age of 45 had a large number of children and a low miscarriage rate. These factors indicated they had a natural ability to escape the aging process of the ovaries. The investigators identified 716 genes that were different in the highly fertile group compared with the controls. They observed: "These women have a distinctive genetic makeup that protects them from the DNA damage and cellular aging that leads to a decline in oocyte quantity and quality."

130 **"So to assess how much longer a woman will remain fertile she should look to her own mother as a guide."** – van Asselt K et al "Heritability of menopausal age in mothers and daughters." *Fertility and Sterility*, Nov; 82(5):1348-51, 2004.
In this study of 164 mother-daughter pairs, a heritability of 44% for natural age of menopause was estimated.

A Case of Bad Eggs? The Age-Old Question

130 **"The older half of my patient population is close to 40 years of age and has failed IVF more than three times."** – January 2006 statistics based on Dr Beer's own data. This figure is analyzed monthly, and has not varied significantly over the past three years.

130 **"According to a 2013 "ART Fertility Clinic Success Rates Report.."**
https://www.cdc.gov/art/pdf/2013-report/art-2013-fertility-clinic-report.pdf

131 **"Consequently, the ovary is considered to be one of the fastest aging organs in a woman's body."** – Brann D and Mahesh V: "The aging reproductive neuroendocrine axis." *Steroids*, Apr; 70(4): 273-83, 2005.
"It is well known that the reproductive system is one of the first biological systems to show age-related decline."

131 **"Researchers at Harvard Medical School discovered, by observing mice, that ovaries harbor a previously undiscovered type of stem cell..."** – Johnson J et al: "Germline stem cells and follicular renewal in the postnatal mammalian ovary." *Nature*, August 26; 430(7003): 1062, 2004.
"Young and adult mouse ovaries possess germ cells that continuously replenish the follicle pool...these data establish the existence of proliferative germ cells that sustain oocyte and follicle production in the post-natal mammalian ovary."
See also:
Bazer F: "Strong science challenges conventional wisdom: new perspectives on ovarian biology." *Reproductive Biology & Endocrinology*, 2 (1):28, 2004.
"...in addition to providing new directions to explore with respect to elucidating the biology of mammalian female germ stem cells, this work has significant

NOTES

clinical implications related to the therapeutic expansion of the follicular reserve as a means to postpone normal and premature ovarian failure."

131 **"In this 2004 study, whose finding have since been confirmed by other research teams..."** – "Making new eggs in old mice" by Maher B, *Nature*, April 2009. *See also*:

Powell K: "Egg-making stem cells found in adult ovaries." *Nature*, Feb 2012

131 **"Associate Professor Ray Rodgers, former President of the Endocrine Society of Australia supports the discovery..."** – Rodgers R and Russell D: "Extracellular matrix of the developing ovarian follicle." *Reproduction, 126*; 415-424, 2003.
"Ovaries can be considered tissues in which endocrine organs – follicles and corpora lutea – continually grow and regress." *See also*:

Rodgers R et al: "Development of the ovarian follicular epithelium." *Molecular & Cellular Endocrinology*, May 25; 151(1-2):171-9, 1999.
In this review, the authors state that the growth and development of ovarian follicles occurs postnatally and throughout adult life. The follicular epithelium has similarities to other epithelia in the body, but is more dynamic.

132 **"The first attempts to analyze the chromosomal content of human female eggs were made in the early 1970s..."** – Pellestor F et al: "The chromosomal analysis of human oocytes: An overview of established procedures." *Human Reproduction Update*, 11(1):15-32, 2005.

132 **"...for women aged 40 to 45, chromosomal defects could affect between 70 and 80% of their eggs..."** – Battaglia D et al: "Influence of maternal age on meiotic spindle assembly in oocytes from naturally cycling women." *Human Reproduction*, Oct; 11(10):2217-22, 1996.
In this study, 79% of the oocytes from the older group (aged 40-45 years) exhibited abnormal chromosomal characteristics while only 17% of the oocytes from the younger age group (aged 20-25 years) have these problems. *See also*:

Miyara F et al: "Multi-parameter analysis of human oocytes at metaphase II stage after IVF failure in non-male infertility." *Human Reproduction*, Vol.18, No.7, 1494-1503, Jul 2003.
The authors observed that the incidence of spindle and chromosome aberrations was strongly influenced by maternal age: 69% for 40- to 45- year-old women versus 35% for 26- to 33-year-olds.

132 **"...later in life, aging and cancer occur because of chromosomal anomalies caused by DNA damage and faulty DNA repair mechanisms."** – Friedberg, EC et al: *DNA Repair and Mutagenesis*. 2nd edition published by ASM Press in 2005. ISBN: 1555813194. *See also*:

Stewart R: "The Nature of a Fatal DNA Lesion." PNNL-SA-30810, June 25, 2001. See:
http://www.pnl.gov/berc/bg/fatal_lesion.html.

- 379 -

NOTES

Levy D et al: "Comparing DNA damage-processing pathways by computer analysis of chromosome painting data." *Journal of Computational Biology*, Vol. 11, No. 4: 626-641, 2004.
"Chromosome aberrations are large-scale illegitimate rearrangements of the genome. They are indicative of DNA damage and informative about damage processing pathways."

Raffoul J et al: "Effect of age on the up-regulation of base excision repair (BER) in response to 2-nitropropane (2-NP)-induced oxidative stress." *The Federation of American Societies for Experimental Biology Journal*, 2002.
"The reduction in DNA repair capacity is a proposed mechanism under-lying aging and cancer phenotypes in mammalian species."

132 **"It is hypothesized that DNA damaging agents…are behind the inability of chromosomes to segregate successfully."** – Takada S et al: "Drosophila checkpoint kinase 2 couples centrosome function and spindle assembly to genomic integrity." *Cell*, Apr 4; 113(1):87-99, 2003.
In this review, it is reported that damaged or incompletely replicated DNA triggers centrosome disruption in mitosis, leading to defects in spindle assembly and chromosome segregation. *See also*:

Sibon et al: "DNA-replication/DNA-damage-dependent centrosome inactivation in Drosophila embryos." *Nature Cell Biology*, Feb; 2(2):90-5, 2000.
During early embryogenesis mutations in the DNA-replication check-point lead to chromosome-segregation failures.

132 **"These same harmful influences are also responsible for DNA fragmentation…"** – Wu J et al: "Maturation and apoptosis of human oocytes in vitro are age-related." *Fertility & Sterility*, Dec; 74(6):1137-41, 2000.
In this study of oocytes in women aged from 21 to 50, the researchers conclude: "DNA fragmentation in oocytes associated with apoptotic death might be one of the reasons for poor oocyte quality and lower fertility in older women." *See also*:

Lim A and Tsakok M: "Age-related decline in fertility: a link to degenerative oocytes?" *Fertility & Sterility*, Aug; 68(2):265-71, 1997.
Unfertilized eggs from 151 women (ages 24 to 44 years) undergoing IVF were analyzed. Oocyte chromosome degeneration, characterized by chromosomes splitting into unassociated chromatids, was observed with increasing age. "…age-related decline in fertility may be due more to degenerative oocytes than to aneuploidy."

132 **"The consensus here is that exposure to TNF-alpha produced by the NK cells is associated with deterioration in egg quality, and poor fertilization results."** – Nikolettos N et al: "Evaluation of leptin, interleukin-1beta, tumor necrosis factor-alpha and vascular endothelial growth factor in serum and follicular fluids of women undergoing controlled ovarian hyperstimulation as prognostic markers of ICSI outcome." *In Vivo*, Sep-Oct; 18(5):667-73, 2004.
The investigators concluded: "…serum TNF-alpha was negatively correlated with fertilization rate." *See also*:

Soto P et al: "Actions of tumor necrosis factor-alpha on oocyte maturation and embryonic development in cattle." *American Journal of Reproductive Immunology*, Vol.50; Issue 5, p.380, Nov 2003.
"TNF-alpha can have deleterious actions on oocyte maturation that compromise development of the resultant embryo."

Kim WW et al: "Relationships between concentrations of tumor necrosis factor-alpha and nitric oxide in follicular fluid and oocyte quality." *Assisted Reproduction & Genetics*, April; 17(4):222-8, 2000.
The concentration of TNF-alpha was measured in 115 follicular fluid samples collected from 43 patients undergoing IVF. TNF-alpha concentrations in follicular fluids were significantly higher in poor quality oocytes. "TNF-alpha levels…influence oocyte quality."

Braverman J: "Follicular fluid cytokine measurements: another window nto diagnosis and therapy for our patients." March 2015.
www.preventmiscarriage.com/follicular-fluid-cytokine-measurements "Many patients with immune issues have altered cytokine levels in the serum and abdominal cavity. Measurement of FF cytokine levels at the time of egg retrieval will allow us to adapt immune therapy in subsequent IVF stimulations, compare changes in FF cytokine composition and assess the efficacy of treatment… Altogether, this will help minimize the rate of failed embryo transfers due to the quality of eggs developed. We are currently developing tailored-strategy therapies to manipulate the follicular fluid components, improve egg quality and increase the chance of a successful pregnancy.

Winger E, Reed J et al: "The preconception TNF-α:IL-10 ratio, an immmuno-logic marker correlated with a marker of poor egg quality." *American Journal of Reproductive Immunology*, Nov;68(5):428-37, 2012
Egg to embryo die-off ratio may offer an additional tool to help improve implantation rate, clinical pregnancy rate, live birth rate, and live birth rate per embryo transferred for an upcoming IVF cycle. Although many mechanisms may contribute to a high die-off ratio's negative effect on IVF success rates, its correlation with elevated preconception TNF-α:IL-10 ratio and correction with Humira suggests a strong immunologic component that may be treatable.

133   **"It has beens shown that the highest IVF success rates are achieved when the last anti-TNF injection is given 61–120 days before the day of IVF transfer"** – Winger E, Reed J et al: "Degree of TNF-α/IL-10 Cytokine Elevation Correlates With IVF Success Rates in Women Undergoing Treatment With Adalimumab (Humira) and IVIG," *American Journal of Reproductive Immunology*, Jun;65(6):610-8, 2011.
In women with TNF/Il1- elevation and infertility, the highest IVF success rates were achieved when the last injection of Humira was given 61–120 days before the day of IVF transfer rather than the closer time point of 0–60 days (although the group with the 0–60 day time point still achieved better success rates than the group using no Humira or IVIG at all). It appears that much of Humira's effect is unrelated to implantation and may be related.

134   **"Women with endometriosis are particularly prone to such problems…"** – El-Hendy U et al: "Peritoneal fluid embryotoxicity and tumor necrosis factor alpha level in endometriosis associated infertility." 2003 report at:

www.gfmer.ch/International_activities_En/El_Mowafi/PF_Endometriosis.html
See also:
Velasco I et al: "Embryotoxicity of peritoneal fluid in women with endometriosis: its relation with cytokines and lymphocyte populations." *Human Reproduction*, Mar; 17(3):777-81, 2002.

Bullimore D: "Endometriosis is sustained by tumor necrosis factor-alpha." *Medical Hypotheses*, Jan; 60(1):84-8, 2003.
This study presents evidence to suggest that abnormal production of TNF-alpha is required for the establishment and maintenance of endometriosis and is responsible for the associated infertility through its effect on sperm motility and function and oocyte development.

12. IMMUNE PROBLEMS AND PREGNANCY

135 **"A quadruple screen...should be performed at approximately 16 weeks' gestation..."** – For more information see:
http://www.dynagene.com/education/patmsqs.html

137 **"Calcification or 'grittiness' is a sign of placental aging and inflammatory immune activity."** – Imad Nadra et al: "Pro-inflammatory activation of macrophages by basic calcium phosphate crystals via protein kinase C and MAP kinase pathways: A vicious cycle of inflammation and arterial calcification?" *Circulation Research,* 96: 1248, 2005. *See also:*

Varma V and Kim K: "Placental calcification: ultrastructural and X-ray microanalytic studies." *Journal of Scanning Electron Micros-copies,* (Pt 4):1567-72, 1985.
In this study, it was shown that calcification is not just a consequence of chronic inflammatory disease but can also promote further inflammation. 11 human placentas were studied to elucidate the mechanism of placental calcification. The pattern of calcification was similar to that seen in other tissues.

The Inherent Risks (and Benefits) of Autoimmunity

139 **"... mental health problems affect approximately 10% of U.S. preschool children"** – Professor A. Angold, Associate Professor of Psychiatry at Duke University Medical Center in North Carolina, presenting the findings of a study of 307 pre-school children at a conference in 2005. Attention deficit disorder was identified in 3.3% of children, depression in 2%, disruptive disorders in 8.4% and anxiety disorders in 9.5%. 11.3% had one or more disorder.

139 **"...anxiety problems like obsessive-compulsive disorder, depression and autism are thought to be autoimmune in origin..."** – Sperner-Unterweger B: "Immunological aetiology of major psychiatric disorders: evidence and therapeutic implications." *Drugs*, 65 (11):1493-520, 2005.
The author states that there is evidence that the immune system might play a role in the development of schizophrenia, affective disorders and infantile autism, with autoimmune mechanisms interrupting neurotrans-mission. *See also:*

Okado N: "Mechanisms for formation and maintenance of synapses mediated by biogenic amines: pathogenesis and therapy of mental retardation and

NOTES

developmental disabilities by genetic and epigenetic factors." *Kaibogaku Zasshi*, Jun; 74(3):351-62, 1999.
Antibodies against the 5-HT2A (serotonin) receptor protein resulted in a 58% decrease of synapses in animal studies.

Singh V et al: "Hyperserotoninemia and serotonin receptor antibodies in children with autism but not mental retardation." *Biological Psychiatry*, Mar 15; 41(6):753-5, 1997.

139 **"...if the mother has untreated autoimmune problems before she conceives there is an eight-fold greater likelihood that her child will suffer from hyperactivity, autism or attention deficit disorder."** – Comi A et al: "Familial clustering of autoimmune disorders and evaluation of medical risk factors in autism." *Journal of Child Neurology*, Jun; 14(6):388-94, 1999.
In this survey of the families of 61 autistic patients and 46 healthy controls, the average number of autoimmune disorders was greater in families with autism. 46% had two or more members with autoimmune disorders. In mothers and first-degree relatives of autistic children, there were more autoimmune disorders (16% and 21%) compared with controls (2% and 4%).

140 **"...genes for autoimmunity may actually do more good than harm."** – Rudi G et al: "Optimizing human fertility and survival." *Nature Medicine*, 7; 873, 2001.
The authors hypothesize that during evolution humans have developed Th1-dominant immunity that favors survival against disease over fertility.

13. COMPREHENSIVE IMMUNE TESTING

141 **"According to a 2008 survey of doctors at 217 fertility clinics..."** – Kwak-Kim J and Fishel F: "Results of the Survey – Reproductive Immunology Practice in IVF"
https://ivf-worldwide.com/survey/reproductive-immunology-practice-in-ivf/results-reproductive-immunology-practice-in-ivf.html

14. IMMUNOTHERAPIES

151 **"Antibodies that react with ovarian tissue may also cause recurrent pregnancy loss and pregnancy failure."** – Kelkar R et al: *Journal of Reproductive Immunology*, Jun; 66 (1):53-67, 2005.
Blood samples from 15 women with premature ovarian failure (POF) were compared with those of seven normally cycling women and eight menopausal women. 10 of the 15 women with POF had antiovarian antibodies. In the control group, only one woman tested positive. *See also*:

Luborsky J et al: *Journal of Clinical Endocrinology & Metabolism*, Jan; 70(1):69-75, 1990
45 patients with premature ovarian failure were tested for ovarian and oocyte antibodies. A combined total of 69% of blood samples were positive for both types of antibodies. Two patients were treated by immunosuppression and became pregnant coincident with a decline in the serum concentration of ovarian antibodies.

NOTES

Luborsky J et al: *Human Reproduction*, May; 15(5):1046-51, 2000 This study concluded: "...in unexplained infertility, ovarian antibodies are an independent marker of potential ovarian failure, and may precede changes in regulatory hormones."

Luborsky J and Pong R: *American Journal of Reproductive Immunology*, Nov; 44(5):261-5, 2000
Blood samples from 47 women undergoing IVF were tested. 25% of women who became pregnant tested positive. 58% of women with ovarian antibodies did not become pregnant. The researchers observed, "Ovarian antibodies may contribute additional information for the prediction of successful IVF outcomes."

Intravenous Immunoglobulin G (IVIG)

158 **"...the remaining clear serum, composed primarily of IgG antibodies, is screened for a range of infections..."** – Boschetti N et al: "Pathogen inactivation and removal procedures used in the production of intravenous immunoglobulins." *Biologicals,* Mar 30, 2006. *See also*:

Schleis T: "The process: New methods of purification and viral safety." *Pharmacotherapy*, Nov; 25 (11 Pt 2):73S-77S, 2005.
"New IVIG products not only provide superior antiviral safety, but also show advances in product purity and manufacturing processes."

158 **"It helps to control activated T cells, which are major producers of Th1 cytokines..."** – Graphou O et al: "Effect of intravenous immunoglobulin treatment on the Th1/Th2 balance in women with recurrent spontaneous abortions." *American Journal of Reproductive Immunology*, January; 49(1):21-9, 2003.
21 women experiencing recurrent miscarriages were treated with IVIG before conception. Th1 and Th2 cells were measured in blood samples taken before, and 5 days after the first IVIG infusion. A decrease in the Th1:Th2 ratio was seen in 76.1% of the cases. *See also*:

Yamada H et al: "Intravenous immunoglobulin treatment in women with recurrent abortions: Increased cytokine levels and reduced Th1: Th2 lympho-cyte ratio in peripheral blood." *American Journal of Reproductive Immunology*, Vol.49, Issue 2, p.84, Feb 2003.

159 **"In addition, there are differences between various IVIG products."** – Clark DA, Coulam C and Stricker R: "Is intravenous immunoglobulins (IVIG) efficacious in early pregnancy failure? A critical review and meta-analysis for patients who fail in vitro fertilization and embryo transfer (IVF)." *Journal of Assisted Reproduction and Genetics*, Jan; 23(1): 1–13, 2006.
"We tested the Bayer Gamimune product (used by Stephenson and Fluker) for the ability to suppress NK cytolytic activity in vitro, and compared the activity to the Baxter Gammagard product used by Coulam. It can be seen in Fig. 2 that both IVIG products suppressed NK activity. However, Gamimune was less potent. Based on the titration curve, it appeared one would require eight times more Gamimune to achieve the suppression achieved by Gammagard.

NOTES

159 **"IGM antibodies... are a much stronger active ingredient than the IGG rich antibody product."** Braverman IVF & Reproductive Immunology, 23 May 2012
http://www.preventmiscarriage.com/antibodies-may-be-important-to-successful-treatm.html

159 **"...APAs have not responded to treatment with heparin, corticosteroids and low dose aspirin."** – Shoenfeld Y and Katz U: "IVIG therapy in autoimmunity and related disorders: our experience with a large cohort of patients." *Autoimmunity*, 38:123-137, 2005.
"...in the presence of a steroid and immunosuppressive-resistant autoimmune disease, IVIG is a rational and safe choice." *See also*:

Piette J et al: "Therapeutic use of intravenous immunoglobulins in the anti-phospholipid syndrome." *Annales de Medecine Interne (Paris)*, May; 151 Supplement, 1:1S51-4, 2000.
"...IVIG therapy probably has a place in the management of selected patients with the antiphospholipid syndrome. It seems effective for the prevention of recurrent pregnancy losses when conventional strategies using subcutaneous heparin and low dose aspirin have failed."

159 **"At present, the most consistently effective treatment for reducing NK cell numbers and activity for both IVF and recurrent miscarriage patients is IVIG."** – De Carolis C et al: "High levels of peripheral blood NK cells in women suffering from recurrent spontaneous abortion are reverted from high dose intravenous immunoglobulins." *American Journal of Reproductive Immunology,* Mar; 55 (3):232-9, 2006.
"High levels of NK cells are detected in women affected by recurrent spontaneous abortion (RSA). IVIGs are capable of decreasing them with a short and long-term efficacy, allowing a very high success rate of pregnancies in RSA women." *See also*:

Clark DA et al: "Is intravenous immunoglobulins (IVIG) efficacious in early pregnancy failure? A critical review and meta-analysis for patients who fail in vitro fertilization and embryo transfer (IVF)." *Journal of Assisted Reproduction and Genetics*, Jan;23(1):1-13, 2006.
"A meta-analysis of three published randomized controlled trials of IVIG in IVF failure patients shows a significant increase in the live birth rate per woman. A rationale for use of IVIG is provided by a review of mechanisms of IVIG action and mechanisms underlying failure of chromosomally normal embryos."

Heilmann L et al: "CD3-CD56+ CD16+ natural killer cells and improvement of pregnancy outcome in IVF/ICSI failure after additional IVIG-treatment." *American Journal of Reproductive Immunology*, 63:263 – 265, 2010.
A total of 188 women with 226 treatment cycles between 2007 and 2009 were evaluated for IVIG therapy. Women with NK cell percentages above 12% were included. In comparison with the meta-analysis of Clark et al., we observed a pregnancy rate of 50.5%, an implantation rate of 21% and a miscarriage rate of 16.8%. In 42% of IVIG- patients we observed a live born baby... In accordance with the study of Kwak et al., we indicate a decrease in the NK cells in patients with improved pregnancy outcome.

NOTES

Hutton B et al: "Use of intravenous immunoglobulin for treatment of recurrent miscarriage: a systematic review." *BJOG*; Feb;114(2):134-42. Epub 2006 Dec 12 2007.

In a systematic review of randomised controlled trials evaluating IVIG for treatment of spontaneous recurrent miscarriage, eight trials involving 442 women using IVIG therapy for recurrent miscarriage were evaluated. There was a significant increase in live births following IVIG use in women with secondary recurrent miscarriage.

143 **"These side effects are usually short lived and often relate to the rate of infusion."** – Shoenfeld Y et al: "Intravenous immunoglobulin: adverse effects and safe administration." *Clinical Reviews in Allergy & Immunology,* Dec; 29 (3):173-84, 2005.

"Immediate adverse effects can be treated by the slowing or temporary discontinuation of the infusion and symptomatic therapy with analgesics, non-steroidal anti-inflammatory drugs, antihistamines and gluco-corticoids in more severe reactions."

Intralipid

160 **"Fertility centers who have adopted this protocol are seeing very impressive results."** –Coulam C et al: "Duration of Intralipid's Suppressive Effect on NK Cell's Functional Activity." *American Journal of Reproductive Immunology,* 2008.

"Intralipid is effective in suppressing in vivo abnormal NK-cell functional activity. The results suggest that intralipid can be used successfully as a thera-peutic option to modulate abnormal NK activity in women with reproductive failure." *See also*:

Lédéé N et al: "Intralipid may represent a new hope for patients with repro-ductive failures and simultaneously an over-immune endometrial activation." *Journal of Reproductive Immunology,*
https://doi.org/10.1016/j.jri.2018.09.050, 2018.

94 patients a history of repeated implantation failures despite multiple embryos transfers received intralipid. The live birth rate was 54% (51/94) at the next embryo transfer.

Meng L et al: "Effectiveness and potential mechanisms of intralipid in treating unexplained recurrent spontaneous abortion." *Archives of Gynecology and Obstetrics,* published online Dec 2015.

"In this prospective, randomized clinical research, we found that... both and intralipid and IVIG could equally lower NK activity to improve pregnancy outcomes. Intralipid can be used as an alternative treatment to IVIG for URSA. The underlying mechanism may be associated with its ability to decrease NK cell activity and regulate trophoblast invasion."

Dakhly D et al: "Intralipid supplementation in women with recurrent sponta-neous abortion and elevated levels of natural killer cells." *International Journal of Gynecology and Obstetrics,* April 2016.

"The present trial showed that intravenous infusion of intralipid is an effective means for increasing the ongoing pregnancy rate and the live birth rate in women with unexplained RSA undergoing IVF/ICSI cycles."

NOTES

Coulam C et al: "Natural Killer Cell Functional Activity Suppression by Intravenous Immunoglobulin, Intralipid and Soluble Human Leukocyte Antigen-G." *American Journal of Reproductive Immunology,* 2007.
"The present data are the first to demonstrate the ability of intralipid to suppress NK cytotoxic activity in peripheral NK cells from women experiencing recurrent reproductive failure."

Coulam C et al: "Pregnancy Outcome After Intralipid Infusion among Women Experiencing Recurrent Pregnancy Loss." *Fertility and Sterility,* Volume 89, Issue 4, April 2008.
"79 patients with elevated NK-cell activity and a history of recurrent pre- or post-implantation pregnancy loss were treated with IV Intralipid. Of the 79 women, 68 had a diagnosis of recurrent implantation failure and 11 experienced recurrent pregnancy loss... Among the 68 women with a history of recurrent implantation failure, 27 became pregnant after in vitro fertilization and embryo transfer with intralipid treatment. Four of the 68 patients were over the age of 40 years and none of these became pregnant. Of 64 women under the age of 40 years who were experiencing recurrent implantation failure with elevated NK-cell activity, the pregnancy rate per cycle was 42%. Ten of the 11 women experiencing recurrent pregnancy loss (91%) had a successful pregnancy."

Mekinian A et al: "Unexplained Recurrent Miscarriage and Recurrent Implantation Failure: Is There a Place for Immunomodulation?" *American Journal of Reproductive Immunology,* 2016.
"Among 200 women with recurrent miscarriages and elevated NK cell activity which were treated with intralipids, the pregnancy rate was 52%, with pregnancy ongoing/live birth rate of 91%."

Allahbadia G: "Intralipid Infusion is the Current Favorite of Gynecologists for Immunotherapy." *Journal of Obstetrics and Gynaecology India* 65(4): 213-217, 2015.
"Evidences from both animal and human studies suggest that intralipid administered intravenously may enhance implantation and maintenance of pregnancy when the patient has an abnormal NK cell level or function."

Neupogen®

162 **"Patients treated with Neupogen® have higher pregnancy rates and higher average pregnancy hormone levels..."** – Aleyasin A et al: "Granulocyte colony stimulating factor in repeated IVF failure, a randomized trial." *The Society for Reproduction and Fertility,* March 2016.
"This multi-centric, prospective, randomized, controlled, trial was con- ducted on 112 infertile women who had repeated IVF failure... In our study subcutaneous administration of GCSF independently improved the successful implantation and pregnancy rates." *See also*:

Santjohanser C et al: "Granulocyte-Colony Stimulating Factor as Treatment Option in Patients with Recurrent Miscarriage." *Archivum Immunologiae et Therapiae Experimentalis.* 61:159–164, 2013.
In 127 patients a pregnancy rate of 47 % was achieved after G-CSF administration, of 27 % in recurrent miscarriage patients with alternative medications and 24 % in cycles without medication.

NOTES

Li J and Chen Y: "The effect of G-CSF on Women Undergoing IVF Treatment." *Reproductive Immunology Open Access*, Vol 1 No.2.33 2017.
"Our latest meta-analysis was conducted to investigate the effect of G-CSF on pregnant outcomes with six studies and 607 patients involved. The results indicated that G-CSF might have the capacity to improve pregnancy outcomes, especially for patients with the thin endometrium or repeated IVF failure."

Davari F et al: "The role of G-CSF in recurrent implantation failure. A randomized double blind placebo controlled trial." *Abstracts / Placenta 45* 63e133, 2016.
100 patients with history of recurrent implantation failure were recruited in the study and received either G-CSF, saline or a placebo. The implantation rate was 12.3% in G-CSF group, 6.1% in the saline group and 4.7% in placebo group.

Mekinian A et al: "Unexplained Recurrent Miscarriage and Recurrent Implantation Failure: Is There a Place for Immunomodulation?" *American Journal of Reproductive Immunology,* 2016.
"In women with infertility, 6% of embryos with low G-CSF in individual follicular fluids had successful implantation vs 36.4% with high G-CSF levels."

Lymphocyte Immunization Therapy (LIT)

164   **"A survey of over 4,500 women who had used LIT from 1996 to 2003 found no incidence of acute side effects."**– Kling C et al: "Adverse effects of intra-dermal allogeneic lymphocyte immunotherapy: acute reactions and role of autoimmunity," *Human Reproduction*, Feb; 21(2):429-35, 2006.
This survey involved a prospective 4-week follow-up of 2,587 couples treated from 2000 to 2003 and 1,914 couples treated from 1996 and 2002. "Local reactions predominantly consisted of redness and itching that lasted for approximately two weeks. Systemic reactions could be attributed to LIT in 6-8%. Blisters at the injection sites were characteristic of LIT but not dependent on the HLA class I mismatch status between cell donor and host. The incidence of autoimmune disease was 0.1%. Four patients developed thromboembolism in pregnancy, which was not ascribed to antiphospholipid syndrome. Acute side effects are comparable to those reported after intradermal vaccination for infectious diseases. Specific risks for anaphylaxis, autoimmune or graft versus host disease were not detected."

Corticosteroids (Prednisone & Dexamethasone)

165   **"Their beneficial effect is associated with a reduction of inflammation..."** – Sibilia, J: "Corticosteroids and inflammation." *La Revue du Praticien-Médecine Générale,* 53(5):495-501, 2003.
"The anti-inflammatory efficacy of corticoids may be explained by their inhibition of the synthesis of numerous cytokines, enzymes and mediators of inflammation or induction of cytokines and anti-inflammatory molecules..."

Agarwal S and Marshall G: "Dexamethasone promotes type 2 cytokine production primarily through inhibition of type 1 cytokines." *Journal of Interferon & Cytokine Research*, Mar; Vol.21, No.3:147-155, 2000. *See also:*

Franchimont D: "Overview of the actions of glucocorticoids on the immune response: A good model to characterize new pathways of immunosuppression

- 388 -

NOTES

for new treatment strategies." *Annals of the New York Academy of Sciences*, 1024:124-137, 2004.
"Glucocorticoids...suppress cellular (Th1) immunity and promote humoral (Th2) immunity."

Shirlow R et al: "The Effects of Adjuvant Therapies on Embryo Transfer Success." *Journal of Reproduction and Infertility*, Oct-Dec; 18(4):368-378, 2017.
In this retrospective cohort study of embryo transfers between January 2010 and April 2015 from a multi-site IVF clinic the authors concluded, "...use of aspirin or steroids demonstrated promising, potentially beneficial outcomes."

165 **"...some moderate suppression of the immune response."** – Beer AE et al: "Immunoglobulin G infusion treatment for women with recurrent spontaneous abortions and elevated CD56+ natural killer cells." *Early Pregnancy*, Apr; 4(2):154-64, 2000.
In this study, the livebirth rates of women with elevated NK cell levels who had post-conception IVIG treatment in addition to anticoagulants and prednisone was 100.0%. In women with elevated NK cell levels who continued with anticoagulants and prednisone the livebirth rate was 33.3%.

165 **"...prednisone or prednisolone, which although not quite identical drugs, are used in the same way."** – See:
http://ratguide.com/meds/endocrine_hormones/prednisone_prednisolone.php
"Though prednisone and prednisolone are used in the same manner and equally as effective, they should not be confused with each other."

165 **"Prednisone does not pass through the placenta easily..."** – Ostensen M and Ramsey-Goldman R: "Treatment of inflammatory rheumatic disorders in pregnancy: what are the safest treatment options?" *Drug Safety*, Nov; 19(5):389-410, 1998.
"Some corticosteroids such as prednisone and prednisolone do not readily cross the placenta and can be safely used during pregnancy as immunosuppressive drugs."

166 **"...prednisone is a moderately effective means of depressing NK cell activity..."** – Vitale C et al: "The corticosteroid-induced inhibitory effect on NK cell function reflects down-regulation and/or dysfunction of triggering receptors involved in natural cytotoxicity." *European Journal of Immunology*, Nov; 34(11): 3028-38, 2004.
NK cells isolated from peripheral blood during methylprednisolone treatment showed a reduction in the expression of activating receptors as well as cytotoxicity. *See also*.

Thum M et al: "Prednisolone suppresses NK cell cytotoxicity in vitro in women with a history of infertility and elevated NK cell cytotoxicity." *American Journal of Reproductive Immunology*, 59:259 – 265, 2008.

Alhalabi M: "Prednisolone improves implantation in ICSI patients with high peripheral CD69 + NK Cells." *Human Reproduction*, 26 (suppl_1):i219, 2011.
This randomized control prospective study was performed between February 2009 and August 2010. The study included 112 women undergoing ICSI treatment elevated levels of CD69+ NK cells. The patients were randomly

divided into two groups: Group1 was given prednisolone 20mg daily. Group2: was not given prednisolone. The pregnancy rate was in the Prednisolone group was 48.28%, compared with the control group at 29.63%.

"The present study indicates that Prednisolone in effectively improved implantation and pregnancy rate in ICSI patient with high peripheral CD69+ NK Cells."

166   **"Dexamethasone is better at restricting NK cell division."** – Piccolella E et al: "Effects of dexamethasone on human natural killer cell cytotoxicity, interferon production, and interleukin-2 receptor expression induced by microbial antigens." *Infection and Immunity*, Feb; 51(2): 712 -714, 1986.

"Dexamethasone inhibits the expression of the interleukin-2 receptor, the synthesis of immune interferon and the development of natural killer cells when added to peripheral blood mononuclear cells cultured with soluble microbial antigens..." *See also*:

Migliorati G et al: "Dexamethasone induces apoptosis in mouse natural killer cells and cytotoxic T lymphocytes." *Immunology*, Jan; 81(1):21-6, 1994.

In this study, it was observed that dexamethasone induced cell death in NK cells and cytotoxic T lymphocytes in vitro.

Hsueh C et al: "Effect of dexamethasone on conditioned enhance-ment of natural killer cell activity." *Neuroimmunomodulation,* Nov-Dec; 1(6):370-6, 1994.

"It is believed that the expression of the conditioned natural killer cell activity is regulated through the hypothalamus-pituitary axis...These studies suggest that treatment with dexamethasone was able to block the expression of the conditioned NK cell activity..."

166   **"Dexamethasone can have a positive impact on ovarian response..."** – Parsanezhad M et al: "Use of dexamethasone and clomiphene citrate in the treatment of clomiphene citrate-resistant patients with polycystic ovary syndrome and normal dehydroepiandrosterone sulfate levels: a prospective, double-blind, placebo controlled trial." *Fertility & Sterility*, Nov; 78(5):1001-4, 2002. *See also*:

Keay S: "Low dose dexamethasone augments the ovarian response to exogenous gonadotrophins leading to a reduction in cycle cancellation rate in a standard IVF programme." *Human Reproduction*, Sep; 16(9): 1861-5, 2001.

290 IVF patients were given either 1 mg dexamethasone or a placebo tablet daily. The group receiving dexamethasone had a lower incidence of poor ovarian response and increased clinical pregnancy rates.

166   **"Early successes for the treatment of immune-induced reproductive failure were reported with high dose corticosteroids (40 mg prednisone daily)..."** – Lubbe W et al: "Fetal survival after prednisone suppression of maternal lupus-anticoagulant." *Lancet*, i: 1361-1363, 1983.

Five out of six women with the lupus anticoagulant and poor obstetric histories gave birth to live infants when they were treated during pregnancy with prednisone (40-60 mg daily) and low dose aspirin (75 mg daily).

166   **"1 mg dexamethasone is equivalent to approximately 7 mg of prednisone."** – For corticosteroid conversions see:

NOTES

http://www.globalrph.com/corticocalc.htm

167 **"In a survey of literature on corticosteroid use and birth defects from 1952 to 1994..."** – Fraser FC and Sajoo A: "Teratogenic potential of corticosteroids in humans." *Teratology*, 51:45-6, 1995.
Fraser and Sajoo surveyed the available literature from 1952-1994 and found 457 exposed patients, in which the frequency of malformations was 3.5%. The two cases of cleft palate observed were higher than the 0.2 cases expected and a possible association could not be excluded.

167 **"The incidence of cleft palate and/or cleft lip is about 1 or 2 per 1,000..."** – Illinois Teratogen Information Service, Newsletter: "Corticosteroids in pregnancy." Vol.8, No.1 May 2000. Available from: http://fetal-exposure.org

Regular Molecular Weight Heparin (Multiparin)

168 **"Regular heparin is also used in some reproductive immunology programs to treat APA positive/inherited thrombophilia negative patients."** – Girardi G: "Heparin treatment in pregnancy loss: Potential therapeutic benefits beyond anticoagulation." *Journal of Reproductive Immunology*, Jun; 66(1):45-51, 2005.
"In addition to direct effects of heparin on the coagulation cascade, heparin might protect pregnancies by reducing the binding of antiphospholipid antibodies, reducing inflammation, facilitating implantation and or inhibiting complement activation." *See also*:

Sher G et al: "High fecundity rates following in vitro fertilization and embryo transfer in antiphospholipid antibody seropositive women treated with heparin and aspirin." *Human Reproduction*, Dec; 9(12): 2278-83, 1994.
APA-positive patients were treated daily with aspirin and heparin during ovarian stimulation. The pregnancy rate was 49% in treated women, 16% in the untreated group and 27% for APA-negative women.

Low Molecular Weight Heparin (Lovenox, Clexane, Fragmin & Arixtra)

169 **"Their main advantage is their...safety in pregnancy."** – Sanson B et al: "Safety of low-molecular-weight heparin in pregnancy: a systematic review." *Thrombosis Haemostatis*, 81: 668-72, 1999.
"Low molecular weight heparins appear to be a safe alternative to unfractionated heparin as an anticoagulant during pregnancy."

170 **"...there is a very low risk of osteoporosis with low molecular weight heparins..."** – Greer I: "Anticoagulants in pregnancy." *Journal of Thrombosis & Thrombolysis*, Feb; 21(1):57-65, 2006.
"Low molecular weight heparins...have clinical and practical advantages... (significantly lower incidence of osteoporosis and heparin induced thrombocytopenia)..." *See also*:

Melissari E et al: "Use of low molecular weight heparin in pregnancy." *Thrombosis Haemostatis*, 68:652-6, 1992.
The use of low molecular weight heparin was evaluated in 11 patients with a severe thromboembolic tendency who had suffered recurrent miscarriages and responded poorly to conventional anticoagulation. All patients gave birth to

NOTES

healthy babies (three for the first time) without complication. Bone density scans also showed normal mineral mass.

170 **"The administration of these anticoagulants in pregnancy is generally considered safe."** – Hoppensteadt D and Bick R: "Recurrent miscarriage syndrome and infertility due to blood coagulation protein/platelet defects: a review and update." *Clinical and Applied Thrombosis/Hemostasis*, Jan; 11(1):1-13, 2005.

351 women with recurrent loss were assessed over a 3-year period. Those with thrombophilia were given low dose aspirin plus heparin or low molecular weight heparin. Only 2 of 312 patients had a further miscarriage. The side effects of therapy were minimal. *See also*:

Regan L et al: "Bone density changes in pregnant women treated with heparin: a prospective, longitudinal study." *Human Reproduction*, 14: 2876-80, 1999.

No significant risk was found in this study of women with APS taking low doses of heparin during pregnancy.

Winger E and Reed J: "A retrospective analysis of Fondaparinux versus Enoxaparin treatment in women with infertility or pregnancy loss." *American Journal of Reproductive Immunology July 2009.*

The pregnancy success rate was 59% for patients receiving fondaparinux (Arixtra) and 58% for patients receiving enoxaparin (Lovenox). No difference was detected in birth weight or gestational age at delivery. No birth defects, severe bleeding-related complications, or serious allergic reactions were observed.

75 mg or 81 mg "Low dose" Aspirin

170 **"A randomized clinical trial carried out at the Harvard Medical School hospital in 2004..."** – Dunoyer-Geindre S et al: "Aspirin inhibits endothelial cell activation induced by antiphospholipid antibodies." *Journal of Thrombosis Haemostatis*, Jul; 2(7):1176-81, 2004.

171 **"...better implantation and pregnancy rates. Improved IVF cycle outcomes have also been seen when it is taken during the ovarian stimulation phase."** – Rubinstein M et al: "Low dose aspirin treatment improves ovarian responsiveness, uterine and ovarian blood flow velocity, implantation, and pregnancy rates in patients undergoing in vitro fertilization: a prospective, randomized, double-blind placebo controlled assay." *Fertility & Sterility*, May; 71(5):825-9, 1999.

149 patients took 100 mg daily of aspirin during the ovarian stimulation phase, starting from day 1. The number of follicles and quantity of eggs retrieved was up to double that of the control group of 149 women. The pregnancy rate was 45% versus 28%, with an implantation rate of 17.8% versus 9.2%. *See also*:

Regan L et al: "Recurrent miscarriage – an aspirin a day?" *Human Reproduction*, Vol.15, No.10, 2220-2223, 2000.

In women with unexplained recurrent miscarriage, the livebirth rate was 68.4% for those who took aspirin compared to 63.5% of controls. In the group with late pregnancy losses the livebirth rate was 64.6% compared to 49.2% who did not take aspirin.

NOTES

171 **"...a beneficial side effect...reducing the incidence of preeclampsia."** – Duley L et al: "Antiplatelet drugs for prevention of preeclampsia and its consequences: systematic review." *British Medical Journal*, 322:329-333, 2001.
In this review of 39 trials involving 30,563 women at risk of preeclampsia, the use of anti-platelet drugs, largely low dose aspirin, was associated with a 15% reduction in the risk of preeclampsia. There was also an 8% reduction in the risk of preterm birth.

Sildenafil Citrate (Vaginal Viagra)

171 **"Viagra has been shown to increase blood flow to the uterus as well as thickening its lining."** – Sher G and Fisch J: "Effect of vaginal sildenafil on the outcome of in vitro fertilization (IVF) after multiple IVF failures attributed to poor endometrial development." *Fertility and Sterility*, Nov;78 (5):1073-6, 2002.
105 infertile women aged with normal ovarian reserve and at least two consecutive prior IVF failures due to inadequate endometrial development, underwent IVF with the addition of sildenafil vaginal suppositories (25 mg, 4 times per day) for up to 10 days. Enhanced endometrial development was seen in 70% of patients along with high implantation and ongoing pregnancy rates. *See also*:

El-Shourbagy S et al: "The role of sildenafil citrate (viagra) suppositories on endometrial response (thickness and mean resistance index of endometrial spiral artery) in cases of unexplained infertility." Menoufia Medical Journal, Vol 30, Issue 2, 343-349, 2017.
50 women with unexplained primary infertility were treated with 25 mg of sildenafil citrate suppositories four times per day for 7 days. Sildenafil citrate treated women showed a statistically significant increase in endometrial thickness, yielding a better conception rate.

Anti-TNF Agents: (Enbrel [Etanercept], Humira and Simponi)

172 **"By blocking the action of TNF-alpha, these drugs tip the immune balance from a Th1 dominated to a more baby friendly Th2 state which encourages successful implantation and reduces miscarriage risk."** – Winger E and Reed J: "Treatment with tumor necrosis factor inhibitors improves live birth rates in women with recurrent spontaneous abortion." *American Journal of Reproductive Immunology*, 60:9-16, 2008. *See also*:

Winger E and Reed J: "Treatment with adalimumab (Humira) and intravenous immunoglobulin improves pregnancy rates in women undergoing IVF." *American Journal of Reproductive Immunology*, Feb;61 (2):113- 20, 2009.
75 women with Th1:Th2 cytokine elevation were divided into 4 groups. Group 1 received both IVIG and Humira, Group 2 received IVIG, Group 3 received Humira, Group 4 received no treatment. The authors concluded, "The use of a TNF-alpha inhibitor and IVIG significantly improves IVF outcomes in young infertile women with Th1/Th2 cytokine elevation."

Clark DA: "Anti-TNFalpha therapy in immune-mediated subfertility: state of the art." *Journal of Reproductive Immunology*, May;85(1):15-24, 2010.
"Anti-TNF alpha drugs may offer a new safe and effective approach to treating patients with Th1-cytokine-dependent infertility and recurrent miscarriages."

- 393 -

NOTES

Jerzak M et al: "Etanercept immunotherapy in women with a history of recurrent reproductive failure," *Ginekologia Polska*, 83:260, 264, 2012
30 women with reproductive failure and increased peripheral NK-cell numbers and/or activity were studied. They received 4 doses (25 mg) of etanercept twice weekly before conception. NK-cell activity was significantly decreased after etanercept therapy in the study women. This effect was significantly higher in women with subsequent pregnancy success but not in those with pregnancy failure.

173 **"The highest IVF success rates are seen in patients when anti-TNF-alpha medications are taken preconception and IVIG is given before the embryo transfer."** – Winger E Reed J et al: "Treatment with adalimumab (Humira) and intravenous immunoglobulin (IVIG) improves pregnancy rates in women undergoing IVF." *American Journal of Reproductive Immunology*, 61:113-120, 2009.
75 pregnancies in patients with a history of recurrent pregnancy loss were retrospectively evaluated. The population was divided into three groups: group I: 21 patients treated with anticoagulants (AC), group II: 37 patients treated with AC and IVIG, and group III: 17 patients treated with anticoagulants, IVIG and the TNF inhibitor Etanercept (Enbrel) or Adalimumab (Humira). The live birth rate was 19% (4/21) in group I, 54% (20/37) in group II, and 71% (12/17) in group III. Side effects of AC, IVIG and TNF inhibitor treatment were minimal in these patients, and no birth defects were identified in their offspring.
"In women with RSA, addition of either IVIG or a TNF inhibitor plus IVIG to the AC regimen appears to improve live birth rates compared to the treatment with AC alone."

174 **"Recent information suggests that these drugs do not affect the fetus in the first trimester..."** – Carter J et al: "A safety assessment of tumor necrosis factor antagonists during pregnancy: a review of the Food and Drug Administration database." *The Journal of Rheumatology*, 36:3. 2009.
"Pregnancy outcome following gestational exposure to TNF-alpha-inhibitors: a prospective, comparative, observational study." *Reproductive Toxicology.* Jan;43:78-84, 2014.
83 anti-TNF-α-exposed-pregnancies were compared with 86 disease-matched and 341 non-teratogenic-exposed pregnancies. The anti-TNF-α group consisted of 35 infliximab-, 25 etanercept-, and 23 adalimumab-exposed pregnancies. The rate of major congenital anomalies did not significantly differ between the three groups."The present study suggests that anti-TNF-α treatment does not pose a major teratogenic risk in humans."

Schnitzler F et al: "Outcome of pregnancy in women with inflammatory bowel disease treated with antitumor necrosis factor therapy." *Inflammatory Bowel Disease*, Sep;17(9):1846-54, 2011.
"This observational study assessed pregnancy outcomes in 212 women with IBD under antitumor necrosis factor alpha (TNF) treatment at our IBD unit.... Direct exposure to anti-TNF treatment during pregnancy was not related to a higher incidence of adverse pregnancy outcomes."

Viktil K et al: "Outcomes after anti-rheumatic drug use before and during pregnancy: a cohort study among 150,000 pregnant women and expectant fathers." *Scandinavian Journal of Rheumatology*, May;41(3):196-201, 2012.

NOTES

In 154,976 singleton pregnancies, 1461 of the women and 1198 of the known fathers were dispensed anti-rheumatic drugs at least once during the study period: 723 had non-steroidal anti-inflammatory drugs, 633 prednisolone, 119 sulfasalazine, 101 azathioprine, 58 hydroxy-chloroquine, 37 etanercept, eight methotrexate, two leflunomide and three adalumimab.
"This study revealed no major malformations of the alert drugs methotrexate, leflunomide, etanercept and adalumimab."

UK Teratology Information Service "Use of Adalimumab in Pregnancy." www.medicinesinpregnancy.org, May 2015"
"Studies investigating the use of anti-TNFα therapies during pregnancy show no compelling evidence of an increase in risk of overall congenital malformation rate, spontaneous abortion,intrauterine death or adverse neurodevelopmental outcome…"

Fasoulakis Z et al: "Common Adverse Effects of Anti-TNF Agents on Gestation." *Obstetrics and Gynecology International,* Article ID 8648651, 2016.
In this comprehensive review of over 1,000 women treated with anti- TNF agents the authors concluded, "To date, there is no evidence that anti-TNF agents are associated with teratogenicity, increased pregnancy loss, or embryo toxicity."

Noriega J et al: "Effect of tumor necrosis factor blocker (infliximab) on blastocyst development in vitro." *Fertility & Sterility,* Vol.81, No.6, June 2004.
"This study provides the first evidence that infliximab (Remicade) does not affect the blastocyst development rate at concentrations similar to the maximum in vivo levels." *See also*:

Katz J et al: "Outcome of pregnancy in women receiving infliximab for the treatment of Crohn's disease and rheumatoid arthritis." *American Journal of Gastroenterology*, 99:2385-92, 2004.
Of 106 pregnancies with exposure to infliximab, outcomes were consistent with those of the U.S. general population.

Khanna D et al: "Safety of tumor necrosis factor-alpha antagonists." *Drug Safety,* 27(5):307-24, 2004.
"At present there is no evidence implicating TNF-alpha antagonists with embryotoxicity, teratogenicity or increased pregnancy loss."

Metformin (Glucophage)

174 **"Metformin can also help to promote ovulation, restore fertility, improve uterine blood flow…"** – Palomba S et al: "Uterine effects of metformin administration in anovulatory women with polycystic ovary syndrome." *Human Reproduction,* Feb, 21(2).457-465, 2006.
37 patients with PCOS were treated with metformin for 6 months. Before treatment, uterine and endometrial blood flows were significantly lower in patients with PCOS than in the control group. Uterine vascularization was also significantly improved and endometrial thickness was restored to normal levels. *See also*:

NOTES

van Santbrink E et al: "Does metformin modify ovarian responsiveness during exogenous FSH ovulation induction in normogonadotrophic anovulation? A placebo controlled double-blind assessment." *European Journal of Endocrinology*, Apr; 152(4):611-7 2005.
Metformin co-treatment in a group of insulin-resistant anovulatory patients resulted in normalization of hormone levels and promoted follicular development.

Sabatini M et al: "Metformin therapy in a hyperandrogenic anovulatory mutant murine model with polycystic ovarian syndrome characteristics improves oocyte maturity during superovulation" *Journal of Ovarian Research*, 2011; 4:8. Published online 2011.
"Our data provide evidence to suggest that metformin may optimize ovulatory performance in mice with a specific reproductive and metabolic phenotype shared by women with PCOS."

Dasari P and Pranahita G: "The efficacy of metformin and clomiphene citrate combination compared with clomiphene citrate alone for ovulation induction in infertile patients with PCOS" *Journal of Human Reproductive Science*, Jan-Jun; 2(1): 18–22 2009.
In 24 patients with PCOS... "the ovulatory rate and the pregnancy rate with the metformin and clomiphene citrate combination was found to be higher when compared with clomiphene citrate (CC) alone. Metformin increased the ovulatory rate in CC failures, also implying increased sensitivity to CC."

174   **"One study has reported an ongoing pregnancy success rate for this patient group of 83% with metformin versus 34% without."** – Glueck C et al: "Pregnancy outcomes among women with polycystic ovary syndrome treated with metformin." *Human Reproduction*, Nov; 17(11):2858-64, 2002. *See also*:

Nestler J et al: "Reduced serum glycodelin and insulin-like growth factor-binding protein-1 in women with polycystic ovary syndrome during first trimester of pregnancy." *Journal of Clinical Endocrinology & Metabolism*, Feb; 89(2):833-9, 2004.
"Because glycodelin inhibits certain responses of the immune system and natural killer cell activity, impaired production of glycodelin could allow a maternal immune response against the embryo."

Jungheim, E: "Fertility treatment in women with polycystic ovary syndrome: a decision analysis of different oral ovulation induction agents" *Fertility Sterility*, December; 94(7): 2659–2664, 2010.
"Combination therapy with metformin and clomiphene citrate should be considered as first-line treatment for infertile women with polycystic ovary syndrome."

FaBB (Folic acid 2.2mg)

175   **"Folic acid supplementation can also reduce the chances of the baby developing neural tube birth defects..."** – Larsen R et al: "Implementation and outcomes of recommended folic acid supplementation in Mexican-American women with prior neural tube defect-affected pregnancies." *Preventative Medicine*, Jun; 40(6):867-71, 2005. *See also:*

NOTES

Blencowe H et al: "Folic acid to reduce neonatal mortality from neural tube disorders." *International Journal of Epidemiology*, April; 39 (suppl_1): i110–i121. Published online March 23 2010.
In this meta-analysis of three randomized controlled trials of folic acid supplementation for women with a previous pregnancy with neural tube defects indicates a 70% reduction in recurrence. A meta-analysis of eight population-based studies examining folic acid food fortification gave an estimated reduction in neural tube defect incidence of 46%.

Honein M et al: "Impact of folic acid fortification of the US food supply on the occurrence of neural tube defects" JAMA. June 20;285(23):2981-6, 2001.
From January 1990 and December 1999 a 19% reduction in NTD birth prevalence occurred following folic acid fortification of the US food supply.

Vitamin D (ergocalciferol-D2, cholecalciferol-D3, alfacalcidol)

176 **"Vitamin D and its receptors are present in the ovaries where they stimulate the production of estrogen and progesterone."** Lerchbaum E et al: "Vitamin D and fertility: a systematic review," *European Journal of Endocrinology*, May;166(5):765-78, 2012.
In this literature search in Pubmed until October 2011 it was estimated that Vitamin D helped increase levels of progesterone and estrogen by 13% and 21% respectively, regulating menstrual cycles and making conception more likely.

176 **"Research has shown that sufficient vitamin D levels reduce the risk of miscarriage in women who have suffered previous losses."** Zakia Mahdy Abolill Z et al: "Role of 1,25-dihydroxyvitamin D (vitamin D3) as immuno-modulator in recurrent missed miscarriage," *Middle East Fertility Society Journal,* 18(3):171–176, September 2013. 40 pregnant women with recurrent miscarriage were randomly assigned to a study group or control group. The study group received vitamin D3 supplementation. The risk of miscarriage was 15% lower among the study group than the control group. Continuing pregnancy rate was 70% in the study group and 55% in the control group.

176 **"A lack of vitamin D also plays a significant role in... other inflammatory disorders such as endometriosis and pre-eclampsia."** Sablok A et al: "Supplementation of vitamin D in pregnancy and its correlation with feto-maternal outcome," *Clinical Endocrinology*, Oct;83(4):536-41, 2015.
In this randomized control trial from years 2010 to 2012, 180 pregnant women were divided randomly into two groups. Group B received vitamin D supplementation and Group A did not.
44% of women in group A and 20.3% of women in group B developed preterm labour, pre eclampsia or gestational diabetes. Newborns of mothers in group A were also of lower birth weight.

Chu J et al: "Vitamin D and assisted reproductive treatment outcome: a systematic review and meta-analysis," *Human Reproduction*, 1;33(1): 65-80. doi: 10.1093/humrep/dex326, 2018.
In this systematic review and meta-analysis of 11 published cohort studies (including 2700 women) investigating the association between vitamin D and IVF outcomes, it was observed that vitamin D deficiency and insufficiency was associated with poor reproductive outcomes when compared to women with normal levels.

NOTES

15. IMMUNE THERAPY: Rejected by a Body of Opinion

181 **"According to data collected from 434 fertility doctors…"** Kwak-Kim J and Fishel S: "Results of the survey – Reproductive Immunology Practice in IVF" 2008 IVF worldwide.com.

186 **"In a 2010 interview for the Guardian newspaper…"** Carpenter L: "Miscarriage: a mother's last taboo," *The Guardian*. www.theguardian.com/lifeandstyle/2010/aug/22/pregnancy-miscarriage-lesley-regan

188 **"The ASRI therefore performed a meta analysis of hundreds of published and unpublished trials…"** – Recurrent Miscarriage Immunotherapy Trialists Group: "Worldwide collaborative observational study and meta analysis on allogeneic leukocyte immunotherapy for recurrent spontaneous abortion." *American Journal of Reproductive Immunology*, 32: pp.55-72, 1994.

188 **"…according to a subsequent 1996 ASRI meta analysis concerning the treatment of recurrent spontaneous abortion…"** – Clark DA, Coulam C et al: "The Recurrent Miscarriage Immunotherapy Trialists Group: Implication of abnormal human trophoblast karyotype for the evidence based approach to the understanding, investigation, and treatment of recurrent spontaneous abortion." *American Journal of Reproductive Immunology*, 35: pp.495-498, 1996.

189 **"Immunological Testing and Interventions for Reproductive Failure"** – Scientific Advisory Committee Paper 5, October 2003. Produced on behalf of the Royal College of Obstetricians and Gynaecologists by Regan L, Backos M and Rai R.

189 **"Professor Regan stated in 2004, 'This center has four purposes…'"** – Regan L: "Overview of recurrent miscarriage." *Gynaecology Forum*, 1997. See: http://www.medforum.nl/gynfo/leading6.htm

190 **"Her resistance… was confirmed in a 2007 interview for The Daily Telegraph newspaper."** Lambert V: "Solving the mystery of recurrent miscarriage," 4th June 2007. www.telegraph.co.uk/women/womens-health/3349488/Solving-the-mystery-of-recurrent-miscarriage.html

190 **"Professor Gab Kovacs, former Medical Director of Monash IVF states, 'That is the key to generating income for an IVF clinic.'"** – *"The Fertility Business"* Amazon movie, 2016.

192 **"…*testing for antibodies other than lupus anticoagulant and anticardiolipin is of clinical significance*:"** – McIntyre J: "Antiphospholipid antibodies in implantation failures." *American Journal of Reproductive Immunology*, Apr; 49(4):221-9, 2003.
This overview confirms that the trophoblast is targeted by antiphospholipid antibodies, especially against serine. Antibodies to ethanol-amine are also said to be significantly associated with very early recurrent pregnancy loss. *See also*:

Rote N and Stetzer B: "Autoimmune disease as a cause of reproductive failure." *Clinical Laboratory Medicine*, Jun; 23(2):265-93, 2003.

NOTES

The authors state that testing for anticardiolipin antibodies and lupus anticoagulant is "inadequate for diagnosis of all patients with autoimmune pregnancy loss." The report also says that many patients with autoimmune-like pregnancy complications are negative in tests for lupus anticoagulant and anticardiolipin antibodies, but may have antibodies against serine or other antigens.

192 *"...thyroid antibodies do affect pregnancy outcome and that screening for them is useful:"* – Bussen S and Steck T: "Thyroid autoantibodies in euthyroid non-pregnant women with recurrent spontaneous abortions." *Human Reproduction*, Nov; 10(11):2938-40, 1995.
"...thyroid antibodies may be a marker for autoimmune-mediated recurrent spontaneous abortions, not dissimilar to, for example, anticardiolipin." *See also*:

Bussen S et al: "Increased prevalence of thyroid antibodies in euthyroid women with a history of recurrent in vitro fertilization failure." *Human Reproduction & Embryology*, 15 (3):545, 2000.
In a study of 24 women with three consecutive IVF failures, the incidence of thyroid antibodies was "significantly increased." The report concludes: "Since these autoantibodies seem to be distinct and independent markers for reproductive failure, their identification provides the opportunity to identify women at risk for an adverse outcome in an IVF embryo transfer programme. Therefore, it is suggested to include the determination of thyroid antibodies in the evaluation of women with recurrent IVF failure."

Dendrinos S et al: "Thyroid autoimmunity in patients with recurrent spontaneous miscarriages." *Gynecological Endocrinology*, Aug; 14(4): 270-4, 2000.
30 recurrent miscarriers aged 25 to 37 were tested for thyroid antibodies and compared with 15 matched controls. The frequency of those with ATAs was 37% versus 13%. "This may represent an additional marker for impaired regulation of the maternal immune system."

Kim C et al: "Influence of antithyroid antibodies in euthyroid women on in vitro fertilization-embryo transfer outcome." *American Journal of Reproductive Immunology*, Jul; 40(1):2-8, 1998.
Cycle outcomes of 79 patients with thyroid antibodies undergoing IVF (the study group) were compared with those of 51 women without antithyroid antibodies (the control group). The pregnancy rate per cycle was significantly lower in the study group (26.3%) compared with in the control group (39.3%). The chemical pregnancy rate per cycle and the miscarriage rate were also significantly higher in the study group.

Lejeune B et al: "Antithyroid antibodies underlying thyroid abnormalities and miscarriage or pregnancy induced hypertension." *British Journal of Obstetrics & Gynaecology*, Jul; 100(7):669-72, 1993.
730 pregnant women were tested for the presence of antibodies to thyroid hormones. The report concludes: "The presence of thyroid autoantibodies during pregnancy constitutes a marker of increased risk of miscarriage and poor obstetric prognosis."

NOTES

Poppe K et al: "Assisted reproduction and thyroid autoimmunity: an unfortunate combination?" *Journal of Clinical Endocrinology & Metabolism*, Vol.88, No.9, 4149-4152, 2003.

234 women were screened for thyroid peroxidase antibodies, among others, before their first IVF cycle. 14% tested positive. The miscarriage rate in this group was 53% compared with 23% of women without thyroid antibodies. The researchers state that women testing positive for thyroid antibodies have a significantly increased risk of miscarriage.

Stagnaro-Green A et al: "Thyroid antibodies and fetal loss: an evolving story." *Thyroid*, Jan; 11(1): 57-63, 2001.

This review of the research papers on thyroid antibodies and miscarriage concludes: "The majority of the studies (67%) reported a statistically significant increase in the incidence of thyroid antibodies in the recurrent abortion group as compared to controls."

197 *"Before 1996, a clear association between antisperm antibodies and recurrent miscarriage had been established. Subsequent studies have confirmed that their presence also affects IVF outcome:"* – Cropp C and Schlaff W: "Antisperm antibodies." *Archivum Immunologiae et Therapice Experimentalis*, (Warsz), 38(1-2):31-46, 1990.

25% of women in 172 infertile couples had antisperm antibodies in their cervical mucus and 12.7% had antisperm antibodies in their sera. The report concludes: "The risk of spontaneous abortion is higher in women whose male partner has antisperm antibodies." *See also*:

Erguven S: "Antisperm and anticardiolipin antibodies in recurrent abortions." *Mikrobiologie Bulgaria*, Jan; 24(1):1-7, 1990.

Antisperm, anticardiolipin and some other autoantibodies were analyzed in 63 cases of habitual abortion, spontaneous abortion and intrauterine fetal death. Antisperm antibodies and anticardiolipin antibodies were positive in 28.5% and 33.3% of the patients respectively. 11.1% were positive for both. The authors speculate: "It can be supposed that, besides other factors, antisperm antibodies may play a role in early abortions."

Putowski L et al: "The immunological profile of infertile women after repeated IVF failure (preliminary study)." *European Journal of Obstetrics & Gynecology*, Feb; 10, 112(2):192-6, 2004.

17 women with repeated IVF failure and 10 non-pregnant women with a history of successful IVF pregnancies were included in this study. The presence of antinuclear antibodies, antithyroid antibodies, antiphospholipid antibodies and antisperm antibodies was evaluated. 82.3% of infertile patients had at least one abnormal result on autoimmune testing. The report concludes: "Our results suggest that immunological alterations may be involved in the etiopathogenesis of unexplained infertility."

Sugi T et al: "Influence of immunotherapy on antisperm antibody titer in unexplained recurrent aborters." *American Journal of Reproductive Immunology*, Mar; 29(2):95-9, 1993.

In this study, the percentage of antibody-positive sperm decreased significantly after immunotherapy. The authors conclude that antisperm antibodies may have potential for use as a marker for deficient immuno-suppressive mechanisms and that immunotherapy could be an effective treatment for women with antisperm antibodies who have unexplained recurrent abortions.

Wang L et al: "Analysis on the treatment of 1,020 patients with immunologic infertility." *Chengdu Zhonghua Fu Chan Ke Za Zhi*, Apr; 34 (4):234-6, 1999.
1,020 women with infertility were evaluated. 25.88% tested positive for antisperm antibodies, 22.86% had antiovarian antibodies, 32.81% had anti-endometrial antibodies and 23.61% tested positive for anti-HCG antibodies. Patients were treated with dexamethasone and vitamins E and C for three consecutive cycles. After one course of treatment, the presence of these antibodies was reduced by over 90%. The pregnancy rate was increased by 30%.

198 **"Furthermore, in a study at St. Mary's Hospital that involved Professor Regan..."** – Clifford K et al: "Endometrial CD56+ natural killer cells in women with recurrent miscarriage: a histomorphometric study." *Human Reproduction,* Nov; 14(11):2727-30, 1999.

199 *"Examples of peer-reviewed data from an extensive collection:"* (on the role of NK cells and reproductive failure) – Beer AE et al: "Immunophenotypic profiles of peripheral blood lymphocytes in women with recurrent pregnancy losses and in infertile women with multiple failed in vitro fertilization cycles." *American Journal of Reproductive Immunology*, Apr; 35(4):376-82, 1996.
The authors state that women with multiple IVF failures have significantly higher levels of CD56+ than normal fertile controls and the conception rate is much higher in those with CD56+ levels below 12%. *See also*:

Beer AE et al: "Status of peripheral blood natural killer cells in women with recurrent spontaneous abortions and infertility of unknown aetiology." *Human Reproduction*, May; 16(5):855-61, 2001.
Blood samples were taken from 40 study patients and 13 normal healthy controls. A significant increase in CD69 expression on CD56+ NK cells was demonstrated in women with recurrent miscarriage and infertility compared with controls. CD94 expression was decreased in women with recurrent miscarriage and infertility. The researchers conclude that unbalanced CD69 and CD94 expression might explain the underlying pathology of these conditions.

Grigor'eva V et al: ["Activity of natural killer cells in various forms of abortion."] *Akush Ginekologia (Moskow)*, Apr; (4):26-8, 1991.
"The activity of Natural Killer cells was found to be significantly higher in females with various miscarriages than that in those with normal pregnancy. The highest NK cell activity was observed in females with interrupted pregnancy."

Matsubayashi H et al: "Preconception peripheral natural killer cell activity as a predictor of pregnancy outcome in patients with unexplained infertility." *American Journal of Reproductive Immunology,* Mar; 53(3):126-31, 2005.
77 patients with fertility problems were followed for two years. 28 eventually conceived but 49 did not. The peripheral NK activity of the group that became pregnant was significantly lower than that of the non-conception group. "Our finding suggests that elevated peripheral NK activity in patients with unexplained infertility is a risk factor for attaining pregnancy success."

NOTES

Rezaei A and Dabbagh A: "T-helper (1) cytokines increase during early pregnancy in women with a history of recurrent spontaneous abortion." *Medical Science Monitor*, Aug; 8(8):CR607-10, 2002.

92 women with at least three pregnancy losses and a control group of 40 women with no history of pregnancy loss were studied. Blood samples from both groups were taken at the end of the first trimester and at the time of abortion. Samples were tested for concentrations of Th1 cytokines. Blood from women with recurrent miscarriage had higher concentrations of TNF-alpha, TNF beta, and IL-2 compared to the control group. Tissue culture from women with recurrent loss also produced higher concentration of these cytokines. The report concludes: "These data may explain the increase in NK cells' cytoxic activity during early pregnancy in recurrent miscarriage group. It may also provide a diagnostic tool to predict the outcome of pregnancy."

Yamada H et al: "High NK cell activity in early pregnancy correlates with subsequent abortion with normal chromosomes in women with recurrent abortion." *American Journal of Reproductive Immunology*, Aug; 46(2):132-6, 2001.

66 pregnant women with a history of miscarriage were assessed for peripheral NK cell activity. NK cell activity in women with subsequent livebirth was significantly decreased compared with that in women with subsequent abortion with normal chromosomes. "High NK cell activity at 6 to 7 gestational weeks correlates with subsequent abortion with normal chromosomes."

202   *"There are numerous other reports that also support the use of LIT as a treatment for recurrent implantation failure..."* – Beer AE et al: "Natural killer cell cytotoxicity and paternal lymphocyte immunization in women with recurrent spontaneous abortions." *American Journal of Reproductive Immunology*, Nov; 40(5):352-8, 1998.

33 women with a history of two or more recurrent spontaneous abortions were prospectively studied. CD56+ NK cell activity was significantly suppressed after LIT and CD3+ pan T-cell were significantly increased. *See also:*

Nonaka T et al: "Results of immunotherapy for patients with unexplained primary recurrent abortions - prospective non-randomized cohort study." *American Journal of Reproductive Immunology,* Dec;58(6):530-6, 2007.

228 recurrent aborters were followed up regarding immunotherapy. Of the 228 patients, 165 underwent immunotherapy using LIT. Of the 140 newly pregnant patients after immunotherapy, the pregnancy continued successfully in 110 (78.6%). The success rate of pregnancy was 30.0% in 18 non-immunized patients. Thus, the success rate was significantly higher among patients with immunotherapy.

Pandey M et al: "Induction of MLR-Bf and protection of fetal loss: a current double-blind randomized trial of paternal lymphocyte immunization for women with recurrent spontaneous abortion." *International Immunopharmacology*, Feb; 4(2):289-98, 2004.

124 women with unknown causes of abortions were registered for immunotherapy in a double-blind, randomized trial. Women with recurrent miscarriage who received LIT showed a significantly increased level of blocking antibodies and a pregnancy success rate of 84% compared to 30 to 44% in women who had received other therapies or a placebo.

NOTES

Ramhorst R et al: "Is the paternal mononuclear cells' immunization a successful treatment for recurrent spontaneous abortion?" *American Journal of Reproductive Immunology*, Sept; 44(3):129-35, 2000.
92 recurrent miscarriers received LIT and 37 couples did not (controls). The pregnancy rates were 58% and 46% respectively. The livebirth rate increased from 71% in the controls to 88% after immunotherapy.

Szpakowski A et al: "The influence of paternal lymphocytes immunization on percentage of peripheral blood CD16+/CD56+ cells in women with primary recurrent spontaneous abortion." *Ginekologia Polska*, 72(12):1063-8, 2001.
48 patients with 3 to 5 consecutive miscarriages were studied. LIT was performed twice prior to conception with a four-week interval. It was found that LIT significantly decreased the percentage of CD16+/CD56+ NK cells in the peripheral blood of women with recurrent miscarriage.

Zhu G et al: ["Immunotherapy by B-lymphocytes in patients with unexplained habitual abortion."] *Zhonghua Fu Chan Ke Za Zhi*, Apr; 35(4):212-3, 2000.
24 women with unexplained recurrent abortion were immunized with their partner's B-lymphocytes for 3 months. 22 saw an increase in anti-paternal lymphocytotoxic antibodies from 8% before immunization to 75%. 20 achieved pregnancy and there were 16 successful deliveries.

204 **"...a survey of over 4,500 women who had been treated with LIT..."** – Kling C et al: "Adverse effects of intradermal allogeneic lymphocyte immunotherapy: acute reactions and role of autoimmunity." *Human Reproduction*, Feb; 21(2):429-35, 2006.

205 **"...A recent report on the results of a 2- to 3-year follow-up of 2,687 IVF couples..."** – Kling C et al: "Transfusion-related risks of intradermal allogeneic lymphocyte immunotherapy: Single cases in a large cohort and review of the literature." American *Journal of Reproductive Immunology*, Vol.56, p.157, Sep 2006.
In this follow-up of couples treated during 1996 to 2002, anaphylaxis or malignancy in recipients of LIT and fetal/newborn alloimmune diseases were not observed in 2,687 and 2,848 cases respectively.

Clark DA et al: "Intravenous immunoglobulins (IVIG) efficacious in early pregnancy failure? A critical review and meta analysis for patients who fail in vitro fertilization and embryo transfer (IVF)." *Journal of Assisted Reproduction & Genetics*, Jan 19; 1-13, 2006.

209 **"In 37 of Dr Beer's patients who refused optimal immunotherapy..."** – Unpublished data as of November 2005. Patients using anticoagulant therapy and baby aspirin used alone (due to voluntary patient non-compliance) gave an ongoing pregnancy success rate of 54% (20/37). When LIT and IVIG were added there was a 75% (24/32) ongoing pregnancy success rate in a similar patient population. (Average patient age: 36.5 years. 44% of these patients had 3 or more miscarriages and 18% had 3 or more IVF failures.)

212 **"Professor Lesley Regan interviewed by Norman Swan for Radio National in 1997:"** – "The Health Report," *Radio National,* Monday 27th January 1997.
Transcript can be found at:
http://www.abc.net.au/rn/talks/8.30/helthrpt/hstories/hr270197.htm

- 403 -

NOTES

215 **"One of these spanned a period of nine years during which the pregnancies of 61 women..."** – Babill A and Stray-Pederson S: "Etiologic factors and subsequent reproductive performance in 195 couples with a prior history of habitual abortion." *American Journal of Obstetrics & Gynecology*, 148: pp.140-46, 1984.

215 **"Similar outcomes have been seen in studies where...she is out of the miscarriage 'danger zone.'"** – Clark DA and Daya S: "Trials and tribulations in the treatment of recurrent spontaneous abortion." *American Journal of Reproductive Immunology*, 25, 18-24, 1991.

215 **"...groups that emerge through a process of self selection, or have been pre-selected..."** – Clifford K, Rai R and Regan L: "Future pregnancy outcome following idiopathic recurrent miscarriage." *Human Reproduction*, 14: pp.2868-71, 1999. *See also*:

Liddell H et al: "Recurrent miscarriage: outcome after supportive care in early pregnancy." *Australian and New Zealand Journal of Obstetrics and Gynaecology*, Nov; 31(4):320-2, 1991.

216 **"...a large percentage of miscarriage patients who tested positive for APA (about 50%) had coexisting NK and/or cytokine issues..."** – Beer AE et al: "Immunophenotypic profiles of peripheral blood lymphocytes in women with recurrent pregnancy losses and in infertile women with multiple failed in vitro fertilization cycles." *American Journal of Reproductive Immunology*, Apr; 35(4): 376-82, 1996. *See also*:
Beer AE et al: "Up-regulated expression of CD56+, CD56+/CD16+, and CD19+ cells in peripheral blood lymphocytes in pregnant women with recurrent pregnancy losses." *American Journal of Reproductive Immunology*, Aug; 34(2):93-9, 1995.

216 **"Three years later, a study at St. Mary's..."** – Rai R et al: "Polycystic ovaries and recurrent miscarriage: a reappraisal." *Human Reproduction*, Mar; 15(3):612-5, 2000.
"The prevalence of polycystic ovaries was 40.7% (895/2199). The livebirth rate was similar amongst women with polycystic ovaries (60.9%; 142/233) compared to that amongst women with normal ovarian morphology (58.5%; 148/253; not significant)."

216 **"Another trial the same year quoted a livebirth rate of 58%..."** – Regan L et al: "Prospective pregnancy outcome in untreated recurrent miscarriers with thyroid autoantibodies." *Human Reproduction*, Jul; 15 (7):1637-9, 2000.
"Amongst the 710 thyroid antibody negative women, 47 of 81 untreated pregnancies resulted in livebirths (58%)."

216 The ARGC sued the BBC for slander and won their case. Link to the original BBC Panorama show transcript:
http://news.bbc.co.uk/2/hi/programmes/panorama/6264997.stm

217 **"...two major concerns regarding women who repeatedly lose their babies..."** – Kwak-Kim J et al: "Recurrent pregnancy loss: A disease of inflammation and coagulation." *Obstetric and Gynaecological Research,* Vol. 35, No. 4: 609–622, August 2009.

NOTES

Han A and Sung K: "Immune modulation of i.v. immunoglobulin in women with reproductive failure," Reproductive Medicine and Biology, Apr; 17(2): 115–124, 2018. In this review, the action of IVIG the authors concluded, "It is obvious that IVIG is effective in recurrent pregnancy losses and repeated implantation failures with immunologic disturbances... including a high natural killer cell proportion and its cytotoxicity or an elevated T helper 1 to T helper 2 ratio."

17. TRIALS ON TRIAL

221 **"In his 2002 article, 'Wars of the Roses: Disagreements among Reproductive Immunologists'..."** – Gleicher N et al: "The immunological 'Wars of the Roses' – disagreements among reproductive immunologists." *Human Reproduction*, Vol.17, No.3, 539-542, 2002.

221 **"...U.S. Congress Office of Technology Assessment..."** –U.S. Congress Office of Technology Assessment: "The impact of randomized clinical trials on health policy and medical practice." p.10, Aug 1983. See: http://govinfo.library.unt.edu/ota/Ota_4/DATA/1983/8310.PDF

224 **"The publication of these discoveries in *Science* in 1973..."** – Beer AE and Billingham RE: "Maternally acquired runt disease: Immune lymphocytes from the maternal blood can traverse the placenta and cause runt disease in the progeny." *Science*, 4070, pp.240-43, Jan 1973.

225 **"Dr W. Page Faulk found four couples with recurrent miscarriage..."** – McIntyre J and Faulk W: "Maternal blocking factors in human pregnancy are found in plasma not serum." *Lancet*, Oct 20; 2(8147):821-3, 1979.
"Autologous pregnancy plasma, but not serum was found to contain a specific allogeneic inhibitor for paternal lymphocytes."

225 **"Professor Mowbray...set up a trial in 1982..."** – Mowbray J et al: "Controlled trial of treatment of recurrent spontaneous abortion by immunization with paternal cells." *Lancet*, Apr 27; 1(8435):941-3, 1985.
17 of 22 women given paternal cells had successful pregnancies, compared with 10 of 27 given their own cells.

225 **"...many studies have reinforced these initial findings with success rates approaching 100% for selected patient groups."** – Daya and Gunby: "The effectiveness of allogeneic leukocyte immunization in unexplained primary recurrent spontaneous abortion." *American Journal of Reproductive Immunology*, 32:294-302, 1994.
In this review the data from randomized controlled trials in eight centers showed that the effectiveness of LIT was close to 100% for those with normal karyotype embryos

225 **"In 2005, a national U.K. newspaper reported..."** – "Baby joy for fertility expert." *Daily Mail*, 8th July 2005.
Embryologist Kathryn Berrisford suffered four miscarriages before her boss at Nottingham's CARE fertility clinic recommended immune therapy to help her become a mother. See:
http://www.dailymail.co.uk/pages/live/articles/health/womenfamily.html?in_article_id=355116&in_page_id=1799

- 405 -

NOTES

226 **"...(approximately 70% of Japanese university hospitals still provide this therapy)..."** – Takeshita T: "Diagnosis and treatment of recurrent miscarriage associated with immunologic disorders: Is paternal lymphocyte immunization a relic of the past?" *Journal of Nippon Medical School*, EN; 715: 308-313, 2004.
"We observed that NK cell activity in women with recurrent miscarriage was higher than that in women without a history of miscarriage... Approximately 70% of Japanese university hospitals are still performing paternal lymphocyte immunization."

226 **"...five-year long Recurrent Miscarriage Study (REMIS)..."** – Ober C et al: "Mononuclear-cell immunisation in prevention of recurrent miscarriages: a randomised trial." *Lancet*, pp.354:365-9, 1999.
Women who had experienced three or more unexplained spontaneous abortions were enrolled in this double-blind, multicenter, randomized clinical trial. 91 received paternal lymphocyte immunization and 92 were given a sterile saline (control). The success rate was 31/86 (36%) in the treatment group and 41/85 (48%) in the control group. In pregnant women only, the corresponding success rates were 31/68 (46%) and 41/63 (65%).

227 **"...the entry criteria were relaxed...to increase the number of patients taking part."** – Clark DA et al: "Unexplained sporadic and recurrent miscarriage in the new millennium: a critical analysis of immune mechanisms and treatments." *Human Reproduction Update*, Vol.7, No.5, pp.501-511, 2001.
"In the study by Ober et al., due to poor accrual, the entry criteria were relaxed such that recruitment increased, and many of these patients may have had subclinical autoimmunity detectable by more extensive testing that included ANA."

227 **"It was known from the 1991 American Society for Reproductive Immunology Ethics Committee study..."** – Coulam C and Clark DA: "Report from the Ethics Committee for Immunotherapy, American Society for the Immunology of Reproduction." *American Journal of Reproductive Immunology*, Sept; 26(2):93-5, 1991.

227 **"...far less of an initial dose than they needed, which means success rates could never be optimal."** – Aoki K et al: *American Journal of Obstetrics & Gynecology*, Sep; 169(3):649-53 1993
Here, 106 primary recurrent aborters were immunized with LIT twice in early pregnancy. A further 38 controls received a reduced cell dosage. The ongoing pregnancy success rate for those immunized with a large number of cells was 83.0%. For those receiving a lesser dose the rate was 55.3%.

227 **"With overnight storage, the CD200 molecule is lost."** – Clark DA and Chaouat G. "Loss of surface CD200 on stored allogeneic leukocytes may impair anti-abortive effect in vivo." *American Journal of Reproductive Immunology*, Jan; 53(1):13-20, 2005.

228 **"It has been reported that $2.2 million of taxpayers' dollars was spent on an abortive trial..."** – Professor David Clark in a reply to a letter from Dr Gerard Chaouat featured in *The American Journal of Reproductive Immunology*, 52:340-343, 2004.

- 406 -

NOTES

228   **"Professor Clark, Dr Coulam and others also produced an analysis of the discrepancies, which was also published."** – Clark DA, Coulam C et al: "Unexplained sporadic and recurrent miscarriage in the new millennium: A critical analysis of immune mechanisms and treatments." *Human Reproduction Update*, 7:501-511, 2001.

The flaws in the Recurrent Miscarriage Study are detailed in this paper and summarized in the following report: Clark DA: "Shall we properly re-examine the status of allogeneic lymphocyte therapy for recurrent early pregnancy failure?" *American Journal of Reproductive Immunology*, 51:7-15, 2004.

229   **"...a 2003 Cochrane Review in 2003 written by Dr Jim Scott, a colleague of Dr Ober..."** – Scott J: "Immunotherapy for recurrent miscarriage." *The Cochrane Database of Systematic Reviews:* 2003.

The report concludes: "Paternal cell immunization, third party donor leukocytes, trophoblast membranes, and intravenous immune globulin provide no significant beneficial effect over placebo in preventing further miscarriages."

This conclusion is reiterated in an updated version of the report in 2006: Scott J et al: "Immunotherapy for recurrent miscarriage." *Cochrane Database Systematic Review*, Apr 1:19; 2:CD000112, 2006.

Professor Clark comments: "The updated review includes a double-blind, randomized controlled trial carried out at the Mayo Clinic in the U.S. in 2004, which showed an ongoing pregnancy rate of 84% in recurrent aborters treated with paternal LIT, compared with 25 to 33% in groups who received other forms of lymphocyte treatment. (Pandey MK and Agrawal S: *International Immunopharmacology,* Feb; 4(2): 289-98, 2004.) However, instead of analysis by intention-to-treat, Scott reduced the odds ratio by using as the denominator only those patients who became pregnant, which is not representative of the true outcome. This same maneuver was used in the 1999 Ober/Lancet paper in a post-hoc analysis to claim LIT was harmful. A referee of this paper came to me and said he had objected, but the Editor did not make the authors remove that statement. In the *Cochrane Review* update, the number of patients in the Illeni et al study is also less than in the published paper in *Human Reproduction*."

229   **"The journalist issuing these warnings was Jon Cohen, the author of *Coming to Term: Uncovering the Truth About Miscarriage.*"** –Published by Houghton Mifflin in 2005. ISBN: 0618277242.

p.75: "I contacted the Food and Drug Administration to clarify how, in the light of the REMIS results, it regulated this supposed therapy."

p.237: "After my calls to the Food and Drug administration about Lymphocyte Immunization therapy apparently led the FDA to contact Beer..."

229   **"...the 1997 article 'Immunotherapy for Recurrent Pregnancy Loss: Standard of Care or Buyer Beware'"** – Hill J: "Immunotherapy for recurrent pregnancy loss: 'Standard of Care or Buyer Beware'" *Society for Gynecologic Investigation*, Nov-Dec; 4(6):267-73, 1997. *See also:*

Hill J: "It's Not What You Don't Know That Makes You Look Like a Fool. It's What You Do Know That Ain't So." *Fertility & Sterility*, 74, 637-638, 2000.
Hill J and Scott R: "Immunologic Tests and IVF: 'Please Enough Already.'" *Fertility and Sterility*, Volume 74, Issue 3, pp. 439-442, Sep 2000.

- 407 -

NOTES

229   **"...a critique that was praised by Professor Regan..."** – *Miscarriage: What Every Woman Needs to Know*, by Regan L. Published by Orion in 2001. ISBN: 0752837575.

p.174: "A colleague of mine in the U.S. [Joseph Hill] published a frank account of immunotherapy for recurrent miscarriers entitled: Immunotherapy for Recurrent Pregnancy Loss: 'Standard of Care or Buyer Beware.' He was brave to do so and I think the title of his article sums up the problem for readers of this book."

230   **"Finally, in January 2002, the FDA sent out a letter..."** – See: http://www.fda.gov/cber/ltr/lit013002.htm

230   **"...the ongoing pregnancy success rate dropped..."** – From a paper presented by Dr Alan E. Beer at the American Society for Reproductive Immunology 23rd Annual Meeting, New Haven, Connecticut, June 18-22, 2003.

231   **"...LIT data from Europe..."** – Christiansen OB et al: "Active or passive immunization in unexplained recurrent miscarriage." *Journal of Reproductive Immunology*, Jun; 62(1-2):41-52, 2004.

This report states that in clinics in Denmark, LIT and IVIG immunotherapies have been tested in placebo controlled trials since 1986. Both are now used routinely. *See also*:

Professor Mowbray's continued use of LIT:
https://www.youtube.com/watch?v=SxhcesGDpYI

Related Studies and Articles (Selection):

Beer AE and Billingham RE: "Histocompatibility gene polymorphisms and maternal-fetal relationships." *Transplant Procedures*, 9:1393-1401, 1977.
Beer AE and Billingham RE: "Maternal immunological recognition mechanisms during pregnancy." *Ciba Foundation Symposium*, (64): 293-322, 1978.
Beer AE et al: "Maternal hamster immune responses to alloantigens of the fetus." *Federal Procedures*, 37: 2054-2056, 1978.

Beer AE: "The paradox of feto-placental units as allografts." *Recent Advances in Reproduction and Regulation of Fertility*, Editor: Talwar G, Elsevier/North Holland Biomedical Press, pp.501-514, 1979. ISBN: 0444801235

Beer AE and Sio J: "Maternal immunoregulation and the immunologically privileged status of the trophoblast." pp.143-154 *Immunological Aspects of Infertility and Fertility Regulation*, Editors: Schumacher G and Dhindsa D, Elsevier/ North Holland, 1980. ISBN: 044400405X

Beer AE and Billingham RE: "Mechanisms of non-rejection of feto-placental allografts." *Folia Biologica (Praha)*, 26: 243-255, 1980.

Beer AE et al: "Immunologically induced reproductive disorders." *Endocrinology of Human Infertility: New Aspects, Proceedings of the Serono Clinical Colloquia on Reproduction,* Editors: Crosignani PG and Rubin BL, Academic Press, London, pp.419-439, 1981. ISBN: 080891393X

NOTES

Beer AE et al: "Major histocompatibility complex antigens, maternal and paternal immune responses, and chronic habitual abortions in humans." *American Journal of Obstetrics & Gynecology*, Dec 15; 141 (8): 987-99, 1981.

Beer AE and Sio J: "Placenta as an immunological barrier." *Biology of Reproduction*, 26:15-27, 1982.

Beer AE et al: "Recurrent abortion: Analysis of the roles of parental sharing of histocompatibility antigens and maternal immunological responses to paternal antigens." *Reproductive Immunology 1983*, pp.185-195. Editors: Isojima S and Billington W, Elsevier Science, 1983. ISBN: 0444805516

Beer AE: "How did your mother not reject you?" *Annals of Immunology, (Institute Pasteur)*, 135 D: 315-318, 1984.
Beer AE and Menge A: "The significance of human leukocyte antigen profiles in human infertility, recurrent abortion, and pregnancy disorders." *Fertility & Sterility*, 43: 693-695, 1985.

Beer AE et al: "Pregnancy outcome in human couples with recurrent spontaneous abortions: HLA antigen profiles; HLA antigen sharing; female serum MLR blocking factors; and paternal leukocyte immunization." *Experimental & Clinical Immunogenetics*, 2(3):137-53, 1985.

Beer AE et al: "Pregnancy outcome in human couples with idiopathic recurrent abortions: The roles(s) of female serum, mixed lymphocyte culture blocking factors, potentiating factors, and local uterine immunity before and after paternal leukocyte immunization." *Immunological Approaches to Contraception and Promotion of Fertility*, pp.393-406. Plenum Publishing. ISBN: 0306422743

Beer AE et al: "Pregnancy outcome in human couples with recurrent spontaneous abortions: The role(s) of HLA antigen sharing, ABO blood group antigen profiles, female serum MLR blocking factors, antisperm antibodies and immunotherapy." *Immunoregulation and Fetal Survival*, Editors: Gill, TJ and Wegmann TG, Oxford University Press, 1987. ISBN: 0195039890

Beer AE: "Immunotherapy in reproductive disorders." *Immunology and Medicine: Immunology of Pregnancy*, Editors: Reeves G and Stern C. Kluwer Academic Publishers, 165-195, 1989. OCLC: 21901078

For a complete listing see: http://repro-med.net/papers/scpapers.php

ADDENDUM

I – FERTILITY UNDER FIRE

261 **"Fewer babies are being born and more couples are resorting to fertility treatment..."** – Daya S et al: "Advances in Fertility and Reproductive Medicine: Proceedings of the 18th World Congress on Fertility and Sterility," held in Montreal, Canada 23-28 May 2004. Elsevier Publication, ISBN: 0444515453. *See also*:

"An Aging World: 2001: The Legacy of Fertility Decline," U.S. Census Bureau. See: www.census.gov/prod/2001pubs/p95-01-1.pdf

- 409 -

NOTES

261 **"The increased number of chromosomal changes that are being seen today coincide with the introduction of chemical products..."** – Huddle A et al: "Generations at Risk – Reproductive Health and the Environment." The MIT Press, Cambridge, Massachusetts and London, England. *See also*:
Andersen AG: "High frequency of suboptimal semen quality in an unselected population of young men." *Human Reproduction*, Vol.15, 366–372, 2000.

Auger J et al: "Decline in semen quality among fertile men in Paris during the past 20 years." *New England Journal of Medicine*, 332, 281-285, 1995.

261 **"Worldwide, over 400 million tons of chemicals are manufactured annually."** WWF: Toxic Chemicals
http://wwf.panda.org/knowledge_hub/teacher_resources/webfieldtrips/toxics/

261 **"Of the several thousand chemicals that are produced in volume, reproductive toxicology data exists for only a hundred or so."** – Sullivan F: "Little is known on the reproductive dangers of chemicals." *Environmental Health Perspectives*, 101(Suppl.2):13-18, 1993.
The Organization for Economic Cooperation and Development (OECD) and the European Economic Community (EEC) prepared lists of several thousand chemicals produced in amounts from 1,000 up to over 10,000 tons per year. The report concludes: "Toxicological data of any type exist for a few hundred and reproductive toxicology data exist for probably 100."

262 **"A 2006 Canadian report has revealed that everyone that took part in their study was contaminated by more than half of the 88 chemicals that were tested."** – See:
http://www.environmentaldefence.ca/toxicnation/resources/publications

262 **"A further investigation found over 500 potentially dangerous man-made chemicals..."** – Data provided by London-based Biolab, a medical laboratory analyzing toxins in blood and fatty tissue. Source: Johnston L and Ingham J: "Cocktail of Toxins in Us All." *Express Newspapers*, Jan 2000.
http://www.gene.ch/info4action/2000/Jan/msg00010.html

262 **"...it has been estimated that each of us consumes around four and a half pounds of pesticides and herbicides..."** – Source: Associazione Italiana per l'Agricoltura Biologica and Legambiente, Oct 2001, as cited in *The Organic Newsline*, Vol.2, Issue 38, Oct 4, 2001.
Consumers in Italy annually consume approximately two kilos of chemicals and pesticides from products grown through conventional farming practices.

262 **"As of 2018, infertility is estimated to affect 15% of the population, and in some countries, it has exceeded 25%."** – Sciarra J: "Infertility: an international health problem." *International Journal of Gynecology & Obstetrics,* 46:155-163, 1994. *See also*:
Sanocka D and Kurpisz M: "Infertility in Poland – present status, reasons and prognosis as a reflection of Central and Eastern Europe problems with reproduction." *Medical Science Monitor*, Mar; 9(3): SR16-20, 2003.

262 **"According to a 2005 report, the rate of infertility in Europe and other developed nations is set to rise to 33%."**– Source: Meikle J: "Expert fears fertility problem for 1 in 3 couples." *The Guardian*, June 21 2005.

- 410 -

NOTES

On Professor Bill Ledger speaking at the European Society of Human Reproduction and Embryology conference in Copenhagen, 2005.

262 **"...endometriosis afflicts upwards of 10% of women of child-bearing age."** – Buck L et al: "Incidence of endometriosis by study population and diagnostic method: the ENDO study." *Fertility and Sterility*; 96(2): 360-5, 2011.

262 **"...by the age of fifty, up to 80% have uterine fibroids."** Uterine Fibroids Fact Sheet. Office on Women's Health. January 15, 2015.

262 **"...the detection of toxins in the follicular fluid surrounding the egg has been associated with increasing levels of fertilization failure."** – Foster W et al: "An overview of some reproductive toxicology studies conducted at Health Canada." *Toxicology & Industrial Health*, Vol.12, Nos.3/4, pp.447-459, 1996.
In six couples undergoing IVF, three of the couples became pregnant and three had embryos that failed to fertilize. The PCB level of the follicular fluid was higher in the group that failed fertilization.

262 **"The sexual development and fertility problems that are seen in both men and women are strongly linked to substances called endocrine disruptors..."** – "International Workshop on the Impact of the Environment on Reproductive Health (1991: Copenhagen)." *Progress in Human Reproduction Research*, (20):1-11, 1991.
"The costs of environmental injury to reproduction include sub-fertility, intrauterine growth retardation, spontaneous abortion, and various birth defects...complications of pregnancy may be related to pollution levels surrounding industrial plants. Reproductive health is affected through chromosome damage and cell destruction, prenatal death, altered growth, fetal abnormalities, postnatal death, functional learning deficits, and premature aging." *See also*:

"Vallombrosa Consensus Statement on Environmental Contaminants and Human Fertility Compromise." Oct 2005. See:
www.healthandenvironment.org/workinggroups/fertility

Pollack A et al: "Exposure to bisphenol A, chlorophenols, benzophenones, and parabens in relation to reproductive hormones in healthy women: A chemical mixture approach." *Environment International*, Volume 120, Pages 137-144, November 2018.
Abnormally high levels of estrogen and progesterone were found in the urine of 100 women out of 143 women tested who were not taking birth control pills. Those with higher levels of chlorophenols in their urine produced more estrogen and FSH, while parabens and BPA increased estrogen.

Leonard J et al: "Hypospadias trends in two U.S. surveillance systems." *Pediatrics*, Vol. 100 No.5, pp.831-834, 1997.
"The Metropolitan Atlanta Congenital Defects Program (MACDP) provided birth prevalence rates from 1968 to 1993. The nationwide Birth Defects Monitoring Program (BDMP) provided rates from 1970 to 1993...Data from both surveillance systems showed an approximate doubling of hypospadias rates in the 1970s and 1980s."

- 411 -

NOTES

Carlsen E et al: "Evidence for decreasing quality of semen during the past 50 years." *British Medical Journal*, Vol.305, pp.609-613, 1992. *See also*:

Kold Jensen T et al: "Poor semen quality may contribute to recent decline in fertility rates." *Human Reproduction*, Vol.17, No.6, 1437-1440, June 2002.

263 **"According to a review of thousands of studies... sperm concentration fell by 52% in Western countries between 1973 and 2011."** – Levine H et al: "Temporal trends in sperm count: a systematic review and meta-regression analysis." *Human Reproduction Update*, 2017.

263 **"...up to 85% of these sperm will be defective."** – "WHO laboratory manual for the Examination and processing of human semen," 2010. ISBN 978 92 4 154778 9
The World Health Organization estimates that the median percentage of normal sperm morphology in fertile men is 15%. The WHO "normal" reference range for healthy sperm was redefined at between 4 and 48% per sample.

263 **"...'some 75% of cancers are due to mutations induced by environmental factors: mainly chemicals.'"** – Professor Belpomme, President of the French "Association for Research on Treatments against Cancer" (ARTAC) speaking at PAN Europe network members' conference in Copenhagen, November 2003.

Organic Mercury

263 **"It interferes with cell division in the developing fetal brain and binds to DNA to disrupt the copying of chromosomes."** – Bakulski K et al: "Prenatal mercury concentration is associated with changes in DNA methylation at TCEANC2 in newborns," International Journal of Epidemiology, Aug; 44(4): 1249–1262, 2015.

Chalfin N: "Reproductive & Developmental Hazards: Spotlight on Mercury." A report for CETOS (Center for Ethics and Toxics). See:
http://www.cetos.org/articles/reprodevel.html

Dioxins

264 **"Laboratory studies have shown that dioxins can adversely affect fertility, pregnancy and fetal growth."** – Hattori Y et al: "Dioxin-induced fetal growth retardation: the role of a preceding attenuation in the circulating level of glucocorticoid." *Endocrine* Apr, 47(2):572-580 2014. *See also*:
Klonisch T et al: "Molecular actions of polyhalogenated arylhydro-carbons (PAHs) in female reproduction." *Current Medicinal Chemistry*, 12(5):599-616, 2005.

264 **"In a study of German women, elevated levels of dioxins were measured in those with endometriosis, fibroids, miscarriage and persistent infertility."** – Gerhard I et al: "Chlorinated hydrocarbons in infertile women." *Environmental Research,* 80; 4:299-310, 1999.
"In women with uterine fibroids, endometriosis, miscarriages, persistent infertility and hormonal disturbances, elevated concentrations of chlorinated hydrocarbons with long half-lives were observed." *See also*:

NOTES

Rier S and Foster W: "Environmental dioxins and endometriosis." *Toxicological Sciences*, 70:161-170, 2002.

Alkylphenols

264   **"Alkylphenols are another group of endocrine disrupting chemicals linked to sexual deformities"** – De Coster S and van Larebeke N: "Endocrine-Disrupting Chemicals: Associated Disorders and Mechanisms of Action": J Environ Public Health. 2012; 2012: 713696, 2012. *See also*:

Seki M et al: "Effects of 4-nonylphenol and 4-tert-octylphenol on sex differentiation and vitellogenin induction in medaka (Oryzias latipes)." *Environmental Toxicology & Chemistry,* Jul; 22(7):1507-16, 2003.
Fish were exposed to various concentrations of two alkylphenols from fertilized eggs to 60 days of age. "...intersex gonads still existed, even after the fish were transferred to clean water for two months."

264   **"...in animals, alkylphenols are associated with reduced sperm counts and testicular size ..."** – Greve T: "Endocrine disrupting compounds: effect of octylphenol on reproduction over three generations." *Theriogenology*, Jan; 55(1): 131-50, 2001. *See also*:
vom Saal F et al: "A physiologically based approach to the study of bisphenol-A and other estrogenic chemicals on the size of the reproductive organs, daily sperm production and behavior." *Toxicology & Industrial Health*, 14(1-2):239-260, 1998.

265   **"In experiments on mice, this chemical induces a similar chromosomal defect to the one that results in Down's syndrome."** – Hunt P et al: "When disaster strikes: rethinking caging materials." *Lab Animal*, 32:24-27, 2003.
Aging polycarbonate cages and drinking bottles in animal laboratories released chemicals which produced "a highly significant increase in chromosomal aneuploidy and other serious meiotic defects" in mice. A 20-fold increase in chromosome misalignment was seen at maximum exposure.

265   **"Other studies have reported elevated levels of Bisphenol A in women with...a history of three or more pregnancy losses."** – Suzumori K et al: "Exposure to bisphenol A is associated with recurrent miscarriage." *Human Reproduction*, 20:2325-2329, 2005.

265   **"Prenatal exposure...shown to increase the Th1 immune response in adulthood."** – Mori Y et al: "Prenatal exposure to bisphenol A up-regulates immune responses, including T helper 1 and T helper 2 responses, in mice." *Immunology*, Jul; 112(3):189 95, 2004.

265   **"A 2005 review of the literature revealed that of 115 published studies involving Bisphenol A..."** – vom Saal et al: "An extensive new literature concerning low dose effects of bisphenol A shows the need for a new risk assessment." *Environmental Health Perspectives*, Vol. 113, No.8, Aug 2005.
"In 31 publications with vertebrate and invertebrate animals, significant effects occurred below the predicted 'safe' or reference dose of 50 mcg/kg/day BPA. An estrogenic mode of action of BPA is confirmed by in vitro experiments, which describe disruption of cell function at 10(-12) M or 0.23 ppt."

- 413 -

NOTES

Phthalates (Plasticizers)

265 **"The Centers for Disease Control and Prevention reported the highest levels of phthalates were found in the urine of women aged between 20 and 40..."** – Blount B et al: "Levels of seven urinary phthalate metabolites in a human reference population." *Environmental Health Perspectives*, 108(10):979-982, 2000.

265 **"...a common type of phthalate called DEHP, which is found in many food products, interfered with male and female fertility, particularly during early life. ..."** – Zhang X et al: "Histo-pathological changes of the crypt-orchid testis and epididymis of mice exposed to DEHP." *Zhonghua Nan Ke Xue*, Nov; 10 (11):807-10, 814, 2004.
This study concludes: "During the critical period of male sexual differentiation, exposure to DEHP may lead to a significantly high incidence of cryptorchidism, testicular damage and fertility impairment in the male offspring." *See also*:

Schettler T et al: "Health risks posed by use of Di-2-ethylhexyl phthalate (DEHP) in PVC medical devices: a critical review." *American Journal of Industrial Medicine,* Jan; 39(1):100-1, 2001.
"In vivo and in vitro research links DEHP or its metabolites to a range of adverse effects in the liver, reproductive tract, kidneys, lungs, and heart. Developing animals are particularly susceptible to effects on the reproductive system."

Duty S et al: "The relationship between environmental exposures to phthalates and DNA damage in human sperm using the neutral comet assay." *Environmental Health Perspectives*, 111:1164-1169, 2003.
In one of the first studies of the effects on humans, researchers found signs of correlation between exposure to phthalates and damage to the DNA of human sperm. The study, conducted at a Massachusetts ferti-lity clinic, analyzed urine and semen samples from 168 men. Results suggested exposure to those phthalates was associated with increased DNA damage in sperm. The scientists are unsure as to whether this damage could leave men infertile or cause birth defects. Four manuscripts describing the findings from this ongoing study were published in peer-reviewed journals in 2003 and 2004.

265 **"...all pthalates undergo hydrolysis in the body to produce compounds which rapidly reduce fetal testosterone production..."** – "Phthalates and Cumulative Risk Assessment: The Tasks Ahead." National Research Council (US) Committee on the Health Risks of Phthalates, Washington (DC): National Academies Press (US); 2008.

266 **"High blood levels of phthalates have also been detected in women with endometriosis."** – Petraglia F: "High plasma concentrations of di-(2-ethylhexyl)-phthalate in women with endometriosis." *Human Reproduction*, Jul; 18(7):1512-5, 2003.

Pesticides

266 **"Organochlorine compounds are known to affect female human reproduction by shortening the menstrual cycle..."** – Windham G et al:

- 414 -

NOTES

"Exposure to organochlorine compounds and effects on ovarian function." *Epidemiology*, Mar; 16(2):182-90, 2005.

During 1997-1999, 50 Southeast Asian immigrant women of reproductive age collected urine samples daily. The samples were tested for metabolites of estrogen and progesterone. All samples had detectable DDT and DDE, with average levels higher than typical U.S. populations. The average menstrual cycle length was approximately 4 days shorter in women whose concentration of DDT or DDE was highest and their progesterone levels during the luteal phase were consistently decreased. "This study indicates a potential effect of DDE on ovarian function, which may influence other end points such as fertility, pregnancy, and reproductive cancers."

266 **"...a 2001 report...exposure to commercially applied agricultural pesticides and fetal death due to congenital defects..."** – Bell E et al: "A case controlled study of pesticides and fetal death due to congenital anomalies." *Epidemiology*, 12:148-156, 2001.

Mothers who lived near crops where certain pesticides were sprayed faced a 40 to 120% increase in risk of miscarriage due to birth defects. The report states: "There appears to be a special 'window of vulnerability' for birth defects, between the 3rd and 8th week of pregnancy." *See also*:

Fernandez-Arguelles R et al: "Risk for congenital malformations in pregnant women exposed to pesticides in the state of Nayarit, Mexico." *Ginecologia Y Obstetricia de Mexico*, Nov; 70:538-44, 2002.

279 newborns from mothers living in rural areas in the northwest of Mexico were studied. 93 had central nervous, face, genital, hip, foot or finger congenital malformations.

267 **"Regular exposure (both indoors and outdoors) to pesticides before pregnancy has also been linked to a 300% greater incidence of cleft palate, cleft lip and stillbirth."** – Midtling J et al: "Congenital anomalies associated with maternal exposure to oxydemetonmethyl." *Environmental Research,* Dec; 50(2):256-61, 1989.

35 people became ill after working in a cauliflower field contaminated with residues of insecticides. One was pregnant with a 4-week-old fetus. The child died 14 days after being born. This case represents the first report of human malformations associated with prenatal exposure to oxydemetonmethyl. *See also*:

Nurminen T: "Maternal pesticide exposure and pregnancy outcome." *Journal of Occupational and Environmental Medicine*, Aug; 37(8):935-40, 1995.

"Orofacial clefts have been related to maternal environmental exposure to pesticides and exposure in agricultural work. Moreover, there is evidence that maternal agricultural occupation and pesticide exposure may be associated with elevated risk of spontaneous abortion and stillbirth."

267 **"...the use of home pesticides during the first two months of pregnancy has also been associated with stillbirth..."** – Pastore L et al: "Risk of stillbirth from occupational and residential exposures." *Occupational and Environmental Medicine,* Vol.54:511-518, 1997.

Women exposed to chemicals such as cockroach and ant insecticides for one month in the home environment during early pregnancy were found to have a

NOTES

70% raised risk for stillbirths due to congenital defects and 2.4 times increased risk for stillbirth.

267   **"It is estimated that 90% of U.S. households use at least one pesticide product indoors...in a year..."** – Louie S et al: "Pesticides." In *Environmental and Occupational Medicine: Third Edition.* Lippincott-Raven Publishers, 83:1157-70, 1998.

267   **"...a major metabolite of DDT has been identified in the follicular fluid of women undergoing IVF..."** – Jarrell J et al: "Levels of environmental contaminants in human follicular fluid, serum, and seminal plasma of couples undergoing in vitro fertilization." *Archives of Environmental Contamination & Toxicology*, Jul; 43(1):121-6, 2002.
"These data reveal that more than 50% of the population of women attending a fertility program have had exposure to environmental chemicals sufficient to produce detectable concentrations in their serum and ovarian follicular fluid. Of the chemical contaminants detected in the serum and follicular fluid of these women, p, p'-DDE was the most frequently detected, had the highest residue levels, and was associated with failed fertilization.

267   **"Methoxychlor...has an estrogenic effect on birds and mammals, disrupting sexual development and reproduction and stimulating the growth of cancer cells."** – Eroschenko V and Cooke P: "Morphological and biochemical alterations in reproductive tracts of neonatal female mice treated with the pesticide methoxychlor." *Biology of Reproduction*, Vol.42:573-583, 1990.
In this study involving newborn mice, the pesticide methoxychlor was shown to interfere with the sexual development and reproductive behavior and to stimulate the growth of cancer cells.

267   **"In animal studies, methoxychlor 'feminized' male embryos..."** – Gray L et al: "A dose-response analysis of methoxychlor-induced alterations of reproductive development and function in the rat." *Fundamental & Applied Toxicology*, 12(1):92-108, 1989.

267   **"...vinclozolin blocked the production of testosterone causing feminization of males and other birth defects."** – Gray L et al: "Developmental effects of an environmental antiandrogen: the fungicide Vinclozolin alters sex differentiation of the male rat." *Toxicology & Applied Pharmacology*, 129(1):46-52, 1994. *See also*:
Kelce W et al: "Environmental hormone disruptors: Evidence that Vinclozolin developmental toxicity is mediated by antiandrogenic metabolites." *Toxicology & Applied Pharmacology*, 126(2):276-285, 1994.

267   **"These changes reduced the sperm counts and sperm motility, not only of those in the generation exposed to the chemical, but also of those in three subsequent generations."** – Skinner M et al: "Epigenetic transgenerational actions of endocrine disruptors and male fertility." *Science*, Jun 3; 308 (5727):1466-9, 2005.
"Transient exposure of a gestating female rat to the endocrine disruptors vinclozolin induced an adult phenotype in the F1 generation of decreased spermatogenic number and viability and increased incidence of male infertility.

- 416 -

NOTES

These effects were transferred through the male germline to nearly all males of all subsequent generations examined."

267 **"...the pesticide chlorpyrifos (Dursban) has been associated with increased autoimmune antibodies in tests on animals."** – Thrasher J et al: "Dangerous autoantibodies higher in pesticide exposed people." *Archives of Environmental Health*, Vol.48 (2), Mar/Apr, 1993.
The pesticide Chlorpyrifos (Dursban) was found to cause increases in autoimmune antibodies. Other references in this report link some cases of male and female infertility to autoimmune disorders in which the immune cells attack either the sperm or egg.

267 **"...lindane...has been shown to accumulate in the ovarian follicles, fallopian tubes and uterus of animals, causing reproductive failure."** – Sircar S and Lahiri P: "Lindane (gamma-HCH) causes reproductive failure and fetotoxicity in mice." *Toxicology*, 59(2):171-177, 1989. *See also*:

Cooper R et al: "Effect of lindane on hormonal control of reproductive function in the female rat." *Toxicology & Applied Pharmacology*, 99 (3):384-394, 1989.

268 **"Data from other laboratory tests have shown that it also retards testicular growth and reduces sperm quality."** – Taddei A et al: "Sperm quality and reproductive traits in male offspring of female rabbits exposed to lindane (gamma-HCH) during pregnancy and lactation." *Reproduction, Nutrition & Development*, May-Jun; 41(3): 217-25, 2001.

268 **"Pentachlorophenol (PCP) is another pesticide is linked to immunodeficiencies."** – Opelz G et al: "Association of elevated blood levels of pentachlorophenol (PCP) with cellular and humoral immuno-deficiencies." *Archives of Environmental Health*, Jan-Feb; 56(1):77-83, 2001.
The possible relationship between blood levels of PCP and immune function was studied in 190 patients who had been exposed to PCP-containing pesticides. The patients suffered from frequent respiratory infections and general fatigue. A dose-response relationship between blood levels of PCP and cellular and humoral immune parameters was seen. The authors concluded: "...increased blood levels of PCP were associated significantly with cellular and humoral immunodeficiencies."

268 **"In animal studies, PCP dramatically reduced levels of thyroid hormone and levels of thyroxine uptake in the fetal brain..."** – Jekat F et al: "Effects of pentachlorophenol (PCP) on the pituitary and thyroidal hormone regulation in the rat." *Toxicological Letters*, 71:9-25, 1994.
In female rats given PCP, "distinct effects on thyroid hormones as well as on thyrotropin (TSH) were observed." *See also*:

Beard A and Rawlings N. "Thyroid function and effects on reproduction in ewes exposed to the organochlorine pesticides lindane or pentachlorophenol (PCP) from conception." *Journal of Toxicology & Environmental Health*, Dec 24; 58(8):509-30, 1999.
Ewe lambs were exposed to lindane and pentachlorophenol (PCP) from conception to 67 weeks of age. "...PCP consistently disrupted thyroid function, most likely through a direct effect on the thyroid gland."

- 417 -

NOTES

268 **"An investigation in the mid-1990s found that around two thirds of the U.S. population had PCP residues in their urine."** – Hill R et al: "Pesticide residues in the urine of adults living in the United States: Reference range concentrations." *Environmental Research*, 71:99-108, 1995.

Polybrominated Diphenyl Ethers (PBDEs or fire retardants)

268 **"Exposure, even at low levels, appears to disrupt brain development..."** – Hooper K: "Learning and developmental disabilities initiative." *Body of Evidence – Report on PBDEs*. Feb 2004. See: http://www.iceh.org/pdfs/LDDI/2004NIHMeeting/LDDIMtgLeaveBehinPBDEr eport.pdf

268 **"PBDE's have also been implicated in reduced conception rates, increased abortion rates, menstrual abnormalities and developmental defects..."** – Klonisch T: "Molecular actions of polyhalogenated arylhydrocarbons (PAHs) in female reproduction." *Current Medicinal Chemistry*, 12(5):599-616, 2005.

Perfluorochemicals (PFCs)

268 **"High blood concentrations (of PFOS and PFOAs) are associated with irregular periods, longer conception times and infertility."** Potera C: "Study Associates PFOS and PFOA with Impaired Fertility." *Environmental Health Perspectives*, Apr; 117(4): A148, 2009.
Blood concentrations of PFOA and PFOS were measured in 1,240 pregnant women from weeks 4 through 14 of pregnancy. Women with higher levels were about twice as likely to have taken longer than 12 months to achieve pregnancy or needed infertility treatments.

268 **"These substances break down very slowly in the soil, air, and/or water they will remain in the environment for decades."** Biomonitoring/ Perfluorochemicals "America's Children and the Environment" Third Edition, Updated August 2017.
www.epa.gov/sites/production/files/2017

Benzene

269 **"...environmental exposure studies have shown that it can cause chromosomal damage."** – Smith M et al: "Use of octochrome fluorescence in situ hybridization to detect specific aneuploidy among all 24 chromosomes in benzene-exposed workers." *Chemical & Biological Interactions*, May 30; 153-154:117-22, 2005.
"...benzene has the capability of producing selective effects on certain chromosomes, which is supported by our in vitro findings showing that chromosomes 5 and 7 are more sensitive to loss than other chromosomes following exposure to benzene metabolites." *See also*:
Holland N et al: "Hydroquinone, a benzene metabolite, increases the level of aneusomy of chromosomes 7 and 8 in human CD34-positive blood progenitor cells." *Carcinogenesis*, Aug; 21(8):1485-90, 2000.

269 **"Benzene has also been linked to neural defects and childhood cancers including leukemia, lymphoma, and brain and urinary tract cancers."** –

- 418 -

NOTES

Knox E: "Childhood cancers and atmospheric carcinogens." *Journal of Epidemiology & Community Health*, Feb; 59 (2): 101-5, 2005.
Areas of of industrial and car exhaust emissions were compared to child cancer addresses. "Significant birth proximity relative risks were found within 1.0 km of hotspots for carbon monoxide, PM10 particles, VOCs, nitrogen oxides, benzene, dioxins, 1,3-butadiene, and benz(a)pyrene... most child cancers and leukaemias are probably initiated by such exposures." *See also*:

Gerin M et al: "Associations between several sites of cancer and occupational exposure to benzene, toluene, xylene, and styrene: Results of a case-control study in Montreal." *American Journal of Industrial Medicine*, Vol.34, 144-156, 1998.

Solvents

269 **"Organic and industrial solvents...are associated with a greater risk of miscarriage."** – Ember L: "Glycol ethers linked to increased miscarriage rate." *Chemical and Engineering News*, June 14, 1993.
This 5-year study found that women working with ethylene glycol ethers in IBM's semiconductor manufacturing clean rooms had an increased rate of miscarriages compared to women who worked in other areas of the plant. *See also*:

Schenker M et al: "Prospective monitoring of early fetal loss and clinical spontaneous abortion among female semiconductor workers." *American Journal of Industrial Medicine,* Dec; 28(6):833-46 1995.
In this 4-year study, University of California researchers found that women who work in fabrication areas of computer chip plants were 40% percent more likely to suffer miscarriages than other female workers in the semiconductor industry. Women exposed to the chemicals also had more difficulty becoming pregnant.

Correa A et al: "Ethylene glycol ethers and risks of spontaneous abortion and subfertility." *American Journal of Epidemiology,* Vol.143, No.7, pp.707-717, 1996.
"Among female manufacturers, potential exposure to mixtures containing Ethylene glycol ether was associated with increased risks of spontaneous abortion...and subfertility..."

269 **"Solvent exposure is also thought to be a 'trigger' for autoimmune disorders..."** – Lacey J et al: "Petroleum distillate solvents as risk factors for undifferentiated connective tissue disease (UCTD)." *American Journal of Epidemiology*, Vol.149, No.8, pp.761-770, 1999.
Information on solvent exposure was obtained from 205 cases of UCTD and 2,095 population-based controls. Occupational involving solvent exposure (e.g., furniture refinishing, perfume, cosmetic, drug or rubber product manufacturing, work in a medical diagnostic or pathology laboratory, painting or paint manufacturing) were significantly associated with connective tissue disease.

269 **"A Canadian study found that women who were exposed to solvents during the first trimester of pregnancy..."** – Khattak S et al: "Pregnancy outcome following gestational exposure to organic solvents." *Journal of the American Medical Association*, Vol.281, No.12, pp.1106-1109, 1999. *See also*:

- 419 -

NOTES

McMartin K et al: "Pregnancy outcome following material organic solvent exposure: A meta-analysis of epidemiologic studies." *American Journal of Industrial Medicine*, Vol.34, pp.288-292 1998.

269 **"...children born to women exposed to solvents through their work ...had learning difficulties and an increased incidence of hyperactivity."** – Koren G et al: "Effects of maternal occupational exposure to organic solvents on offspring visual functioning: a prospective controlled study." *Teratology*, Sep; 64(3): 134-41, 2001.

32 children whose mothers were exposed occupationally to organic solvents during pregnancy were compared with 27 non-exposed children. Solvent-exposed children had significantly higher error scores on color discrimination tests as well as poorer visual acuity compared with the control group. *See also:*

Koren G et al: "Child neurodevelopmental outcome and maternal occupational exposure to solvents." *Archives of Pediatrics & Adolescent Medicine,* Oct; 158(10):956-61, 2004.

The children of 32 pregnant women occupationally exposed to organic solvents were tested for cognitive functioning (IQ), language, visual-motor functioning, and behavioral functioning and were compared with an unexposed control group. "...children exposed in utero to organic solvents obtained lower scores on subtests of intellectual, language, motor, and neurobehavioral functioning."

Electro Magnetic Field (EMF) Non-Ionizing Radiation

270 **"Multiple studies have confirmed a link between EMF radiation and diabetes, heart disease and autoimmune disorders,"** Marshall T and Rumann T "Electrosmog and autoimmune disease," *Immunology Research*. 65(1): 129–135, 2017.

"Electrosmog immunomodulation may soon become necessary for successful therapy of autoimmune disease."

270 **"EMF exposure during pregnancy is associated with abnormal fetal development,"** "Radiation and Pregnancy: A Fact Sheet for Clinicians," Reviewed: April 4, 2018

https://emergency.cdc.gov/radiation/prenatalphysician.asp

"...the human embryo and fetus are particularly sensitive to ionizing radiation, and the health consequences of exposure can be severe, even at radiation doses too low to immediately affect the mother. Such consequences can include growth retardation, malformations, impaired brain function, and cancer.

270 **"...EMF exposure during pregnancy and an increased risk of miscarriage."** Wang, Q. et al. "Residential exposure to 50 Hz magnetic fields and the association with miscarriage risk: a 2-year prospective cohort study." PLoS One 8, e82113, 2013.

270 **"Male fertility is also under threat..."** Gorpinchenko I: "The influence of direct mobile phone radiation on sperm quality," *Central European Journal of Urology*, 67(1): 65–71, Apr 17, 2014.

"Long–term semen exposure... leads to a significant decrease in the number of sperm with progressive movement and an increase in those with non–progressive movement. Prolonged direct mobile phone exposure may bring about sperm DNA fragmentation."

NOTES

Avendano C et al, "Use of laptop computers connected to internet through Wi–Fi decreases human sperm motility and increases sperm DNA fragmentation," *Fertility and Sterility,* 2012;97:39–45, 2012.

For links to hundreds of peer-reviewed scientific studies & reports showing the impacts of EMF exposures on male fertility, pregnancy and health visit: **www.emfresearch.com**

II – THE LEGACY OF A TOXIC PREGNANCY

271 **"The baby's central nervous system is especially sensitive to toxic substances."** – Rice D and Barone S: "Critical periods of vulnerability for the developing nervous system: Evidence from humans and animal models." *Environmental Health Perspectives*, 108:511-533, 2000.
"Of critical concern is the possibility that developmental exposure to neurotoxicants may result in an acceleration of age related decline in function." *See also*:

Schettler T: "Toxic threats to neurologic development of children." *Environmental Health Perspectives*, Dec; 109 Suppl. 6:813-6, 2001.

271 **"With a body that is ill equipped to rid itself of manmade chemicals, the developing baby is extremely vulnerable to toxic exposure."** – In 1993, the National Academy of Sciences and Environmental Protection Agency (EPA) concluded that unborn babies and children are much more vulnerable to the effects of environmental toxins. *See also*:

Perera F et al: "Biomarkers in maternal and newborn blood indicate heightened fetal susceptibility to pro-carcinogenic DNA damage." *Environmental Health Perspectives*, 112, 1133-1136, July 2004.
This study demonstrates that the developing fetus is more susceptible than the adult to carcinogenic effects of polycyclic aromatic hydro-carbons (widespread air contaminants released by transportation vehicles and power generation).

Parkin R et al: "Children's susceptibility to chemicals: a review by developmental stage." *Journal of Toxicology & Environmental Health*, Part B: Critical Review. Nov-Dec; 7(6):417-35, 2004.

del Rio Paredes S: "Chemical contamination of the child: bioaccumulation and potential effects." *Revista Española de Salud Pública*, Mar-Apr; 79(2):221-8, 2005.
This study focuses on alkylphenols, bisphenol A, brominated flame retardants, organotins, phthalates, chlorinated paraffins and artificial musks. The report identifies the different illnesses and diseases that are now being linked to exposure and the specific health impacts of these chemicals.
Shelby M et al: "Center for the evaluation of risks to human reproduction – the first five years." *Birth Defects Research Part B: Developmental and Reproductive Toxicology*, Feb; 74(1):1-8, 2005.

"In 2011, researchers found traces of dozens of harmful chemicals…" – Woodruff J et al: "Environmental Chemicals in an Urban Population of Pregnant Women and Their Newborns from San Francisco." *Environmetnal Science and Technology*, 50, 22, 12464-12472, 2016.

- 421 -

NOTES

271 **"In 2003 the EPA concluded that carcinogens have around ten times the potency for babies compared to adults."** – "Adjusting for youth: Updated cancer risk guidelines." *Environmental Health Perspectives*, Vol.111, No.13, Oct 2003. *See*:
http://www.ehponline.org/members/2003/111-13/EHP111pa708PDF. PDF

271 **"The report by the Environmental Working Group was based on tests of samples of umbilical cord blood, which were found to contain 287 chemicals."** – Environmental Working Group (EWG): "Body Burden: The Pollution in Newborns" September 2004. *See:*
www.ewg.org/reports/bodyburden2/

272 **"3 to 5% of babies in the U.S. are born with birth defects, which are now the leading reported cause of infant mortality..."** – Trasande L and Landrigan P: "The National Children's Study: a Critical National Investment." *Environmental Health Perspectives,* Oct; 112 (14): A789-90, 2004. *See also*:

Luster M et al: "Consensus workshop on methods to evaluate developmental immunotoxicity." *Environmental Health Perspectives*, 111(4): 579-583 2003.
This study of data gathered by the Centers for Disease Control from 1989 to 1996, found that rates of birth defects, preterm births and low birthweight babies have been rising steadily since the mid-1980s. The report concludes: "...birth defects are the biggest cause of infant mortality in the first 12 months of life as we enter the 21st century."

272 **"...scientists in the Netherlands have discovered that, with exposure to PCBs during gestation, boys tend to engage in more 'feminine' behavior..."** – Vreugdenhil H et al: "Effects of perinatal exposure to PCBs and dioxins on play behavior in Dutch children at school age." *Environmental Health Perspectives*, Vol.1, No.10, 2002.
In boys, higher prenatal PCB levels were related with less masculinized play. Girls with higher PCB levels were associated with more masculinized play. These effects suggested prenatal steroid hormone imbalances were caused by prenatal exposure to environmental levels of PCBs, dioxins, and other organochlorine compounds.

272 **"They may also be prone to developing breast cancer later in life."** – Warner M et al: "Serum dioxin concentrations and breast cancer risk in the Seveso Women's Health Study." *Environmental Health Perspectives*, 110:625–628, 2002.
In this study researchers found that a 10-fold increase in dioxin levels was associated with a 2.1 increase in risk for breast cancer and that breast cancer incidence increased steadily with age, with the most rapid increase between ages 40 and 55 years.

272 **"...scientists have given them the generic name of 'testicular dysgenesis syndrome.' "** – Fisher J et al: "Human testicular dysgenesis syndrome: a possible model using in-utero exposure of the rat to dibutyl phthalate." *Human Reproduction*, Vol.18, No.7, 1383-1394, 2003.
This study states: "The disorders comprising human 'testicular dysgenesis syndrome' (TDS) may be increasing in incidence." The study investigated whether male rats exposed in utero to dibutyl phthalate would provide a suitable model for human TDS.

- 422 -

NOTES

272   **"According to the EPA's 'Guidelines for Carcinogen Risk Assessment,' children receive 50% of their lifetime cancer risks during their first two years of life."** – EPA "Guidelines for Carcinogen Risk Assessment (Cancer Guidelines)" and "Supplemental Guidance for Assessing Susceptibility from Early-Life Exposure to Carcinogens (Supplemental Guidance)." 2003. Both documents and additional information are available at: http://www.epa.gov/cancerguidelines

272   **"Confirmation of the harmful effects of pollution on children's health was published in January 2005."** – Knox E: "Childhood cancers and atmospheric carcinogens." *Journal of Epidemiology & Community Health*, 59:101-105 2005. The study analyzed the records of 22,500 children born between 1953 and 1980 who died from leukemia or other cancers before age 16. The findings corresponded with the results of earlier studies, indicating that many childhood cancers start in early infancy or in the womb. The children at greatest risk appear to be those living within 0.2 miles of a bus station, who are 12 times more likely to die of cancer.

273   **"...the skin of infants is thinner and more permeable than an adult's, and as a result, more toxins are able to pass through it."** Information from the Canadian Association of Physicians for the Environment, 2000. Visit: http://www.cape.ca/children/derm8.html

273   **"The seeds for many adult diseases, including cancer and reproductive failure, can be sown in childhood."** – Landrigan P et al: "Assessing the effects of endocrine disruptors in the National Children's Study." *Environmental Health Perspectives*, Vol. 111, No.13, Oct 2003.
"Children are undergoing rapid growth and development, and their developmental processes are easily disrupted by exposures to xenobiotics. Because children have more future years of life than most adults, they have more time to develop chronic diseases that may be triggered by early exposures."

273   **"A 2004 report by the wildlife charity WWF..."** – On October 8th 2004 the World Wildlife Fund U.K. and the Co-Operative Bank released a report entitled "Contamination: The Next Generation" detailing the results of blood tests for 104 man-made chemicals carried out on families in England, Scotland and Wales.

EMF Radiation Exposure During Pregnancy

274   **"Wireless radiation can cause DNA breakages in the developing fetus even at low levels."** – Pall M. "Wi-Fi is an important threat to human health," *Environmental Research*, Volume 164, pages 405-416, July 2018.
This paper features the results of 23 controlled, scientific studies of the effects of EMF exposure in animals, human cells in culture and in human beings. Adverse outcomes included: sperm/testicular damage, male infertility, cellular DNA damage, endocrine changes, abnormal postnatal development, cardiac changes and blood pressure disruption.

274   **"... children absorb 60% more electro magnetic field (EMF) radiation than an adult"** – The Stewart Report, by The Independent Expert Group on Mobile Phones, ISBN 0-85951-450-1, Published in May 2000. *See also*:

- 423 -

NOTES

Morris R et al: "Children Absorb Higher Doses of Radio Frequency Electromagnetic Radiation From Mobile Phones Than Adults,"*IEEE Access,* September 16, 2015.

274 **"...offspring that are more likely to be anxious, hyperactive, unable to focus and display other traits within the autistic spectrum.."** – Sudan M et al: "Pregnancy & Wireless Radiation Risks: Prenatal maternal cell phone use linked to lower child cognition at 5 years of age: 3 birth cohorts," *Environ International*, Nov;120:155-162, 2018.
In this study of over 3,000 children the authors reported, "We observed patterns of lower mean cognition scores among children in relation to high frequency maternal prenatal cell phone use." *See also*:

Wang Kai et al: "Effect of 1.8 GHz radiofrequency electromagnetic radiation on novel object associative recognition memory in mice," *Scientific Reports*, 7: 44521, 2017.
"Mounting evidence suggests that exposure to radiofrequency electro-magnetic radiation (RF-EMR) can influence learning and memory in rodents."

Kane R: "A possible association between fetal/neonatal exposure to radiofrequency electromagnetic radiation and the increased incidence of autism spectrum disorders," *Medical Hypotheses*, 62(2):195-7, 2004.
"This study shows that EMF radiation may be particularly harmful during pregnancy because the embryo or fetus is not always fully protected by amniotic fluid and can absorb radiation which can damage its development."

274 **"There is also a three times greater risk of miscarriage with high EMF exposure."** De Kun Li et al: "Exposure to Magnetic Field Non-Ionizing Radiation and the Risk of Miscarriage: A Prospective Cohort Study, *Scientific Reports* volume 7, Article number: 17541, 2017.
In this study we found an almost three-fold increased risk of miscarriage if a pregnant woman was exposed to higher MF levels compared to women with lower MF exposure.

274 **"Symptoms related to high EMF exposure include headaches, difficulty concentrating, sleep problems, depression and fatigue."** Belyaev I et al: "EUROPAEM EMF Guideline 2016 for the prevention, diagnosis and treatment of EMF-related health problems and illnesses," *Reviews on Environmental Health*, Sep 1;31(3):363-97, 2016.
"Common EHS symptoms include headaches, concentration difficulties, sleep problems, depression, a lack of energy, fatigue, and flu-like symptoms."

Further reading:
Disconnect: The Truth About Cell Phone Radiation, by Devra Davis, November 21, 2013. ISBN 9780991219902.

III – THE TOXINS EATING AT OUR HEALTH

275 **"MSG has been linked to many health problems..."** – "Processed free glutamic acid (MSG): Selected references sufficient to demonstrate that MSG places humans at risk." (Around 70 references.) See:
http://www.truthinlabeling.org/additional.html

- 424 -

NOTES

275 **"It has also been shown to cause infertility in animals."** – Pizzi W et al: "MSG greatly reduces pregnancy success." *Neurobehavioral Toxicology*, Vol.2:1-4, 1979.
Male rats fed MSG before mating had less than a 50% success rate (5 of 13 animals), whereas male rats not fed MSG had over a 92% success rate (12 of 13 animals). Offspring of the MSG-treated males had a shorter body length, reduced testes weights and evidence of being over-weight at 25 days.

275 **"A regular intake of aspartame has been linked to brain tumors, migraines, epilepsy, chronic fatigue syndrome, diabetes and joint pains."** – Olney J: "Brain damage in mice from voluntary ingestion of glutamate and aspartate." *Neurobehaviour, Toxicology & Teratology*, 2:125-129, 1980. *See also*:

Green-Waite R et al: "Adverse reactions to aspartame; double-blind challenge in patients from a vulnerable population." *Biological Psychiatry*, 34(1-2):13-17, 1993.

Gums J et al: "Relief of fibromyalgia symptoms following discontinuation of dietary excitotoxins." *Annals of Pharmacotherapy*, Jun; 35 (6):702-6, 2001.
"Four patients diagnosed with fibromyalgia had a complete, or nearly complete, resolution of their symptoms within months after eliminating monosodium glutamate (MSG) or MSG plus aspartame from their diet.

275 **"Industry-funded studies have all suggested that aspartame is safe for consumption..."** – Walton R: "Survey of aspartame studies: Correlation of outcome and funding sources." www.dorway.com/peerrev.html
Studies of aspartame in the peer reviewed medical literature were surveyed for funding source and study outcome. Of the 166 studies relevant to human safety, 74 received Nutrasweet® industry-related funding and 90 were independently funded. 100% of the industry- funded research attested to aspartame's safety, whereas 92% of independently funded research programs identified a problem.

275 **"The results of a two-year independent study suggest that aspartame may interact with other common food additives..."** – Howard V et al: "Synergistic interactions between commonly used food additives in a developmental neurotoxicity test." *Toxicological Sciences*, 0: 731, Dec 2005.

276 **"In the U.S., the Environmental Working Group has found that commercially grown fruits and vegetables contain the highest levels of pesticide contamination."** – Wiles R et al: "How 'bout them apples? Pesticides in children's food ten years after alarm." *Environmental Working Group Report*, 1999.

276 **"Traces of pesticides were found in 34% of the 1,089 food samples tested in 2004..."** – "Pesticide Residues Monitoring: Second Quarter Results April to June 2004." See:
http://www.pesticides.gov.uk/uploadedfiles/Web_Assets/PRC/PRC_2004_Q2_Report.pdf
Pesticides were found at more than three times the safe level for children, according to this report. Overall, traces of pesticides were found in 34% of the 1,089 samples tested between April and June 2004.

NOTES

276 **"There are many books and online resources to help people establish a toxin reduced lifestyle."** – Source: *Better Basics for the Home: Simple Solutions for Less Toxic Living* by Berthold-Bond A. Published by Three Rivers Press in 1999. ISBN: 0609803255. *See also*:

Green Clean: The Environmentally Sound Guide to Cleaning Your Home by Hunter ML and Halpin M. Published by Melcher Media in 2005. ISBN: 1595910042.

The Safe Shopper's Bible: A Consumer's Guide to Non-Toxic House-hold Products by Steinman D and Epstein S. Published by Wiley in 1995. ISBN: 0020820852.

Further Reading:
Pesticides and the Immune System, by Repetto R and Baliga S. Published by World Resources Institute in 1996. ISBN: 1569730873.

How Everyday Products Make People Sick: Toxins at Home and in the Workplace, by Blanc P, Published by University of California Press in 2007. ISBN: 0520248821.
"...a critical and disquieting perspective on the relationship between industrial development and its adverse health consequences."

Our Stolen Future: How We Are Threatening Our Fertility, Intelligence, and Survival – A Scientific Detective Story, by Colborn T et al. Published by Plume; Reprint edition 1996. ISBN: 0452274141
The authors of this book describe how endocrine hormone-disrupting environmental pollutants are linked to altered sexual development of the fetus, infertility, immune system disorders and behavioral problems.

Environmental Causes of Infertility, by Pressinger R and Sinclair W. *See full report at:*
http://www.chem-tox.com/infertility/download/index.htm

IV – NATURAL IMMUNOTHERAPY FOR LIFE: A Baby-Friendly Diet and Lifestyle: for Optimal Health and Fertility by Zita West

280 **"...a holistic fertility clinic in London... we now have one of the top success rates in the country"** Source: www.zitawest.com
"Our latest independently validated published results (2016) show a Clinical Pregnancy Rate of 68.8% for women under 35 years of age per fresh embryo transfer and 50% per fresh embryo transferred... which is the highest in London."

284 **"A number of foods...have been shown, with substantial scientific evidence, to increase inflammation in the body due to their high lectin content.**

284 **"These indigestible proteins stick to the cell membranes in the digestive tract and cause bloating, gastric discomfort and even chronic illnesses."** Van Damme E et al: "Handbook of plant lectins: properties and biomedical applications." London: Wiley; pp. 31–50. 1998.

285 **"...caffeine has been linked to increased rates of miscarriage and low birth weight"** – Fernandes O et al: "Moderate to heavy caffeine consumption during

- 426 -

NOTES

pregnancy and relationship to spontaneous abortion and abnormal fetal growth: a meta-analysis." *Reproductive Toxicology*, Jul-Aug; 12(4):435-44, 1998.
This analysis of 32 studies led the researchers to conclude: "...there is a small but statistically significant increase in the risks for spontaneous abortion and low birthweight babies in pregnant women consuming more than 150 mg caffeine per day" (about one and a half cups of coffee). *See also*:

Cnattingius S et al: "Caffeine intake and the risk of first trimester spontaneous abortion." *New England Journal of Medicine*, Dec; 1,343 (25):1839-45, 2000.
562 women who had spontaneous abortion at 6 to 12 weeks of gestation and 953 women with successful pregnancies were compared. "Among nonsmokers, more spontaneous abortions occurred in women who ingested at least 100 mg of caffeine per day than in women who ingested less than 100 mg per day, with the increase in risk related to the amount ingested..."

285 **"...cocaine's strong association with infertility..."** – Mueller B et al: "Recreational drug use and the risk of primary infertility." Division of Public Health Sciences, Fred Hutchinson Cancer Research Center, Seattle, WA 98104, *Epidemiology*, May; 1(3):195-200, 1990.

285 **"...women who use this drug [cocaine] in first three months of pregnancy are at twice the risk of placental abruption and premature delivery..."** – Addis A et al: "Fetal effects of cocaine: an updated meta-analysis." *Reproductive Toxicology*, Jul-Aug; 15(4):341-69, 2001.
The risk of placental abruption and premature rupture of membranes was increased with cocaine use.

286 **"The chances of a successful IVF cycle are also severely reduced as exposure to toxic hydrocarbons cuts the number of viable eggs, lessens the likelihood of implantation, and increases the risk of chromosomal abnormalities in the fetus."** – Man L and Chang B: "Maternal cigarette smoking during pregnancy increases the risk of having a child with a congenital digital anomaly." *Plastic Reconstructive Surgery,* Jan; 117(1):301-8, 2006.
"This is the largest study to date to investigate specifically the association between maternal cigarette smoking and the risk of having a newborn with a congenital digital anomaly...smoking during pregnancy may be an important preventable risk factor for these common congenital differences." *See also*:

Braat D et al: "Effects of subfertility cause, smoking and body weight on the success rate of IVF." *Human Reproduction & Embryology*, Human Reproduction, 20(7):1867-1875, 2005.
The success rate of IVF was examined in 8,457 women. Smoking was associated with a significantly lower delivery rate and a higher abortion rate compared to non-smoking delivery rates. "The devastating impact of smoking on the livebirth rate in IVF treatment is comparable with an increase in female age of more than 10 years from age 20 to 30 years."

de Mouzon J and Belaisch-Allart J: "Consequences on women's fecundity and on assisted reproductive technology." *Journal of Gynecology, Obstetrics & Biological Reproduction (Paris)*, Apr; 34 Spec No.1:3S112-8, 2005.
"In assisted reproductive technology...the deleterious effects of smoking on fertility have been clearly demonstrated: lower estradiol levels, decreased pregnancy and implantation rates, and poorer oocyte morphology."

NOTES

285 **"Smoking can also have a pro-inflammatory effect, leading to thrombo-philia..."** – Miyaura S et al: "Effect of a cigarette smoke extract on the metabolism of the pro-inflammatory autacoid, platelet-activating factor." *Circulation Research,* Feb; 70(2):341-7, 1992.
Platelet-activating factor (PAF) is a potent pro-inflammatory agent. The researchers conclude that increase in PAF concentrations in smokers may contribute to the increased incidence of cardiovascular and lung diseases known to be present in smokers.

285 **"...smokers have far more pregnancy complications compared to non smokers."** – Castles A et al: "Effects of smoking during pregnancy: Five meta-analyses." *American Journal of Preventative Medicine,* Apr; 16(3):208-15, 1996.
"Smoking was found to be strongly associated with an elevated risk or placenta previa, abruptio placenta, ectopic pregnancy and preterm premature rupture of the membranes..."

286 **"The THC...in cannabis is known to be toxic to the developing egg..."** – Morishima A: "Effects of cannabis and natural cannabinoids on chromosomes and ova." *National Institute on Drug Abuse Research Monogram,* 44:25-45, 1984.
In this study, it was discovered that ova could be damaged by exposure to delta-tetrahydrocannabinol (THC), the main active ingredient of cannabis.

286 **"Alcohol stimulates the production of TNF-alpha..."** – Perez L et al: "Relation of tumor necrosis factor (TNF) gene polymorphisms with serum concentrations and in vitro production of TNF-alpha and interleukin-8 in heavy drinkers." *Alcohol,* Oct-Nov; 34 (2-3):273-7, 2004.
Researchers found that in comparison with control subjects, "heavy drinkers showed higher TNF-alpha production, higher IL-8 production, and higher serum IL-8 concentrations."

286 **"One drink a day for a year prior to an IVF attempt has been associated with fewer eggs and lower pregnancy rates."** – Klonoff-Cohen H et al: "Effects of maternal and paternal alcohol consumption on the success rates of in vitro fertilization and gamete intrafallopian transfer." *Fertility & Sterility,* Feb; 79(2):330-9, 2003.
Among 221 couples with female infertility, female alcohol consumption was associated with 13% decrease in the number of eggs aspirated for each additional drink per day a year before the IVF attempt. The chance of not achieving pregnancy was 2.86 times higher and miscarriage 2.21 times higher. *See also:*

Kaufman M: "A hypothesis regarding the origin of aneuploidy in man: indirect evidence from an experimental model." *Journal of Medical Genetics,* Jun; 22(3):171-8, 1985.
"Recent studies have clearly demonstrated that aneuploidy may be induced in about 10 to 20% of oocytes and recently ovulated eggs when female mice are given an intragastric injection of a dilute solution of ethanol...it is suggested that attention should also be drawn to the potentially greater hazard to the (human) conceptus which could result from maternal alcohol consumption at, and shortly before, conception."

NOTES

286   **"Other research has also linked gum disease in men to poor sperm quality."** Klinger A and Hain B: "Periodontal status of males attending an in vitro fertilization clinic" *Journal of Clinical Periodontology*, Jun; 38 (6): 542-6, 2011.

286   **"...bacteria triggered inflammation is also associated with miscarriage, low birth rate and premature birth."**
Klinger A et al, "Periodontal status of males attending an in vitro fertilization clinic," *Journal of Clinical Periodontology,* Jun;38(6):542- 6. 2011

286   **"[Gum disease] can delay a positive pregnancy test by two months..."**
Hart R: "Gum disease can increase the time it takes to become pregnant," *European Society of Human Reproduction and Embryology*, (ESHRE) August 1, 2011.
In a study of 3737 women, those with gum disease took an average of just over seven months to become pregnant, two months longer than the average of five months that it took women without gum disease. *See also*:

Hart R et al: "Periodontal disease: a potential modifiable risk factor limiting conception," *Human Reproduction,* May;27(5):1332-42, 2012.

287 **"...bacteria-triggered inflammation which can result in late miscarriage."**
Harris et al: "Is poor periodontal oral health in pregnancy a risk factor for spontaneous abortion or stillbirth?" Evidence-Based Practice: September, Volume 21, Issue 8, p.47, 2018.
"Periodontal disease...is associated with an increased risk of late miscarriage or stillbirth."

Non-Baby Friendly Foods

287   **"...on average we consume around 66lbs of refined sugar a year..."** –
United States Department of Agriculture, Economic Research Service. (2012). USDA Sugar Supply: Tables 51-53: US Consumption of Caloric Sweeteners. Retrieved from http://www.ers.usda.gov/data-products/sugar-and-sweeteners-yearbook-tables.aspx

287   **"...soda and energy drinks being the single biggest source in the American diet."** – Watson E: "What are the biggest contributors of added sugars to the American diet?" *Food Navigator USA.com. July 2014.*
"Soft drinks are the largest food group sources of added sugars (34.4%)."

287   **"...the insulin that is released to lower blood sugar levels also promotes the release of serotonin in the brain."** – Wurtman R and Wurtman J: "Serotoninergic mechanisms and obesity." *Journal of Nutritional Biochemistry*, 9:511-515, 1998.
Carbohydrates release insulin and leave tryptophan circulating in the blood. Trytophan enters the brain where it is transformed into serotonin. The increase in serotonin release by the dietary carbohydrates creates a "good mood" and people become reliant on this dietary method to induce a content state of mind, which in turn causes them to develop carbohydrate cravings. Obese patients given serotonergic anti-obesity drugs reduced their consumption of carbohydrate-rich meals.

NOTES

287 **"High consumption can also lead to the loss of the trace mineral chromium..."** – Clodfelder B et al: "A comparison of the insulin-sensitive transport of chromium in healthy and model diabetic rats." *Journal of Inorganic Biochemistry*, Mar; 98(3):522-33, 2004.
This study states, "In response to insulin, chromium is moved from the blood to the tissues where it is ultimately lost in the urine."

287 **"...which further fuels the craving for sugars."** – Docherty J et al: "A double-blind, placebo controlled, exploratory trial of chromium picolinate in atypical depression: effect on carbohydrate craving." *Journal of Psychiatric Practice,* Sep; 11(5):302-14, 2005.
"The results of this study suggest that the main effect of chromium was on carbohydrate craving and appetite regulation in depressed patients and that 600 mug of elemental chromium may be beneficial for patients with atypical depression who also have severe carbohydrate craving."

287 **"A study involving 25,000 people has shown that consuming large amounts of steak, burgers and lamb maybe an independent risk factor for arthritis."** – Pattison D et al: "Dietary risk factors for the development of inflammatory polyarthritis: evidence for a role of high level of red meat consumption." *Arthritis & Rheumatism*, Dec; 50(12): 3804-12, 2004.

288 **"A high intake of red meat, especially processed meat, is also linked to a higher incidence of bowel, breast and pancreatic cancer."** – Bouvard V et al: "Carcinogenicity of consumption of red and processed meat," The Lancet Oncology, Vol. 16, issue 16, pp1599-1600, December 01, 2015.

288 **"Barbequed beef is particularly bad as it combines burnt meat with oxidized sugar..."** – Fenech M and Neville S: "Micronucleus induction in bone-marrow cells following consumption of cooked beef in mice. Preliminary investigations." *Mutation Research*, Jan; 281(1):3-10, 1992.
In this experiment, well-done, pan-fried and charcoal-barbecued meat produced significant increases in genetic damage. *See also*:

Sinha R et al: "Well-done, grilled red meat increases the risk of colorectal adenomas." *Cancer Research,* Sep; 1:59(17):4320-4, 1999.
"Red meat or meat-cooking methods...have been associated with an increased risk of colorectal and other cancers...carcinogenic compounds formed by high-temperature cooking techniques...may contribute to the risk of developing colorectal tumors."

288 **"Today's diets are often low in omega-3 essential fatty acids (EFAs) and have excessive amounts of omega-6 EFAs."** – Simopoulos A: "The importance of the ratio of omega-6/omega-3 essential fatty acids." *Biomedical Pharmacotherapy*, Oct; 56 (8):365-79, 2002.
This review concludes: "A lower ratio of omega-6/omega-3 fatty acids is more desirable in reducing the risk of many of the chronic diseases of high prevalence in Western societies..."

288 **"Omega-3 EFAs are vital for good health and there is strong evidence to show that they can help moderate inflammatory immune activity."** – Calder P: "N-3 polyunsaturated fatty acids and immune cell function." *Advances in Enzyme Regulation*, 37:197-237, 1997.

NOTES

This report concludes that omega-3 polyunsaturated fatty acids may be of use as a therapy for acute and chronic inflammation, for disorders that involve an inappropriately activated immune response and for the enhancement of graft survival. *See also*:

Zhang P et al: "Dietary (n-3) polyunsaturated fatty acids modulate murine Th1/Th2 balance toward the Th2 pole by suppression of Th1 development." *Journal of Nutrition*, Jul; 135(7):1745-51, 2005.
In this animal study, a fish oil diet suppressed the Th1 immune response.

288 **"Organic dairy produce including cheese, cream and butter all contain more omega-3 EFAs than non organic varieties;"** – Dewhurst R et al: "Comparison of grass and legume silages for milk production; 1: Production responses with different levels of concentrate." *Journal of Dairy Science*, Vol.86, pp.2598-2611, 2003.
It is reported here that samples of milk from organic cows contained at least 64% and up to 240% more omega-3 EFAs than conventional milk. *See also*:

Communications Team, Office of External Affairs, University of Aberdeen. "Organic milk – good alternative source of omega-3s." University of Aberdeen Press Release, December 8, 2004.
According to the results of this research project, organic milk was found to contain up to 71% more omega-3 and to have a better ratio of anti-inflammatory omega-3 to pro-inflammatory omega-6 fatty acids compared with conventional milk.

288 **"A diet that is heavy on saturated transfats or hydrogenated fats can have a pro-inflammatory effect…"** – Han S et al: "Effect of hydrogenated and saturated, relative to polyunsaturated, fat on immune and inflammatory responses of adults with moderate hypercholesterolemia." *Journal of Lipid Research*, Mar; 43(3):445-52, 2002.
The researchers conclude that consumption of a diet high in hydrogenated fat increases production of inflammatory cytokines that are associated with the onset of atherosclerosis.

De Souza C et al: "Consumption of a fat-rich diet activates a pro-inflammatory response and induces insulin resistance in the hypothalamus." *Endocrinology*, 146:4192-4199, 2005.
"Here we show…a hyperlipidic diet induces the expression of several pro-inflammatory cytokines and inflammatory responsive proteins in hypothalamus."

Boosting Fertility by Balancing the Immune System

289 **"…a protein dominated diet can harm fertility by producing toxins that disrupt the development of the embryo."** – Gardner D et al: "High protein diets reduce fertility in mice." Study results presented at the European Society of Human Reproduction and Embryology Conference in Berlin, Germany, June 2004.
A control group was given a diet consisting of 14% protein and a test group of 25% protein. After one month, embryos from mice in the high protein group experienced four times as much cell death – thought to be due an accumulation of ammonium in the reproductive tract.

NOTES

289 **Complex carbohydrates that are more resistant to digestion, also referred to as "resistant starches" enable the body to produce the mood boosting hormone serotonin more consistently..."** – Des-Maisons K: *Potatoes Not Prozac: A Natural Seven-Step Dietary Plan to Control Your Cravings and Lose Weight: Recognize How Foods Affect the Way You Feel and Stabilize the Level of Sugar in Your Blood.* Published by Simon & Schuster in 1999. ISBN: 034544132X.

262 **"Certain vegetables and fruits also contain antioxidants and folate which help to slow blood clotting..."** – Noguchi T et al: "Nutritional prevention on hypertension, cerebral hemodynamics and thrombosis in stroke-prone spontaneously hypertensive rats." *Cellular and Molecular Neurobiology*, Oct; 24(5):599-638, 2004.
The authors conclude: "...antioxidative nutrients are beneficial in the prevention of hypertension and stroke and that the nutritional science is very important for prediction and prevention medicine."

290 **"Dehydration can make the blood more viscous..."** Tikhomirova I: "The effect of dehydration on macro- and microrheological blood properties..." *Clinical Hemorheology Microcirculation*, 26(2):85-90, 2002.
"The results of our study indicated that water deprivation caused progressive reduction of blood and plasma fluidity." See also:
Kaibara M et al: "Clinical studies on flow properties of blood in the gynecological patients with potentially hypercoagulable state." *Nippon Sanka Fujinka Gakkai Zasshi*, Aug; 33(8):1173-9, 1981.
"...dehydration and infection should be avoided to prevent thrombus formation in the gynecological patients with potentially hypercoagulable state."

Food for Special Thought

Omega-3 Essential Fatty Acids (EFAs)

291 **"Scientists have discovered that a diet rich in omega-3 EFAs can significantly decrease natural killer cell activity and suppress the production of TNF cytokines..."** – Thies F et al: "Dietary supplementation with eicosapentaenoic acid, but not with other long-chain n-3 or n-6 polyunsaturated fatty acids, decreases natural killer cell activity in healthy subjects aged over 55 years." *American Society for Clinical Nutrition*, 73, No.3, 539-548, March 2001. *See also*:

Caughey G et al: "The effect on human tumor necrosis factor alpha and interleukin 1 beta production of diets enriched in n-3 fatty acids from vegetable oil or fish oil." *American Journal of Clinical Nutrition*, Jan; 63(1):116-22, 1996. In this study, the use of flaxseed oil for 4 weeks inhibited TNF-alpha and IL-1 beta production by approximately 30%. Fish oil supplementation continued for a further 4 weeks reduced TNF-alpha and IL-1 beta levels by 74% and 80% respectively.

291 **"...a diet rich in omega-3 EFAs can...moderate the symptoms of rheumatoid arthritis..."** – Elham Rajaei E et al: "The Effect of Omega-3 Fatty Acids in Patients With Active Rheumatoid Arthritis Receiving DMARDs Therapy: Double-Blind Randomized Controlled Trial," *Global Journal of Health Sciences*, Jul; 8(7): 18–25, 2016.

- 432 -

NOTES

"Daily supplementation with omega-3 results has significant clinical benefit..."

291 **"...a diet rich in omega-3 EFAs can...moderate the symptoms of endometriosis..."** – Hopeman M, "Serum Polyunsaturated Fatty Acids and Endometriosis," *Reproductive Sciences*, Sep;22(9):1083-7, 2015.

291 **"...a diet rich in omega-3 EFAs can...moderate the symptoms of psoriasis..."** – Márquez Balbás G: "Study on the use of omega-3 fatty acids as a therapeutic supplement in treatment of psoriasis," *Clinical, Cosmetic and Investigational Dermatology*. 4: 73–77, 2011.
"Supplementary treatment with omega-3 fatty acids... makes a significant contribution to reducing... scalp lesion and pruritus, erythema, scaling, and infiltration of the treated areas."

291 **"...a diet rich in omega-3 EFAs can...moderate the symptoms of depression."** – Grosso G: "Omega-3 Fatty Acids and Depression: Scientific Evidence and Biological Mechanisms," Oxidative Medicine and Cellular Longevity, Published online doi:[10.1155/2014/313570] Mar 18, 2014.
"...proper intake of omega-3 PUFA and dietary interventions including omega-3 PUFA supplement can result in substantial benefits for the general population." *See also*:

McCrone P et al: "Efficacy of ethyleicosapentaenoic acid in bipolar depression: randomised double-blind placebo controlled study." *British Journal of Psychiatry*. Jan; 188:46-50, 2006.
In this 12-week study, individuals with bipolar depression were ran-domly assigned to adjunctive treatment with placebo or ethyl-EPA. "Significant improvement was noted with ethyl-EPA treatment compared with placebo..."

291 **"Omega-3 fish oil is also a good choice for women with blood clotting tendencies who have suffered recurrent miscarriage..."** – Haghiac M et al: "Dietary Omega-3 Fatty Acid Supplementation Reduces Inflammation in Obese Pregnant Women: A Randomized Double-Blind Controlled Clinical Trial," *PLoS One*, Sep 4;10(9): e0137309, 2015.

Leghi G and Muhlhausler B: :The effect of n-3 LCPUFA supplementation on oxidative stress and inflammation in the placenta and maternal plasma during pregnancy," Prostaglandins, Leukotrienes and Essential Fatty Acids, Oct; 113:33-39, 2016.

291 **"A daily fish oil supplement during pregnancy can reduce the chance of a premature birth by up to 42%."** Middleton P et al: "Omega-3 fatty acid addition during pregnancy," *Cochrane Review*, 15 November 2018.
In this review of 70 studies, oily fish like salmon and mackerel lowers the risk of having a baby born before 37 weeks by 11% and the risk of giving birth before 34 weeks drops by 42%.

291 **"Even small amounts of omega-3 EFAs can assist in protecting against these outcomes [pregnancy complications] by decreasing the production of Th1 cytokines..."** – Wallace F et al: "Dietary fatty acids influence the production of Th1 but not Th2-type cytokines." *Journal of Leukocyte Biology*, Mar; 69 (3):449-57, 2001.

- 433 -

NOTES

"Polyunsaturated fats inhibited the production of Th1-type cytokines, with n-3 fatty acids being particularly potent." *See also*:

Olsen S and Secher N: "Low consumption of seafood in early pregnancy as a risk factor for preterm delivery: prospective cohort study." *British Medical Journal*, Feb; 23; 324(7335):447, 2002.
8,729 pregnant women were studied. The results showed that in women with zero or low intake of fish, small amounts of n-3 fatty acids, provided as fish or fish oil, might protect against preterm delivery and low birthweight.

291 **"Even small amounts of omega-3 EFAs can assist in protecting against these outcomes [low birthweight] by improving placental blood flow."** – Saldeen P and Saldeen T: "Women and omega-3 fatty acids." *Obstetrical & Gynecological Survey*, Oct; 59(10):722-30, 2004.
"An increased prostacyclin/thromboxane ratio induced by omega-3 fatty acids can facilitate pregnancy in women with infertility problems by increasing uterine blood flow. Supplementation with omega-3 fatty acids during pregnancy lowers the risk of premature birth and can increase the length of pregnancy and birthweight by altering the balance of eicosanoids involved in labor and promote fetal growth by improving placental blood flow."

291 **"The benefits of these nutrients are then passed on to the baby..."** – Larque E et al: "Perinatal supply and metabolism of long-chain polyunsaturated fatty acids: importance for the early development of the nervous system." *Annals of the New York Academy of Sciences*, Jun; 967:299-310, 2002.
"From the available data, we conclude that long-chain polyunsaturated fatty acids are conditionally essential substrates during early life that are related to the quality of growth and development."

291 **"Choose a variety with between 500 and 1000mg of omega-3 fats and at least 500mg of DHA."** – Professor Middleton, author of the 2018 Cochrane Review, "Omega-3 fatty acid during Pregnancy, "Our review found the optimum dose was a daily supplement containing between 500 and 1000 milligrams (mg) of long chain omega-3 fats (containing at least 500mg of DHA)."

292 **"...there is some evidence that omega-3's from vegetable sources are not as health promoting as the fish oil."** – Fokkema M et al: "Short-term supplementation of low dose gamma-linolenic acid (GLA), alpha-linolenic acid (ALA), or GLA plus ALA does not augment LCP omega-3 status of Dutch vegans to an appreciable extent." *Prostaglan-dins Leukotrienes & Essential Fatty Acids*, Nov; 63(5):287-92, 2000.

292 **"...fish oil has a slight blood thinning effect (1g of fish oil has the anticoagulant effect of one sixteenth of a full strength aspirin pill)."** – *The Omega Rx Zone: The Miracle of the New High dose Fish Oil,* by Sears B. Published by Regan Books in 2002. ISBN: 0060393130.

Flavonoids (Antioxidants)

292 **"Such changes can trigger the production of damaging TNF-alpha cytokines..."** – Dick C et al: "The role of free radicals in the toxic and inflammatory effects of four different ultra fine particle types." *Inhalation Toxicology*, Jan; 15(1):39-52, 2003.

NOTES

In this study, a role for free radicals and reactive oxygen species in mediating inflammation was supported by the ability of antioxidants to block the release of tumor necrosis factor-alpha (TNF-alpha) from macrophages in vitro.

292 **"A study of 256 women at Massachusetts General Hospital Fertility Center from 2004 to 2014..."** – Messerlian C et al: Urinary Concentrations of Phthalate Metabolites and Pregnancy Loss Among Women Conceiving with Medically Assisted Reproduction." *Epidemiology*, Volume 27, Issue 6, November 2016.

292 **"...oxidative stress can also influence a woman's entire reproductive lifespan..."** – Agarwal A and Allamaneni S: "Role of free radicals in female reproductive diseases and assisted reproduction." *Reproductive Biomedicine Online*, Sep; 9(3):338-47, 2004.
"Treatments that reduce oxidative stress may help infertile women with diseases that are caused by this imbalance." *See also*:

Sharma R et al: "Role of oxidative stress in female reproduction." *Reproductive Biology & Endocrinology*, Jul; 14:3(1), 2005.
In this review, the author describes how oxidative stress can affect every stage of reproduction from oocyte maturation and fertilization, to embryo development and pregnancy. Strategies to overcome oxidative stress and enhance fertility, both natural and assisted, are outlined.

292 **"...if levels of oxidative stress are not within a low range, pregnancy will usually not occur."** – Dirnfeld M et al: "Oxidative stress indices in follicular fluid as measured by the thermochemiluminescence assay correlate with outcome parameters in in vitro fertilization." *Fertility & Sterility*, Oct; 82 Supplement, 3:1171-6, 2004.
"Oxidative stress indices in follicular fluid as measured by the thermo-chemiluminescence assay correlate with outcome parameters in in vitro fertilization."

292 **"Antioxidant and pro-oxidant nutrients reduce levels of free radicals and modulate the inflammatory response by promoting the production of Th2 cytokines."** – George A et al: "Inhibition of NF-kappaB and oxidative pathways in human dendritic cells by antioxidative vitamins generates regulatory T-cells." *Journal of Immunology*, Jun; 15:74(12):7633-44 2005.
Researchers investigated the effects of antioxidants vitamin C and vitamin E on dendritic cells. Following treatment, levels of intracellular oxygen radical species were reduced. T-cells also secreted higher levels of Th2 cytokines and IL-10 than cells incubated with control dendritic cells. *See also*:
Lyu S and Park W: "Production of cytokine and NO by RAW 264.7 macrophages and PBMC in vitro incubation with flavonoids." *Archives of Pharmaceutical Research*, May; 28(5):573-81, 2005.
The study concludes: "...flavonoids have the capacity to modulate the immune response and have a potential anti-inflammatory activity."

292 **"Quercetin, an antioxidant found in grape and cranberry juices has virtually the same clot preventing benefits as low dose aspirin but without the side effects."** – J et al: "Select flavonoids and whole juice from purple grapes inhibit platelet function and enhance nitric oxide release." *Circulation*, June 12; 103(23):2792-8, 2001.

NOTES

292 **"Resveratrol...has anti-inflammatory, antioxidant, anti-tumor and immunomodulatory properties."** – Martin A et al: "The effects of resveratrol, a phytoalexin derived from red wines, on chronic inflammation induced in an experimentally induced colitis model." *British Journal of Pharmacology,* Feb 13, 2006.
"Resveratrol...significantly attenuated the damage score and corrected the disturbances in morphology associated to injury. In addition, the degree of neutrophil infiltration and the levels of TNF-alpha were significantly ameliorated."

293 **"Fresh ginger is widely used in Ayurvedic medicine to treat autoimmune illnesses by decreasing the activity of pro-inflammatory cytokines such as TNF-alpha."** – Frondoza C et al: "Ginger extract components suppress induction of chemokine expression in human synoviocytes." *Journal of Alternative Complementary Medicine,* Feb; 11(1):149-54, 2005. *See also*:

Peng W et al: "Analgesic and anti-inflammatory activities of [6]-gingerol." *Journal of Ethnopharmacology,* Jan 4; 96(1-2):207-10, 2005.

293 **"[Ginger] interferes with the formation of blood clots and lowers cholesterol; it can help guard against thrombosis."** – Ali M et al: "The use of ginger (Zingiber officinale Rosc.) as a potential anti-inflammatory and antithrombotic agent." *Prostaglandins, Leukotrienes & Essential Fatty Acids,* Dec; 67(6):475-8, 2002.
Raw extract of ginger was administered daily to rats for a period of 4 weeks. Considering the results, the researchers concluded: "...ginger could be used as a cholesterol lowering, antithrombotic and anti-inflammatory agent." *See also*:

Frondoza C et al: "An in vitro screening assay for inhibitors of pro-inflammatory mediators in herbal extracts using human synoviocyte cultures." *In Vitro Cellular & Developmental Biology Animal,* Mar-Apr; 40:95-101, 2004.
In this study, ginger extract significantly inhibited the activation of TNF-alpha and suppressed its production. "...ginger extract-HAPC offers a complementary and alternative approach to modulate the inflammatory process involved in arthritis."

293 **"Spinach is a wonderful immune modulator..."** – Bissonnette E et al: "PCT-233, a novel modulator of pro- and anti-inflammatory cytokine production." *Clinical & Experimental Immunology,* Mar; 135 (3): 440-7, 2004.
The modulatory activity of PureCell Complex (PCT)-233, a molecular complex of Spinacia oleacea was studied. "TNF/IL-10 production by LPS-stimulated AM was reduced significantly in the presence of PCT-233 an active molecular complex from mesophyll tissue of spinach ...PCT-233 possesses some anti-inflammatory properties, even when added during the inflammatory process, and could potentiate the effect of other anti-inflammatory agents..."

293 **"Avocados also contain ingredients that can help alleviate inflammation, and have long been used to treat the symptoms of osteoarthritis."** – Ernst E: "Avocado-soybean unsaponifiables (ASU) for osteoarthritis; a systematic review." *Clinical Rheumatology,* Oct; 22(4-5):285-8, 2003.
Four randomized, placebo controlled, double-blind trials of avocado oil were assessed. The majority suggested that avocado oil is effective for the symptomatic treatment of osteoarthritis.

- 436 -

NOTES

293   **"Citrus fruits...contain a substance called nobiletin, which has an anti-inflammatory properties, which, according, according to one report, is similar to those of cortisteroids such as dexamethasone."** – Lin N et al: "Novel anti-inflammatory actions of nobiletin, a citrus poly-methoxy flavonoid, on human synovial fibroblasts and mouse macrophages." *Biochemical Pharmacology,* Jun 15; 65(12):2065-71, 2003.

The researchers found that nobiletin suppressed the interleukin induced production of PGE(2) and the expression of pro-inflammatory cytokines including IL-1alpha, IL-1beta, TNF-alpha and IL-6 in mouse macrophages and concluded: "These anti-inflammatory actions of nobiletin are very similar to those of anti-inflammatory steroids such as dexamethasone..." *See also*:

Murakami A et al: "Suppressive effects of citrus fruits on free radical generation and nobiletin, an anti-inflammatory polymethoxyflavonoid." *Biofactors*, 12 (1-4):187-92, 2000.

"Citrus fruit intake is known to be associated with a reduction of cancer incidence...In addition, nobiletin, a polymethoxyflavonoid isolated from C. nobilis showed a higher anti-inflammatory activity than indomethacin in a TPA-induced edema formation test in mouse ears. These results indicate that citrus fruits could be notable sources of anti-oxidative, anti-inflammatory and cancer preventive compounds."

293   **"Rhubarb...can help to relax the blood vessels and suppress the vascular inflammatory process."** – Moon M et al: "Vasodilatory and anti-inflammatory effects of the aqueous extract of rhubarb via a NO-cGMP pathway." *Life Sciences,* Feb 28; 78(14):1550-7, 2006.

293   **"...onions and garlic are potent sources of selenium, which is a powerful antioxidant and immunomodulator."** – Baraboi V and Shestakova E: "Selenium: the biological role and antioxidant activity." *Ukrainian Biochemical Journal*, Jan-Feb; 76(1):23-32, 2004.

"Selenium is active immunomodulator, much more potent antioxidant than vitamins E, C and A, beta-carotene...Selenium is a serious factor of biological and antioxidant protection of vascular endothelium, of low-density lipoproteins, protection of DNA, chromosomes. As food component selenium is an exceptional agent of protection from atherosclerosis, coronary ischemic disease and cancer."

293   **"In addition, garlic is known to reduce elevated blood sugar levels and protect against environmental toxins."** – Ziamajidi N: "Effects of garlic extract on TNF-α expression and oxidative stress status in the kidneys of rats with STZ + nicotinamide-induced diabetes," *Pharmaceutical Biology*, Dec,55(1).526-531, 2017.

"...garlic extract has hypoglycaemic, antioxidant and anti-inflammatory properties; therefore, it can be useful for the alleviation of diabetic complications." *See also*:

Gedik N et al: "Chronic nicotine toxicity is prevented by aqueous garlic extract." *Plant Foods for Human Nutrition*, Jun; 60(2):77-86, 2005.

294   **"Broccoli "zapped" in some water loses 97% of its flavonoids..."** – Vallejo F et al: "Phenolic compound contents in edible parts of broccoli inflorescences

NOTES

after domestic cooking," Journal of the Science of Food and Agriculture, 15 October 2003.

Detoxification and Rejuvenation

295 **"Chelation is a process in which a substance binds to certain molec-ules to remove them from the body."** – Anderson R et al: "Acute pro-oxidant effects of vitamin C in EDTA chelation therapy and long-term antioxidant benefits of therapy." *Free Radical Biological Medicine*, Jun 15; 38(12):1565-70, 2005.
Chelation therapy is thought not only to remove contaminating metals, but also to decrease free radical production. This study illustrated how multiple sessions of EDTA chelation therapy protected lipids against oxidative damage. *See also*:

Mehta A et al: "Beneficial effect of combined administration of some naturally occurring antioxidants (vitamins) and thiol chelators in the treatment of chronic lead intoxication." *Chemico-Biological Interactions*, Jun 15; 145(3):267-80, 2003.
Rats were exposed to lead acetate in drinking water for three months. Vitamin C plus meso-2, 3-dimercaptosuccinic acid and monoisoamyl DMSA was of significant benefit in reducing oxidative stress levels. The addition of vitamin E was recommended for achieving optimum effects of lead chelation therapy.

296 **"...toxic metals, such as mercury, which promote autoantibody production."** – Podzimek S et al: "Effect of heavy metals on immune reactions in patients with infertility." *Casopis Lekaru Ceskych (Praha)*, 142(5):285-8, 2003.
"Heavy metals can negatively influence reproduction because in sensitive persons they are able to alter the immune reactions including autoantibodies production. The altered immune reaction can then cause infertility." *See also*:

Haggqvist B and Hultman P: "Interleukin-10 in murine metal-induced systemic autoimmunity." *Clinical & Experimental Immunology*, Sep; 141(3):422-31, 2005.

296 **"Fresh cilantro (otherwise called coriander and Chinese parsley) is known to be an effective mobilizer of mercury, lead, aluminum and tin..."** – Omura Y and Beckman S: "Role of mercury (Hg) in resistant infections & effective treatment of Chlamydia trachomatis and Herpes family viral infections (and potential treatment for cancer) by removing localized Hg deposits with Chinese parsley and delivering effective antibiotics using various drug uptake enhancement methods." *Acupuncture Electrotherapy Research*, 20(3-4):195-229, 1995.

296 **"Green tea, plus vitamins A, C and E, is powerfully anti-mutagenic..."** – Chen Q et al: "Pharmacologic ascorbic acid concentrations selectively kill cancer cells: action as a pro-drug to deliver hydrogen peroxide to tissues." *Proceedings of the National Academy of Sciences U.S.A.*, 20; 102(38):13604-9, 2005.

296 **"Green tea has even been shown to reduce DNA damage in human eggs."** – Glei M and Pool-Zobel B: "The main catechin of green tea, epigallocatechin-3-gallate (EGCG), reduces bleomycin-induced DNA damage in human leucocytes." *Toxicology in Vitro*, Sep 28, 2005.

NOTES

In this study, the EGCG in green tea was found to reduce DNA damage and act as a protective agent for human cells.

Baby Friendly Micronutrients

297 **"Research has shown that over a period of 14 months, women who took nutritional supplements conceived earlier than those who did not."** – Czeizel A et al: "The effect of preconceptional multivitamin supplementation on fertility." *International Journal for Vitamin & Nutrition Research*, 66(1):55-58, 1996.
3,953 participants took a daily nutritional supplement containing 12 vitamins, 4 minerals and 3 trace elements. Another 3,952 women were given a preparation that only contained the three trace elements and vitamin C. During the 14-month research period, women taking the multivitamin/mineral preparation became pregnant more quickly.

297 **"Studies also indicate that nutritional supplements such as antioxidants, multivitamins and amino acids can help balance hormones, encourage egg production and improve sperm quality."** – Westphal L et al: "A nutritional supplement for improving fertility in women: a pilot study." *Journal of Reproductive Medicine*, Apr; 49 (4): 289-93, 2004.
This report concludes: "Nutritional supplementation may provide an attractive alternative or complement to conventional fertility therapy." *See also*:

Williams M: "Vitamin C increases fertility in women with luteal phase defect." *Fertility & Sterility*, 80:459–61, 2003.
150 women with luteal phase defect and infertility received either 750 mg of vitamin C per day or no treatment. Progesterone and estrogen levels increased in women receiving vitamin C but did not change in women receiving no treatment. 25% of the women receiving vitamin C became pregnant within six months of starting treatment, while only 11% of untreated women became pregnant.

Greco E et al: "Reduction of the incidence of sperm DNA fragmentation by oral antioxidant treatment." *Journal of Andrology*, May-Jun; 26(3):349-53, 2005.
64 men with unexplained infertility and an elevated percentage of DNA-fragmented spermatozoa were given either vitamin C and E or a placebo daily for two months. The percentage of DNA-fragmented spermatozoa was markedly reduced in the antioxidant treatment group.

297 **"Going Gluten Free to Help Calm Your Immune Response"** – Bustos D et al: "Autoantibodies in Argentine women with recurrent pregnancy loss." *American Journal of Reproductive Immunology*, Mar; 55 (3):201-7, 2006.
118 women with a history of three or more consecutive abortions were analyzed for the presence of auto antibodies. The prevalence of anticardiolipin antibodies was significantly higher than controls. "We recommended the screening of... antibodies in pregnancy, because of the high prevalence of subclinical celiac disease in RPL and the chance of reversibility through consumption of a gluten free diet.

NOTES

Acupuncture

298 **"This therapy has proved to be particularly beneficial to those undergoing IVF..."** – Sterzik K et al: "Influence of acupuncture on the pregnancy rate in patients who undergo assisted reproduction therapy." *Fertility & Sterility*, Apr; 77(4):721-4, 2002.
160 patients who were undergoing ART and who had good quality embryos were divided into the following two groups of 80: one group to undergo embryo transfer with acupuncture and one group to undergo embryo transfer without acupuncture. Acupuncture was performed in the treatment group 25 minutes before and after embryo transfer. Clinical pregnancies were documented in 42.5% of the acupuncture group, whereas the pregnancy rate was only 26.3% in the control group. *See also*:

Liu Z et al: ["Controlled study on acupuncture for treatment of endocrine dysfunctional infertility."] *Zhongguo Zhen Jiu*, May; 25(5):299-300, 2005.
240 infertile women were randomly treated with acupuncture and clomiphene. The pregnancy rates were 65.0% and 45.0% respectively.

298 **"Studies have shown that it [electro-acupuncture] improves blood flow to the ovaries and pelvic area."** – Wikland M et al: "Reduction of blood flow impedance in the uterine arteries of infertile women with electro-acupuncture." *Human Reproduction*, Jun; 11(6):1314-7, 1996.

298 **"Studies have shown that it...could be helpful for women with PCOS."** – Stener-Victorin E: "Effect of electro-acupuncture on ovarian expression of alpha (1)- and beta (2)-adrenoceptors and p75 neuro-trophin receptors in rats with steroid-induced polycystic ovaries." *Reproductive Biology & Endocrinology*, Jun 7; 3(1):21, 2005.
This study indicates that electro-acupuncture might be a possible complementary therapeutic approach to help overcome sympathetic-related anovulation in women with PCOS.

Manual Lymphatic Massage (MLD)

299 **"Manual lymphatic drainage (MLD) assists the body with this pro-cess by encouraging the lymphatic vessels to contract."** – Olszewski W and Engeset A: "Intrinsic contractibility of prenodal lymph vessels and lymph flow in the human leg." *American Journal of Physiology,* 239, H775, 1980.
In this study involving 13 patients with tumors in the upper body. it was observed that filling of the lymphatics with lymph by external massage to the leg evoked intrinsic contractions that propelled lymph even during rest.

299 **"MLD can help restore the balance of hormones and neurotrans-mitters...and reduce the symptoms of premenstrual syndrome."** – *Lymphatic Therapy for Toxic Congestion – Selected Case Studies for Therapists and Patients,* by McCarthy M. Published by Churchill Livingstone in 2002. ISBN: 0443073546. *See also*:

Sulman F et al: "Effect of manual lymph drainage massage on blood compo-nents and urinary neurohormones in chronic lymphedema." *Angiology,* Feb; 32(2):119-27, 1981.

NOTES

"...that histamine and serotonin were released from the edematous tissue and that circulation improved through increased output of adrenaline and noradrenaline."

Mind-Body Therapy

300 **"Mind-body therapy together with healthy nutrition and lifestyle choices can really help to reduce your immune system's stress burden."** – Vitella L et al: "Mind-body medicine: stress and its impact on overall health and longevity." *Annals of the New York Academy of Sciences,* 1057:492–505, 2005.
"Advances in mind-body medicine research together with healthy nutrition and lifestyle choices can have a significant impact on health maintenance and disease prevention and hence the prolongation of the human life span."

300 **"Physical activity, particularly when combined with deep breathing, has a wonderful anti-inflammatory effect"** – Petersen A and Pedersen B: "The anti-inflammatory effect of exercise." *Journal of Applied Physiology,* Apr; 98(4):1154-62, 2005.
In this article, the authors describe how TNF-alpha is the driver behind insulin resistance and that during exercise, IL-6 is produced by the muscles, which stimulates the appearance of other anti-inflammatory cytokines. *See also*:

Bruunsgaard H: "Physical activity and modulation of systemic low-level inflammation." *Journal of Leukocyte Biology,* July 2005.
The author describes how regular muscle contractions send signals via cytokines that suppress inflammatory activity.

Karacabey K et al: "The effects of exercise on the immune system and stress hormones in sportswomen." *Neurological and Endocrinological Letters,* Aug 30; 26(4) 2005.
In this study of 40 sportswomen and 20 sedentary women, it was concluded that, as well as reducing cortisol levels, "...regular and moderate exercise has favorable effects on the immune system by increasing immunoglobulins which are potent protective factors."

NOTES

GLOSSARY

GLOSSARY

Addison's disease: A disorder caused by a poorly functioning or damaged adrenal gland, which leads to a deficiency of cortisol and aldosterone hormones (that help control blood pressure, salt and water balance and immune responses to stress and illness). Symptoms include fatigue, weight loss, low blood pressure, depression, nausea and darkening of the skin. When the cause is autoimmune, half of these patients will develop a secondary autoimmune disease, often involving the thyroid.

Adrenal glands: A pair of hormone-producing glands (located on top of each kidney) that produce epinephrine and norepinephrine (adrenaline) that help control heart rate and blood pressure as well as the steroid hormones that control other important body functions.

Allergen: Any substance that induces an allergic response.

Allergy: An extreme immune response against a non-harmful substance (allergen). IgE antibodies combine with the allergen to cause inflammation.

Allele: An alternative form of a gene that may occur at a given locus (position) on a chromosome. Two different alleles make up an individual's genotype, one from each parent. In the case of DQ alpha genes, the alleles are designated with numbers such as 0101, 0201 etc., which represent the proteins or "antenna" on the surface of the cell.

Alloimmunity: A condition in which a person gains immunity from another person's (non-self) cells; e.g., LIT produces an alloimmune response in the woman against the male partner's T and B lymphoctyes.

Alopecia areata: An autoimmune disease in which the immune system attacks the hair follicles, causing hair loss on the scalp, face and other parts of the body. As the stem cells that supply the follicle are not targeted, the hair often grows back after treatment.

Anaphylaxis: An acute, potentially fatal allergic immune reaction.

Aneuploidy: Too few or too many chromosomes.

Antibodies: Proteins used by the immune system to identify foreign objects like bacteria and viruses. Also known as immunoglobulins (Ig).

Antigen: Any substance capable of eliciting an immune response (including the production of antibodies).

Antinuclear antibody (ANA): An autoantibody that targets the DNA or DNA accessory components within a cell's nucleus.

Antiphospholipid antibody (APA): An antibody that attaches to phos-pholipids (the fatty molecules on the surfaces of all cells). A positive APA test often correlates with a higher risk of developing blood clots.

Antiphospholipid Antibody Syndrome (APLS or APS): A syndrome defined by the presence of antiphospholipid antibodies, thrombosis, recurrent pregnancy loss and/or a decrease in the number of blood platelets. It is also known as Hughes' Syndrome, after the rheumatologist Dr Graham R.V. Hughes (St Thomas' Hospital, London, U.K.)

GLOSSARY

Apoptosis: Orderly cell death where the cell is prompted to self destruct by implosion. The cell shrinks, develops blebs on its surface and its DNA undergoes fragmentation.

Assay: A biological test for determining the concentration of a component contained in a mixture.

Autoimmunity: A condition in which the immune system attacks the body's own tissues.

Blastocyst: A fertilized egg after several days of cell division. It consists of a sphere of cells with an outer cell layer that forms the placenta and a cluster of cells inside that forms the embryo.

Blighted ovum: An abnormal pregnancy in which the placenta develops but no embryo is visible on ultrasound.

Blocking antibodies: These are produced during pregnancy to protect the placenta from rejection and encourage it to grow.

Cardiolipin: A type of phospholipid.

CD (clusters of differentiation): A designation system that is used to define the surface molecules of lymphocytes. It describes the type of cell and how activated it is.

Chromosomes: Protein strands that hold the DNA that contain hereditary material. There are 23 pairs of chromosomes (46 in total). Two of these chromosomes are the sex chromosomes that are called X and Y. Girls have two X chromosomes and boys have one X and one Y chromosome.

Corpus luteum: The progesterone secreting tissue formed by a follicle after it releases an egg. *Corpus* means "body" and *Luteum* is derived from the Latin word for "yellow."

C-reactive protein (CRP): One of the proteins that increase during systemic inflammation. CRP is believed to play a role in the initiation and progression of cardiovascular disease.

Cytogenesis: The origin, development and variation of cells.

Cytokines: These are "messenger molecules" produced by the white blood cells (lymphocytes). They communicate with other cells of the immune system and recruit them to perform aggressive roles in fighting off infection or rejecting foreign tissue from the body.

Cytotoxic: Producing a toxic effect on cells.

Decidua: The lining of the endometrium during pregnancy that is shed with the placenta at delivery. It is also expelled during a miscarriage.

Dilation and curettage (D&C): Surgical procedure to remove pregnancy tissue after a miscarriage. A narrow instrument inserted through the cervix scrapes or suctions away the tissue in the uterus.

- 445 -

GLOSSARY

DNA (Deoxyribonucleic Acid): Genetic instructions for the biological development of all cellular forms of life. DNA is responsible for the propagation of most inherited traits and is replicated during reproduction.

DQ alpha: A type of HLA antenna present on certain white blood cells (lymphocytes) that help cells to recognize each other. Each individual contains two DQ alpha alleles (genes) represented as numbers (for example 1.2, 4.1 or 0102, 0501). One number is inherited from each parent. When couples are compatible for these factors (share the same numbers), it is often unfavorable for pregnancy.

Eclampsia: A life threatening condition in late pregnancy when very high blood pressure leads to seizures.

ELISA (Enzyme-Linked Immunosorbent Assay): A test method used to detect the presence of an antigen or antibody. ELISA tests are primarily used to detect proteins. Some of these include hormones, bacterial antigens and antibodies.

Embryo: Product of conception from the time of implantation through the eighth week of pregnancy.

Endometriosis: A condition where endometrial tissue grows outside the uterus elsewhere in the body.

Endometrium: The lining of the uterus. During the monthly cycle, the endometrium thickens to provide a nourishing place for the embryo to attach and begin its development.

Endorphins: "Natural pain killers." Endorphins are peptides produced by the pituitary gland and the hypothalamus, which have an effect similar to morphine.

Endothelial cells: The thin, flat cells that line the interior surface of blood vessels and form an interface between the circulating blood and the vessel wall. These cells line the entire circulatory system, from the heart to the smallest capillary.

Eosinophil: A type of leukocyte that is responsible for combating parasites in the body.

Epstein Barr virus (EBV): A member of the herpes virus family. EBV remains dormant or latent in a few cells in the throat and blood for the rest of the person's life and can reactivate without symptoms of illness. It is a major cause of infectious mononucleosis and has been associated with chronic fatigue syndrome and the development of certain cancers.

Estrogen: A family of three hormones (Estrone (E1), Estradiol (E2) and Estriol (E3)) which are produced by the ovaries and are responsible for the development of the female sex characteristics. Estrogens, along with progesterone, also help prepare the endometrium for pregnancy.

Fibrin: A protein necessary for blood clotting. Fibrin forms a "mesh" that traps platelets and red blood cells and holds the clot together.

Fibroid: A benign tumor that can grow in the uterus.

Fibrosis: The formation of fibrous tissue (scar tissue).

GLOSSARY

Flow cytometry: A lab test technique for counting microscopic particles suspended in a stream of fluid. A beam of light of a single frequency is directed onto the stream of fluid and particles (usually cells) are counted and sorted by type.

Follicle-stimulating hormone (FSH): A hormone produced in the pituitary gland that stimulates the development of the ovarian follicles that produce the eggs.

Genes: Located in the cell's nucleus, genes are the structural units of inheritance in living organisms.

Graves' disease: An autoimmune thyroid disease in which an excessive amount of the thyroid hormone, thyroxine (T4) is produced. Symptoms include weight loss, increased appetite, elevated heart rate, high blood pressure, tremors, depression, anxiety and diarrhea. Women are seven times more likely to be affected than men, and often have a family history of thyroid disease.

Granulocytes: A division of white blood cells that includes basophils, neutrophils and eosinophils that attack and destroy foreign invaders.

Glycodelin A: An immunosuppressive glycoprotein that is secreted into the endometrial lining.

Hashimoto's disease: An autoimmune disease in which the immune system destroys the thyroid gland. Low levels of thyroid hormone cause fatigue, weight gain, depression, hair loss, coarsening of the skin, goiter (a swelling of the neck due to the enlarged thyroid gland) and sensitivity to cold. The disease is 50 times more common in women than men. It is most prevalent in women in their 30s and 40s.

HELLP syndrome: (**H**emolyticanemia **E**levated **L**iver **E**nzymes and **L**ow **P**latelet count): A life threatening complication of preeclampsia that occurs during the latter stages of pregnancy, and often results in the rapid deterioration of the mother's and baby's health. Symptoms can include edema, excess protein in the urine, high blood pressure, and fetal growth restriction.

Heparin: A natural substance produced by the liver and lungs. As a drug, it acts to prevent the blood from clotting too fast.

Heterozygous: Having two different alleles of a particular gene.

Histocompatibility: Having the same, or mostly the same, alleles of a set of genes (a factor considered for all donors and recipients of organ trans-plants to avoid rejection). In the context of pregnancy, close histocompati-bility between mother and fetus can be detrimental to pregnancy survival.

Histones: Proteins associated with DNA in chromosomes.

Homocysteine: An amino acid that can damage the inner lining of arteries and promote blood clots, leading to stroke and vascular disease.

Homozygous: Having two of the same allele of a particular gene, a similar one inherited from each parent.

GLOSSARY

Human chorionic gonadotropin (HCG): A hormone produced by the cells of the placenta in pregnancy. Its detection is the basis of all pregnancy tests.

Human leukocyte antigens (HLA): These are molecules on the surface of human cells that determine a person's white blood cell type. They are defined as A, B, C, DR or DQ. One type of antigen comes from the mother the other one comes from the father. Couples with infertility and recurrent pregnancy losses often share too many DR and DQ HLA antigens.

IgG (Immunoglobulin G): The most abundant type of antibody class in the blood. IgG can indicate a recent or remote infection. This antibody is produced by B lymphocytes (CD19) and is present primarily in the lymph system.

Immunoglobulins: Also known as antibodies. Immunoglobulins are produced by the B cells to bind to foreign antigens. There are five different classes of immunoglobulins: IgM is the first antibody produced when an immune response is initiated. IgG lives in the lymphatic system and is made by IgM. IgA lives in the organs and protects them. IgD is present as a "memory antibody" in the blood once a person is immune or immunized. IgE causes allergies and asthma and is present throughout the body.

Interferons (IFNs): These are cytokines produced by the cells of the immune system in response to viruses, bacteria, parasites and tumor cells. Interferon-gamma (IFN-λ) is a protein that acts as an antiviral agent.

Interleukins (IL): A class of cytokines produced by white blood cells that allow these cells to communicate with each other. For example, IL-2 is produced by activated CD4 cells to promote the proliferation and activity of T cells and natural killer cells.

Intralipid: Intralipid is an emulsion of essential fatty acids Omega 3 and Omega 6 that helps remove the danger signals that over activate the immune system and contribute to implanation failure. Made from a mixture of soybean oil, egg yolk phospholipids glycerin and water, intralipid is around 10 times less expensive than IVIG.

Intravenous immunoglobulin G infusion (IVIG): A preparation of antibodies pooled from many different blood donors. The serum is washed and processed so that it is free of infection. IVIG takes approximately 2-4 hours to administer through the vein.

In vitro fertilization (IVF): A method of assisted reproduction that involves combining an egg with a sperm in a laboratory environment. If the egg fertilizes, the resulting embryo is transferred back into the woman's uterus where it may implant and develop.

Karyotype: A complete set of human chromosomes.

Lectins: Found in many plant-based foods, these are toxins that plants emit to discourage animals and insects from eating them.

Leukocytes: Consist of granulocytes (neutrophils, basophils and eosinophils), lymphocytes (B cells, T cells and natural killer cells), monocytes and macrophages.

Leukocyte antibody detection (LAD or "Crossmatch"): This is the assay used to measure the blocking antibody response of the woman against her partner's lymphocytes. In a normal pregnancy, LAD levels are usually high. In women with recurrent pregnancy losses or infertility, LAD levels are often low.

- 448 -

GLOSSARY

Luteal phase: The time in a woman's reproductive cycle between ovulation and menstruation. Luteal phase defects (abnormally short luteal phases) can arise when there is a lack of estrogen or progesterone, which prevents the uterine lining from developing properly.

Luteinizing hormone (LH): A hormone that stimulates the ovaries to produce and release an egg each month during the menstrual cycle.

Lymph: This is the fluid-like plasma in blood that contains the lympho-cytes of the immune system.

Lymph node: One of a number of small, bean-shaped glands that are part of the lymphatic system. They are found in the groin, armpit, neck, abdomen and other sites. The immune response starts in this gland. These glands can start to swell when lymphocytes increase in number to elimi-nate a foreign invader.

Lymphocyte immunization therapy (LIT): A vaccine made by extracting the white cells from blood donated by the male partner or an unrelated donor. The white blood cells that are isolated by centrifugion are CD3 T cells and CD19 B cells. The final volume of prepared cells is injected under the surface of the skin. Immunization will usually result in the formation of blocking antibodies in the recipient, reducing the killing power of the NK cells and creating a shift to a more favorable Th2 immune response.

Lymphocytes: B cells, T cells and natural killer cells.

Lymphokines: Cytokines produced by T cells.

Major histocompatibility complex (MHC): A genetic system that determines the antennae (cell surface molecules) on lymphocytes that are responsible for antigen presentation to T lymphocytes in the elicitation and the expression (the beginning) of an immune response. This genetic system is responsible for the rejection of grafts between individuals and of embryos and fetuses in individuals that are too closely matched at the DR and DQ alleles.

Morphology: The configuration or structure of an organism or its parts.

MTHFR (Methylene-Tetra-Hydro-Folate-Reductase): An enzyme needed to metabolize and eliminate homocysteine. A mutation in the gene that codes this enzyme (C677T) often increases homocysteine levels, which can lead to increased miscarriage rates, neural tubes defects or cardiovascular disease. Individuals who are heterozygous for the mutation carry one copy of the gene (inherited from one parent). Individuals who are homozygous for the mutation carry two genes (inherited from both parents).

Multiple sclerosis: A slowly progressive autoimmune disease in which the body's immune system attacks the myelin sheath that surrounds the nerve cells, resulting in disrupted impulse transmission. Symptoms can include numbness, paralysis, seizures, tremors, lack of coordination, muscle weak-ness and vision problems.

Mutagen: An agent that can increase the rate of cell mutation, e.g., toxic chemicals and UV light.

- 449 -

GLOSSARY

Monocytes: a type of leukocyte, or white blood cell (e.g. macrophages and dendritic cells). Monocytes influence the process of adaptive immunity, destroying invaders and facilitating healing and repair. They are formed in the bone marrow and comprise about 5-10% of circulating white blood cells.

Myasthenia Gravis: A chronic autoimmune disorder where the nerve-muscle junctions are attacked, causing gradual muscle weakness that usually starts in the face. Symptoms include drooping eyelids, double vision, and difficulty breathing, talking and swallowing. The disorder most commonly affects women under 40.

Natural killer cells (NK cells): A type of lymphocyte and a component of the innate immune response. They contain granules with enzymes that can kill infected or cancerous cells. Also called large granular lymphocytes.

Natural killer T cells (NK T cells): Natural killer T cells share properties of both T cells and natural killer cells.

Necrosis: The localized death of cells, tissue or an entire organ often caused by the deprivation of blood supply.

Neupogen®: a form of granulocyte colony-stimulating factor (G-CSF), which is naturally produced by the body. It stimulates the production of neutrophils, a type of white blood cell important in the body's fight against infection. It is used to increase the number of good quality eggs during an IVF cycle and can help prevent immunologic miscarriage in some cases.

Neurotransmitter: A chemical used to relay an electrical signal between a neuron and another cell (usually another neuron). Neurotransmitters act in the brain and the nervous system.

Neutrophil: A type of white blood cell making up approximately 40 – 60% of the white blood cells in our bodies.

Nidation: Implantation of the embryo in the endometrium.

Oocyte: An egg still developing in the ovary.

Peptides: Chains of amino acids that combine to make proteins, including antigens.

Phospholipid: The main molecular component of all cell membranes; composed of glycerol, phosphate and fatty acid residues.

Pituitary gland: A pea-sized hormone producing gland at the base of the brain that regulates many body processes, including reproduction.

Placental abruption (abruptio placenta): Early detachment of the placenta from the uterus often caused by a blood clotting disorder, an infection or an inflammatory immune reaction. This condition may cause severe bleeding that is life threatening to both the pregnant woman and fetus.

Platelets: Platelets play a crucial part in the blood clotting process by binding to the site of the wound and binding to each other, forming a plug. This plug combined with fibrin

GLOSSARY

helps to stop the bleeding and allows injuries to heal. 2% of the body's serotonin is stored in platelets.

Polycystic ovary syndrome (PCOS): Also known clinically as Stein-Leventhal syndrome. An endocrine disorder often manifested by multiple cysts on the ovaries, insulin resistance, elevated male hormones, anovulation, weight gain and infertility.

Preeclampsia: A condition that precedes eclampsia. It can occur in the second half of pregnancy and is characterized by high blood pressure, hypertension, excessive swelling of the hands, feet and ankles and exces-sive protein in the urine (proteinuria).

Premature ovarian failure (POF): Loss of ovarian function in women prior to the age of 40 that may be due to genetic, autoimmune, developmental, and/or environmental causes.

Progesterone: A female hormone secreted by the ovary after ovulation during the luteal phase. Produced by the corpus luteum, progesterone is essential for the success of all pregnancies.

Pronucleus: Nucleus of the sperm or the egg prior to fertilization.

Reiter's disease: An autoimmune disease that includes symptoms of arthritis, urethritis (inflammation of the urethra) and conjunctivitis (inflammation of the lining of the eye). It occurs most commonly after infection with chlamydia.

Reproductive endocrinologist (RE): A medical specialist dedicated to the treatment of infertility.

Reproductive immunophenotype: A specialized blood test in which eight of the most important white blood cell types are counted by flow cytometry.

Reproductive immunologist (RI): A medical specialist dedicated to the treatment of immune disorders in pregnancy.

Rh negative: 15% of women do not have the Rh antigen on their red blood cells and are therefore Rh negative. If the woman becomes pregnant with an Rh-positive child, she may make antibodies against the baby's Rh- positive antigens and destroy its red blood cells. The situation is prevented by giving the women Rh immunoglobulin (Rhogam) during pregnancy.

Rheumatoid factor: An antibody found in the blood of most, but not all, people with rheumatoid arthritis or other rheumatic diseases.

Scleroderma ("sclero" means hard and "derma" means skin): A rare systemic illness caused when immune cells attack connective tissue to produce inflammation and scar tissue (fibrosis) in the skin, internal organs and small blood vessels. Symptoms can include skin ulcers on the fingers, joint stiffness, sore throat and diarrhea. Scleroderma is up to eight times more prevalent among women than in men. The peak age of onset is between 30 and 55 years old.

Serotonin (5-hydroxytriptamine or 5-HT): A key neurotransmitter, present in many tissues, especially blood and nervous tissue. It regulates the delivery of messages between nerve cells (neurons) and stimulates a variety of smooth muscles. Serotonin is

GLOSSARY

believed to play an important role in the regulation of mood, sleep, sexuality and appetite.

Serum: The clear, yellowish liquid component of blood that remains when blood cells, platelets and fibrinogen have been removed.

Sjögren's syndrome (pronounced "show-grens"): An autoimmune disorder in which the immune system attacks the glands that produce tears and saliva.

Steroids: This term usually refers to a group of powerful molecules that are related chemically to testosterone, the male sex hormone. However, in reproductive immunology, the term can also refer to corticosteroids (medications like prednisone and dexamethasone used to reduce inflammation).

Subchorionic hemorrhage or hematoma: A collection of blood (seen on a pregnancy ultrasound scan) that can cause the placenta to prematurely separate from the uterine wall. The blood collects and creates a clot. A clot very near the placenta can be more dangerous than a clot further away from the placenta.

Syncytium: A cell-like structure formed when the membranes of two or more cells fuse together.

Testosterone: Primarily a male hormone produced by the testicles, testos-terone is responsible for the development and the release of sperm, male characteristics and sex drive. Small amounts of testosterone are also produced by a woman's ovaries and adrenal glands.

Thrombosis: Formation of a clot or "thrombus" inside a blood vessel.

Tumor necrosis factor alpha (TNF-α): A cytokine that attaches to a cell's TNF receptor to promote inflammation. It is often found at high levels in autoimmune diseases like Crohn's, psoriasis and rheumatoid arthritis as well as in some patients who suffer from recurrent miscarriage and infertility.

Turner syndrome: Instead of the normal XX sex chromosomes for a female, only one X chromosome is present at birth, which means female sexual characteristics are present, but are underdeveloped.

Trophoblast: The membrane that forms the outside wall of the blastocyst in early development. The trophoblast aids implantation in the uterine wall and serves as a nutritive filter for the embryo.

Vasculitis: Inflammation of small arteries or veins that can sometimes result in fibrosis and thrombi formation.

Vitiligo: An autoimmune disease characterized by the destruction of skin pigment cells, resulting in white patches of skin and hair loss.

Zona pellucida: The thick, transparent layer that surrounds the oocyte.

RESOURCES

RESOURCES

U.S. Centers that Specialize in Reproductive Immunology

Braverman IVF & Reproductive Immunology,
Jeffrey Braverman, M.D.
Long Island address:
800 Woodbury Rd G,
Woodbury, NY 11797
http://preventmiscarriage.com

Reproductive Medicine and Immunology,
Joanne Kwak-Kim, M.D.
Reproductive Immunologist,
830 West End Court, Suite 400,
Vernon Hills,
IL 60061
www.rfuclinics.com

Reproductive Medicine Institute,
Carolyn B. Coulam, M.D.
233 E. Erie St. Suite 307,
Chicago,
Illinois 60611
www.reproductivemedicineinstitute.com

Sher Institute for Reproductive Medicine,
Geoffrey Sher, M.D.
Kathy Trumbull, M.D.
5401 N. Knoxville Ave. Suite 102
Peoria, IL 61614
www.haveababy.com

Center for Human Reproduction,
Norbert Gleicher, M.D.
21 E. 69th Street,
New York, NY 10021,
www.centerforhumanreprod.com

Columbia Fertility Associates,
Rafat A. Abbasi, M.D.& Preston C. Sacks, M.D.
2440 M Street NW, Suite 401
Washington, DC 20037
www.columbiafertility.com

- 454 -

RESOURCES

Zouves Fertility Center,
Christo Zouves, M.D.
1241 E Hillsdale Blvd,
Foster City, CA 94404,
Phone: (650) 378-1000
www.goivf.com

Fertility Centers with Access to Reproductive Immunology

Alabama

ART Fertility Program of Alabama,
Kathryn Honea, M.D.
Women's Medical Plaza,
2006 Brookwood, Medical Center Drive, Suite 508,
Birmingham, AL 35209
www.fertilityprogramalabama.com

From website: *"We offer advanced diagnostic procedures such as...male factor evaluation including sperm antibody evaluation and autoimmune antibody testing to identify problems with egg and sperm production."*

Arizona

IVF Phoenix,
John Couvaras, M.D.
9817 N. 95th Street Bldg 1 – Ste 107,
Scottsdale, AZ 85258
www.ivfphoenix.com

From website: *"Dr. Couvaras systematically sets out to reduce sources of inflammation through his Immune Balancing Protocol. It's important to investigate an immunity imbalance in so-called unexplained infertility cases before skipping straight to in-vitro fertilization, as is the typical strategy of most other reproductive endocrinologists."*

California

The Fertility Institutes,
Jeffrey Steinberg, M.D.
16030 Ventura Blvd Suite 404,
Encino, CA 91436
www.fertility-docs.com

From website: *"We offer complete couple tissue type compatibility testing through our association with a leading immunology laboratory. We work closely with the country's leading immunology experts, and offer full laboratory testing that includes preparation for and administration of paternal leukocyte immunization, aspirin/heparin/prednisone protocols as well as a variety of cutting edge methods to both improve pregnancy*

- 455 -

RESOURCES

outcome associated with advanced fertility procedures, as well as to prevent pregnancy loss from occurring."

Fertility Matrix,
Melissa McNamara, M.D.
2301 Camino Ramon, Suite 286,
San Ramon, CA 94583
www.fertilitymatrix.com

Comment: Melisssa McNamara, MD is a Reproductive Immunologist and board certified Rheumatologist with expertise in immunology and diseases related to reproductive immune dysregulation such as implantation failure and endometriosis.

Reproductive Partners Medical Group,
Carrie Melissa Wambach, M.D.
Beverly Hills / Los Angeles,
6330 San Vicente Blvd, Suite 408,
Los Angeles, CA 90048
www.reproductivepartners.com

Comment: "Dr Wambach's current interests in the field include recurrent miscarriage, premature ovarian failure and reproductive immunology. Her work has been published in 'Reproductive Immunology.'"

Acacio Fertility Centers,
Brian Acacio, M.D.
27882 Forbes Road, Suite 200,
Laguna Niguel, CA 92677

Also at:
26800 Crown Valley Parkway, Suite 560,
Mission Viejo, CA 92691
2205 19th Street ,
Bakersfield, CA 93301
www.acaciofertility.com

Doctor comment: "Immunologic problems are treated with immunotherapy. If the cause is related to activated immune cells and their cytokines, treatments include: IVIG and Intralipid. If either acquired or inherited thrombophilia is causing clotting of the placental vessel and subsequent pregnancy loss, then heparin and aspirin are the treatments of choice. If the blood clotting is the result of an immune process, steroids can be used."

The Fertility Institutes
Jeffery Steinburg, M.D.
16030 Ventura Blvd,
Suite 404, Encino, CA 91436
www.fertility-docs.com

Center comment: "We have been offering Reproductive Immunology services for many years. Dr Steinberg did a fellowship with Dr Alan Beer in Chicago and become very involved in the workup and process. We provide access to NK cell evaluations and a large range of additional assays: (antihistone anitbodies, antinuclear antibodies, Anti

- 456 -

RESOURCES

Sm, Anti RNP, AntiSS-B, AntiSS-A, antiphospholipid antibodies, Leukocyte antibody detection - crossmatch, B Cell IgG, T Cell IgG, thyroid antibodies, Immunophenotypes, NK Cell activation, HLA testing and many more as well as all of the blood clotting disorders. We refer to Reproductive Immunologists and have our own M.D., Ph.D. doctor, William Freije from UCLA who has a Ph.D. in Reproductive Genetics. We see many patients with recurrent reproductive failure and have really great outcome data for the great majority."

Zouves Fertility Center,
Christo Zouves, M.D.
1241 E Hillsdale Blvd,
Foster City, CA 94404,
Phone: (650) 378-1000
www.goivf.com

Patient comment: "Strongly believes in Dr Beer's immune treatments. Will prescribe IVIG and Enbrel. Very compassionate and caring."
Very knowledgeable on reproductive immunology. Very high success rates. Recommended by Dr Kwak and Dr Beer. Wrote the preface for "Is Your Body Baby Friendly?"

Colorado

CU Advanced Reproductive Medicine,
Edward Illions, M.D.
3055 Roslyn Street, Suite 230,
Denver, CO 80238
www.arm.coloradowomenshealth.com

Comment from Dr Illions, "Our work up for patients with recurrent pregnancy losses and failed implantation cycles during IVF does include testing for APLS (Lupus anticoagulant, B2GP-1 Ab's and Anticardiolipin Ab's). We will test for the typical blood clotting agents when indicated and these include; Leiden V (or activated Protein C resistance as the initial screening test), Prothrombin II Gene mutation. MTHFR is no longer considered part of the tests required for RPL or failed implantation cycles since the literature does not support that test. I would rather rely on a fasting homocysteine level. We will test for protein S,C, and anti-thrombin III IF the patient's history for clotting supports those tests, but again these are not part of the panel that is required for RPL or failed implantation patients. We do not test for NK activity (uterine or peripheral) since the literature yields conflicted evidence at best and/or no benefit in other studies. We typically also obtain thyroid antibodies (TPO) in this population. We do not have any specific reproductive immunologists that we typically work with but I do have some experts in the area of RPL and failed implantation whose advice I typically seek for difficult cases."

- 457 -

RESOURCES

Florida

Mark Denker, M.D.
7015 Beracasa Way, Suite 201,
Boca Raton, FL 33433

Also at:
4671 South Congress Ave, Suite 101,
Lake Worth, FL 33461
www.palmbeachfertility.com

From website: "Dr. Denker's special areas of interest are the immunology of infertility and pregnancy loss, and treatment of recurrent implantation failure."

IVF MD,
Kenneth Gelman, M.D.
9900 Stirling Rd,
Suite 222,
Hollywood, FL 33024

Also at:
7300 SW 62nd Place,
4th Floor
Miami, FL 33143

9960 Central Park Blvd,
Suite 275
Boca Raton, FL 33428

1265 Creekside Parkway,
Suite 202
Naples, FL 34108
www.ivfmd.com

Comment: "Dr Gelman is a member of the American Society of Reproductive Medicine and the American Society of Reproductive Immunology. This clinic is up to speed with all the latest tests and treatments for immune related pregnancy failure and has just introduced a Systemic Inflammation Fertility Test (SIFT). This advanced assessment examines multiple key circulating blood factors known to induce inflammation. An individualized plan is then formulated to increase the patient's good health and reproductive success."

Illinois

Roumen Roussev, M.D.
Alpha Fertility,
8635 Lemont Road,
Downers Grove, IL 60516
www.alphafertility.com

RESOURCES

Comment: "*Dr Roussev managed the Reproductive Immunology Laboratory at the Center for Human Reproduction in Chicago. He joined the Sher Institute for Reproductive Medicine in 2000 and became Managing Director of Millenova Immunology Laboratories, Chicago. He has dedicated his professional life to analyzing the role of immune system on infertility, IVF or implantation failures as well as recurrent pregnancy loss.*"

Reproductive Medicine Institute,
Carolyn B. Coulam, M.D.
233 E. Erie St. Suite 307,
Chicago,
Illinois 60611

Oak Brook Office:
2425 W 22nd St,
Ste 200,
Oak Brook, IL 60523

Chicago Office:
233 E Erie St,
Ste 307, Chicago, IL 60611
Evanston Office:
2500 Ridge Ave,
Ste 308,
Evanston, IL 60201

Oak Lawn Office:
5851 W 95th St
Ste 117
Oak Lawn, IL 60453

Bloomingdale Office:
471 W. Army Trail Rd
Ste 105
Bloomingdale, IL 60108

Northbrook Office:
1535 Lake Cook Rd
Ste 102
Northbrook, IL 60062
www.reproductivemedicineinstitute.com

From website: "*Dr Coulam is known for the devoted care she provides to her patients and enjoys an international reputation for her contributions to medical/scientific education and research. As one of the first female Reproductive Immunologists in the field, she has also set other 'firsts' while simultaneously raising ten children of her own. She has more than 200 publications in peer-reviewed journals to her credit. Dr Coulam has special expertise in the area of Recurrent Pregnancy Loss, and is an internationally-sought speaker on the topic as well as issues involving reproductive immunology.*"

- 459 -

RESOURCES

Sher Institute for Reproductive Medicine,
Geoffrey Sher, M.D.
Kathy Trumbull, M.D.
5401 N. Knoxville Ave. Suite 102
Peoria, IL 61614
www.haveababy.com

Comment: Dr Sher is an internationally renowned authority on immunologic causes of infertility and the pioneer of many "firsts" in the field of IVF. 60% of his patients travel from out of state to visit his centers.

From website: "There are numerous non-embryologic factors that can be responsible for failed IVF. There are two types of immunologic reactions or immune factors involved in conception and infertility: 1. Autoimmune disorders are more common, implicated in over 90% of immune-related infertility... This is an abnormal reaction that is associated with several non-pregnancy related diseases. 2. Alloimmune disorders, where antibodies against tissue associated with the male partner (e.g. paternal sperm proteins) are produced. Alloimmune problems are associated with less than 10% of implantation failure or recurrent pregnancy loss."

Reproductive Medicine and Immunology,
Joanne Kwak-Kim, M.D.
Reproductive Immunologist,
830 West End Court, Suite 400,
Vernon Hills,
IL 60061
www.rfuclinics.com

Comment: Dr Kwak-Kim is a highly respected authority on the subject of reproductive immunology. Her protocols are not overly aggressive and therefore they can be applied speedily (important for women over 40) for positive results where all else has previously failed.

Indianapolis

Indiana Fertility Institute,
John Jarrett, M.D.
10610 N Pennsylvania St #101,
Indianapolis, IN 46280
www.fertilityindy.com

Comment: This center recognizes autoimmune disorders as one of the causes of recurrent miscarriage and unexplained infertility. Will offer testing and treatment where necessary.

Men's and Women's Specialty Health Centers,
David McLaughlin, M.D.
9660 E 146th St #300,
Noblesville, IN 46060
www.familyjoy.net

RESOURCES

Patient comment: "Offers testing for immune issues before couples opt for expensive and possibly unnecessary IVF treatment."

From website: "Laboratory tests may be ordered to evaluate the possibility of an immune response in relation to your history of pregnancy loss... Our goal is to identify possible explanations to recurrent pregnancy loss and offer individualized medical treatment options."

Iowa

Abey Eapen, M.D.
Reproductive Endocrinologist,
University of Iowa,
Department of Obstetrics and Gynecology,
704 Foster Road,
Iowa City, IA 52245
www.medicine.uiowa.edu/obgyn

Comment: "Tests for immune hyperactivity and uses corticosteroids to mod-erate the immune system when necessary."

Kansas

The Center for Reproductive Medicine
9300 East 29th St N #102,
Wichita, KS 67226
www.cfrm.net

Louisiana

Phillip Rye, M.D.
Fertility Institute of New Orleans,
4770 S I-10 Service Rd W #201,
Metairie, LA 70001
www.fertilityinstitute.com

Patient comment: "Dr Rye highly recommends IVIG and LIT. He recommended I do the LAD test to begin with. He is not against working with reproductive immunologists and quotes Coulam a lot."

Maryland

Rafat Abbasi, M.D.
Columbia Fertility Associates,
10215 Fernwood Rd,
Suite 301A,
Bethesda, MD 20817
www.columbiafertility.com

- 461 -

RESOURCES

From website: "Columbia Fertility Associates is one of a select group of ART centers in the nation that specializes in reproductive immunology."

Maine

The Bangor, ME Fertility Center
12 Stillwater Avenue
Bangor, Maine 04401

Also at:
The Portland Fertility Center
778 Main Street, Suite 2
S. Portland, Maine 04106
www.bostonivf.com

Doctor's comment: "Boston IVF uses evidence based guidelines as the basis for treatment and collaborate with colleagues in related and unrelated fields of medicine as dictated by the needs of our patients, including autoimmune and blood clotting problems."

Massachusetts

Boston IVF,
Michael Alper, M.D.
Steven R. Bayer, M.D.
The Tufts Medical Fertility Center,
800 Washington Street,
Boston, MA 02111

Alan Penzias, M.D.
130 2nd Ave,
Waltham, MA 02451

Kerri Luzzo, M.D.
The Dartmouth Fertility Center,
Healthcare for Women,
531 Faunce Corner Road,
N. Dartmouth, MA 02747
www.bostonivf.com

Patient comment: "My wife and I went through IVF at Boston IVF and it was discovered that she had Factor 5, which contributed to her miscarriage at 17 weeks. It was remedied and we are expecting in September! Boston IVF uses evidence based guidelines as the basis for treatment and collaborate with colleagues in related and unrelated fields of medicine as dictated by the needs of our patients, including autoimmune and blood clotting problems."

Doctor comment: "Boston IVF uses evidence based guidelines as the basis for treatment and collaborate with colleagues in related and unrelated fields of medicine as dictated by the needs of our patients, including autoimmune and blood clotting problems."

- 462 -

RESOURCES

Michigan

IVF Michigan Flint & Rochester Hills,
3950 S Rochester Rd Ste 2300,
Rochester Hills, MI 48307
www.michiganinfertilityexpert.com

Center comment: *"We order testing for clotting disorders and antibody tests for recurrent pregnancy loss. Dr Abuzeid will typically refer to Dr Joanne Kwak-Kim in Chicago for any further immunology testing and follow up."*

Minnesota

Reproductive Medicine and Infertility Associates,
Romaine Bayless, M.D.
2101 Woodwinds Dr Ste 100,
Saint Paul, MN 55125
www.rmia.com

Comment: *"Provides access to tests and treatments for immune issues."*

Missouri

Peter Ahlering, M.D.
Missouri Center for Reproductive Medicine,
17300 N. Outer Forty Road,
Chesterfield, MO 63005
www.mcrmfertility.com

Comment: *"Dr Ahlering founded this center. He previously worked at The Sher Institute for Reproductive Medicine (SIRM). His centers provide the full spectrum of immunology tests and treatments."*

Sher Institute for Reproductive Medicine,
Anthony Pearlstone, M.D.
Molina Dayal, M.D.
555 N New Ballas Rd,
Suite 150, St. Louis, MO 63141
stlouisfertilitycenter.com

Comment: Dr Sher is an internationally renowned authority on immunologic causes of infertility and the pioneer of many "firsts" in the field of IVF.

Fertility Partnership,
Elan Simckes, M.D.
5401 Veterans Memorial Pkwy #201,
St Peters,
MO 63376
http://fertilitypartnership.com

- 463 -

RESOURCES

Comment from Dr Simckes: "*We provide investigative service and treatment of recurrent pregnancy loss. We test for all the recognized and significant causes of antibody mediated infertility and loss. We can test for natural killer cells also and if it is appropriate we do that. I will work with anybody who can help my patients have a baby. Recurrent pregnancy loss really stinks and I spend 20 to 25% of my time battling it.*"

Nevada

Sher Fertility,
Geoffrey Sher, M.D.
Executive Medical Director,
5320 S Rainbow Blvd, Suite 302,
Las Vegas,
NV 89118
www.drgeoffreysherivf.com

Comment: Sher Fertility Centers are internationally renowned for the identification and treatment of immunologic causes of infertility and recurrent miscarriage.

New Hampshire

The Bedford NH Fertility Center
18 Constitution Drive, Ste: 2,
Bedford, New Hampshire 03110
(Also has centers in Rye and Salem.)
www.bostonivf.com

Doctor comment: "*Boston IVF uses evidence based guidelines as the basis for treatment and collaborate with colleagues in related and unrelated fields of medicine as dictated by the needs of our patients, including autoimmune and blood clotting problems.*"

New Jersey

Sher Fertility,
171 NJ-173,
Asbury, NJ 08802
https://haveababy.com

Comment: Sher Fertility Centers are internationally renowned for the identification and treatment of immunologic causes of infertility and recurrent miscarriage.

Princeton IVF,
Robin Hilsenrath, M.D.
2 Princess Rd,
Lawrence Township, NJ 08648
www.princetonivf.com

- 464 -

RESOURCES

Center comment: "We provide access to tests for autoimmune and blood clotting disorders."

Cooper Center for Reproductive Hormonal Disorders,
Jerome Check, M.D.
17000 Commerce Pkwy,
Mt Laurel, NJ 08054
http://ccivf.com

Comment: Dr Check contributed to the 2017 book "Immune Infertility: Impact of Immune Reactions on Human Fertility" and produced a presentation about regulating abnormal immune system activity in early pregnancy, "Non Invasive Methods to Improve Embryo Implantation" which is available online.

Diana Alecsandru, M.D.
Reproductive Immunologist,
Reproductive Medicine Associates of New Jersey,
495 Iron Bridge Rd # 10,
Freehold, NJ 07728
www.rmanj.com

The Fertility Institutes
51 East 67th Street,
New York, NY 10021
www.fertility-docs.com

From website: "We offer complete couple tissue type compatibility testing through our association with a leading immunology laboratory. We work closely with the country's leading immunology experts, and offer full laboratory testing that includes preparation for and administration of paternal leukocyte immunization, aspirin/heparin/prednisone protocols as well as a variety of cutting edge methods to both improve pregnancy outcome asso-ciated with advanced fertility procedures, as well as to prevent pregnancy loss from occurring."

Reproductive Specialists of New York,
Richard Bronson, M.D.
2500 Nesconset Hwy,
Building 23,
Stony Brook, NY 11790
https://rsofny.com

Comment: Dr Bronson is a past President of the American Society for Reproductive Immunology.

Braverman IVF & Reproductive Immunology,
Jeffrey Braverman M.D.
Long Island address:
800 Woodbury Rd G,
Woodbury, NY 11797

Also at:
888 Park Ave., Suite 1B
(Entrance on 78th Street)

- 465 -

RESOURCES

New York City, NY 10075
http://preventmiscarriage.com

Comment: Dr. Braverman runs the only practice in the state of New York that is fully staffed by qualified experts in the field of Reproductive Immunology. Accepted at the age of 14 into New York University, he was honored as their youngest graduate. He attended medical school at the Mount Sinai Medical Center in Manhattan and went on to complete his internship at The Albert Einstein School of Medicine in New York.

From website: "If immune issues are diagnosed we prescribe additional therapy. We do not want our patients to go through the cycle of repetitive IVF failures without quickly diagnosing and treating the underlying causes.
Voted #1 fertility clinic four years in a row."

CNY Fertility
195 Intrepid Lane,
Syracuse, NY 13205

Also at:
38A Old Sparrowbush Road
Latham, NY 12110

2244 East Avenue
Rochester, NY 14610
www.cnyfertility.com

Center comment: "This center provides state-of-the-art fertility treatments for the most difficult IVF cases and incorporate customized immunological treatment for all patients. Reproductive immunology is an important part of their treatment for recurrent pregnancy loss, unsuccessful IVF attempts and unexplained infertility. We have been offering Intralipid therapy since 2009."

Center for Human Reproduction,
Norbert Gleicher, M.D.
21 E. 69th Street,
New York, NY 10021,
www.centerforhumanreprod.com

From website: "We take on the toughest infertility cases. At CHR, because autoimmunity plays a significant role in female fertility, we test a range of autoimmune markers to screen women for clinical and subclinical autoimmunity."

Sher Institute for Reproductive Medicine,
Drew Tortoriello, M.D.
Jeff Wang, M.D.
425 Fifth Ave., 3rd Floor
(5th Ave. & 38th St.)
New York, NY, 10016

Also at:
1126 Park Ave, New York, NY 10128
www.haveababy.com

- 466 -

RESOURCES

Patient comment: "*Dr Tortoriello spent over an hour on the phone with me discussing my case and even offered to work with my local RE. I had previously undiagnosed partial DQ Alpha and had been trying to conceive for 3 years. We ended up doing two IVFs with Dr. T and now I am 18.5 weeks preg-nant with a singleton. He is very caring and compassionate for his patients and tailors protocols based on history and response. They also treat with intralipid.*"

From website: "*Dr Jeff Wang has a special interest in unexplained infertility, recurrent miscarriages, and repeated implantation failure following IVF.*"

North Carolina

UNC Fertility,
Stephen Young, M.D.
7920 ACC Blvd.,
Suite 300,
Raleigh, NC 27617
https://uncfertility.com

Comment: "*Dr. Young has served as President of the Reproductive Immunology Special Interest Group and is currently Vice-Chair of the Endometriosis Special Interest Group of the American Society for Reproductive Medicine.*"

Oregon

The Fertility Center of Oregon,
Douglas Austin, M.D.
590 Country Club Road, Ste A,
Eugene, OR 97401,
www.womenscare.com

Center comment: "*We test for immune issues in recurrent loss. There are many known causes that account for pregnancy loss including... immunological defects and blood clotting abnormalities. Correction of abnormalities significantly increases the possibility of a successful pregnancy.*"

Pennsylvania

ARC Fertility,
Scott Kauma, M.D.
4815 Liberty Ave, Pittsburgh, PA 15224
www.arcfertility.com

Comment: Dr. Kauma has served as clinical section editor for the Journal of Reproductive Immunology and on the editorial boards for the Journal of Reproductive Immunology.

- 467 -

Rhode Island

The Providence Fertility Center
49 Seekonk Street,
Providence, Rhode Island 02906
www.bostonivf.com

Doctor comment: "Boston IVF uses evidence based guidelines as the basis for treatment and collaborate with colleagues in related and unrelated fields of medicine as dictated by the needs of our patients, including autoimmune and blood clotting problems."

Women and Infants Hospital of Rhode Island,
Surendra Sharma, M.D.
Professor of Pediatrics,
101 Dudley St, Providence, RI 02905
Phone: (401) 274 1100

Comment: "Dr. Sharma's research focuses on the biology of pregnancy complications with emphasis on immunobiology, predictive and diagnostic biomarkers, inflammation and vascular pathogenesis. He is co-chair of The American Society for Reproductive Immunology."

South Carolina

Coastal Fertility Specialists,
Heather Cook, M.D.
1375 Hospital Drive,
Mount Pleasant, SC 29464
www.coastalfertilityspecialists.com

Patient comment: "This doctor is open to the idea of immunotherapy being useful in cases of unexplained reproductive failure."

South Dakota

CNY Fertility Center
(Satellite Location)
677 Cathedral Drive, Rapid City, SD
www.winfertility.com

From website: "This center provides state-of-the-art fertility treatments for the most difficult IVF cases and incorporate customized immunological treatment for all patients. Reproductive immunology is an important part of their treatment for recurrent pregnancy loss, unsuccessful IVF attempts, and unexplained infertility."

RESOURCES

Tennessee

Fertility Associates of Memphis
80 Humphreys Center, Suite 307,
Memphis, TN 38120
www.fertilitymemphis.com

Comment: This center offers tests for immune issues for recurrent miscarriage.

Texas

Houston Fertility Institute,
Jason Griffith, M.D.
2500 Fondren, Suite 300
Houston, Texas 77063
www.hfi-ivf.com

Texas Center for Reproductive Health,
Samuel Marynick, M.D.
3600 Gaston Ave, Dallas, TX 75246
https://ivfandfertility.com

Comment: Dr. Marynick is the medical director for The Texas Center for Reproductive Health. He is an active member of the American Society for Reproductive Immunology.

Austin Fertility Institute,
Kenneth K. Moghadam, M.D.
2200 Park Bend Dr Bldg 1 Suite 402,
Austin, TX 78758
www.austinfertilityinstitute.com

From website: "Similar to the thought process behind administration of antibiotics, the use of steroids (prednisone, dexamethasone, or methyl-prednis-olone) around the time of embryo transfer may reduce inflammation at the site of implantation."

Cohen Center Dallas' Advanced Women's Healthcare Institute,
Brian Cohen M.D.
7777 Forest Lane,
Dallas, TX 75230
www.briancohenmd.com

From website: "Our center tests for immunological disorders, when the medical and familial history indicate, include anti-phospholipid antibodies, lupus anti-coagulant, anti-nuclear antibodies, anti-thyroid antibodies, rheumatoid factor, natural killer cells, embryo toxic antibodies, factor V leiden and sticky platelets."

IVF Institute,
Noel Peng, M.D.
7777 Forest Ln Ste C108,
Dallas, TX 75230
www.dallasinfertilitymd.com

- 469 -

RESOURCES

Patient comment: *"Provides testing for immunological causes of infertility and recurrent miscarriage."*

Fertility Center of Dallas,
Michael Putman, M.D.
3900 Junius St #610,
Dallas, TX 75246,
https://fertilitycenterofdallas.com

Patient comment: *"He does some immune testing and says he uses Dr. Carolyn Coulam as R.I.. He prescribes IVIG. He was familiar with ATA, APA, ANA and NK cells.*

Sher Institute for Reproductive Medicine of Dallas,
Walid A. Saleh, M.D.
Medical City Dallas Hospital,
7777 Forest Ln Suite C-638,
Dallas, TX 75230
www.haveababy.com/fertility-clinics/dallas

Comment: Sher Fertility Centers are internationally renowned for the identification and treatment of immunologic causes of infertility and recurrent miscarriage.

Utah

The Fertility Institutes
11762 South State Street, Suite 160,
Draper, UT 84020
www.fertility-docs.com

From website: *"We work closely with the country's leading immunology experts, and offer full laboratory testing that includes preparation for and administration of paternal leukocyte immunization, aspirin/heparin/prednisone protocols as well as a variety of cutting edge methods to both improve pregnancy outcome associated with advanced fertility procedures, as well as to prevent pregnancy loss from occurring."*

Virginia

Columbia Fertility Associates,
Rafat Abassi, M.D.
1005 North Glebe Road, Suite 470,
Arlington, VA 22201
www.columbiafertility.com

From website: *"Columbia Fertility Associates is one of a select group of ART centers in the nation which specializes in reproductive immunology."*

Washington D.C.

Columbia Fertility Associates,
Rafat A. Abbasi, M.D.
Preston C. Sacks, M.D.
2440 M Street NW, Suite 401
Washington, DC 20037
www.columbiafertility.com

Wisconsin

Wisconsin Fertility Institute,
David L. Olive, M.D.
3146 Deming Way,
Middleton, WI 53562
http://wisconsinfertility.com

Comment: Dr Olive has extensive knowledge in the field of reproductive immunology.

University of Wisconsin School of Medicine,
Aleksandar Stanic-Kostic, M.D.
Generations Fertility Care,
365 Deming Way,
Madison, WI 53562
www.obgyn.wisc.edu

From website: Dr. Stanic is an assistant professor in the Department of Obstetrics and Gynecology divisions of Reproductive Endocrinology and Infertility and Reproductive Sciences. He has a PhD in Immunology andspecializes in female infertility, recurrent pregnancy loss and reproductive immunology research.

Note: If you operate, work or attend a fertility center in the U.S.A that provides immune testing and immune therapy for infertility and recurrent loss, or if you wish to amend any of the information here, please contact jkantecki@gmail.com to be listed in the next re-print of this publication.

- 471 -

RESOURCES

International Centers with Access to Reproductive Immunology

Argentina

Fertility Argentina,
Demian Glujovsky, M.D.
Viamonte 1432,
Buenos Aires, Argentina
www.fertilityargentina.com

Comment: Collaborates with other fertility centers in the US and Canada.

IVI Buenos Aires
Av. del Libertador 5.962,
C1428ARP Ciudad Autónoma de Buenos Aires
https://ivi-fertility.com/clinics

Australia

Atef Saba, M.D.
Fertility and Pregnancy Specialist,
31 Arnisdale Rd, Duncraig,
WA 6023, Australia
www.gynae-clinic.com.au

From website: "When the immune system is the cause of miscarriage, the chances of the mother having a successful pregnancy after 3 miscarriages without treatment such as intralipid or/and intravenous immunoglobulin (IVIG) is 30%, after 4 miscarriages 25% and after 5 only 5%. With the proper treatment, the overall success is 80%."

Lyn Burmeister M.D.
Level 8, Suite 8.1,
89 Bridge Road,
Richmond 3121, Victoria
www.drlynnburmeister.com.au

Patient comment: "She will test for NK cells and prescribe prednisone if required. You don't have to do IVF to see her. She takes every precaution and covers all bases. She gave me prescription for Clexane, prednisone and progesterone."

Professor Gamal Matthias
Reproductive Immunologist,
Sydney Reproductive Immunology,
Obstetrics & Gynaecology,
83 Gallipoli St, Bankstown NSW 2200
Tel: (02) 9791 6057

Patient comment: "Dr Matthias trained with Dr Beer. He is not linked with IVF which means he can concentrate on immune issues to help you become pregnant naturally and avoid further losses and expense with failed IVF cycles. He is also an obstetrician so

- 472 -

can monitor you through pregnancy. He does a thorough endometrial biopsy and sends bloods to Chicago. He offers IVIG, intralipids and LIT."

Gavin Sacks M.D.
Suite 1601, Westfield Tower 2,
101 Grafton Street,
Bondi Junction,
NSW 2022

Also at:
Level 3, St George Private Hospital,
1 South Street,
Kogarah,
NSW 2217
www.ivf.com.au

From website: *"We work in association with Dr Braverman in New York. "Under carefully controlled conditions, blood samples are rapidly transported overseas to a specialised laboratory in Boston, USA. They are analysed and the results are presented to Dr Braverman's Reproductive Immunology team in New York, USA. Their detailed interpretation is sent back to Dr Sacks in Australia for guidance in planning immune therapy for IVF cycles or pregnancy management."*

Repromed Fertility Specialists,
Professor Kelton Tremellen,
180 Fullarton Road Dulwich,
South Australia 5065

Centers also at: Mawson Lakes, Darwin and Clovelly Park
http://repromed.com.au

Comment: *"Dr Tremellen completed a PhD in reproductive immunology at the University of Adelaide in 1999. The focus of his studies was on why some women's immune systems "reject" their baby, leading to miscarriage and IVF failure. As such, Dr Tremellen has a keen clinical interest in investigation and management of recurrent miscarriage and IVF failure."*

Azerbaijan

Paul Armstrong, M.D.
The Caspian International Hospital and XMSK,
Baku, Azerbaijan

Tel: ++994 (0) 5198 04485
email: parmstrong365@gmail.com

Comment: *"Previously at The Portland Hospital in London. He is a strong advocate of immune testing and related treatments. He has particular expertise in the area of repeated miscarriage."*

RESOURCES

Barbados

Barbados Fertility Center
Seaston House,
Hastings, Christ Church,
Barbados
http://barbadosivf.com

From website: *"Barbados Fertility Center has been treating women for many years and is one of the leaders of Reproductive Immunology practice within the IVF field."*

Belgium

Centrum voor Reproductieve Geneeskunde (CRG)
UZ Brussel,
Laarbeeklaan 101 - B- 1090,
Brussels, Belgium
www.brusselsivf.be

Brazil

Ginecologia e Obstetrícia Imunologia da Reprodução Medicina Fetal,
Ricardo Barini M.D.
R. Antônio Lapa, 280 - Cambuí,
Campinas - SP, 13025-240, Brazil
http://www.barini.med.br

Comment: *"Dr Barini trained with Dr Beer."*

IVI Clinic Salvador
Avenida Paulo VI, 868,
41810-001 Salvador de Bahía
https://ivi-fertility.com/clinics

Canada

Astra Fertility Group,
Essam Michael, M.D.
300 Main St. N.,
Brampton,
ON L6V 1P6

(6 locations in Ontario)
www.astrafertility.com

From website: *"One of the missed diagnoses for recurrent implantation failure and recurrent early pregnancy loss is an underlying female immune system disorder... To try and identify the cause of recurrent pregnancy loss, genetic testing for both partners, sperm testing, evaluation for clotting and immune disorders is performed."*

- 474 -

RESOURCES

Victoria Fertility Centre,
Stephen Hudson, M.D.
#207 - 4400 Chatterton Way,
Victoria,
BC V8X 5J2
www.victoriafertility.com

Comment: "Provides full range of immune testing and all the latest treatments (including IVIG and intralipids) for unexplained infertility and IVF failure and pregnancy loss."

Carl Laskin, M.D.
Reproductive Immunology Specialist,
Trio Fertility,
655 Bay Street,
Toronto, Ontario

(6 locations in Ontario)
http://triofertility.com

Comment: Dr. Carl Laskin is an internationally recognized expert in the field of reproductive immunology and autoimmune diseases in pregnancy.

OriginElle Fertility Clinic & Women's Health Centre,
Seang Lin Tan, M.D.
2110 Decarie Blvd, Montreal,
QC H4A 3J3
https://originelle.com

Patient comment: "Immune educated, Dr Tan is a great fan of Dr Beer's work"

The Markham Fertility Centre,
Michael R. Virro, M.D.
379 Church Street, #5
Markham, Ontario,
ON L6B 1A1
www.markhamfertility.com

From website: "Over the years, Dr Virro's focus has been on identifying problems for couples with multiple IVF failures, specifically the… immunology of pregnancy, implantation and recurrent pregnancy loss. MFC treatment plans for immunology now include Intravenous Immunoglobulin (IVIG), intralipids (IL) and Leukocyte Immunization Therapy."

Chile

IVI Clinic Santiago de Chile
Avenida Alonso de Córdova, 5153, Local 103
Las Condes,
Santiago de Chile
https://ivi-fertility.com/clinic

China

Laboratory for Reproductive Immunology
Institute of Obstetrics and Gynecology,
Shanghai Medical College,
Fudan University, China
www.fudan.edu.cn

Reproductive Partners Medical Group
Beijing, China
北京市朝阳区东三环北路2号南银大厦1507
www.rpmgchina.com

Department of Gynaecology and Obstetrics,
Doctors Yan Zhang, Min Hu, Liu Liu,
Renmin Hospital of Wuhan University,
Wuhan, China
wsm70.whu.edu.cn

Institute of Biological Medicine,
Dr Xiao-Ling Cheng,
Wuhan University of Science and Technology,
Wuhan, Hubei, China

Department of Gynaecology and Obstetrics,
Dr Jing Cai,
Wuhan Medical and Health Care Center for Women and Children,
(Wuhan Children's Hospital Wuhan Women and Children Care Hospital),
China

Wuhan University of Science and Technology,
Dr Tao Wang, Medical School,
Wuhan, Hubei, China

Renji Hospital,
145 Shandong Middle Rd,
Huangpu Qu,
Shanghai Shi,
China, 200000
Phone: +86 21 5388 2125

Bernard Chan Clinic
Reproductive Immunologist,
Address16B Entertainment Building,
30 Queen's Road Central,
Hong Kong
Phone: 852 2849 4459

Dr Chan Tai Kwong
813 Medical Centre, 16/F, Central Building,
1-3 Pedder Street, Central,
Hong Kong
Phone: 2813 8823

RESOURCES

Hong Kong Reproductive Medicine Centre,
Dr Louis Chan,
Suite 1228-30, 12/F, Ocean Centre,
Tsim Sha Tsui, Hong Kong
http://www.reprodmed.com

Comment: "Works in collaboration with Dr Braverman in New York."

Colombia

CECOLFES,
Elkin Lucena, M.D.
Calle 102 No. 15-15,
Aparta Aereo 56769,
Santafe de Bogota, Colombia
Phone: 011-571-6101569

Asociados en Reproduccion Humana,
Jeanette Cubillos M.D.
Calle 134 no.13-83 Piso 7 Edificio El Bosque,
Bogota, DC, Colombia
http://asociadosenreproduccion.com

Comment: "Student/colleague of Dr Beer."

Cyprus

Pedieos IVF Center,
K.M. Trokoudes M.D.
8 Karaoli and Byron Avenue Corner,
"ANEMOMYLOS" Bldg.
Suite 201, Nicosia, 1095
email: trokoude@spidernet.com.cy

Doctor comment: "We offer the LIT treatment. Three weeks after the last LIT we do the LAD test to check effect."

Czech Republic

Genetika Plzeň, s.r.o. Ltd.
Parková 1254/11a ,
Plzeň, Černice
Czech Republic
www.genetika-plzen.cz/reproductive-immunology
www.ulcovagallova.cz

From website: "Erudition in gynaecology and obstetrics with immunology fully respects the complex neuroendocrine-immune relationships among couples with impaired

- 477 -

RESOURCES

fertility and provides more options for a comprehensive view of diagnosis and mainly of adjustment and the method of the existing therapy."

Denmark

Fertility Clinic 4071,
Ole B. Christiansen,
Rigshospitalet,
Blegdamsvej 9,
DK-2100 Copenhagen, Denmark
email: obchr@post5.tele.dk

Also at:
Clinic for Recurrent Pregnancy Loss and Reproductive Immunology,
c/o Clinic for Gynaecology by Elisabeth Carlsen
Jægersborg Alle 19, 3. sal
DK-2920 Charlottenlund • Denmark
http://www.pregnancyloss.dk.

Patient comment: "He is a miscarriage specialist and also into immune problems, but he is not as far along as Dr Beer. He prescribes IVIG, LIT and prednisolone mostly."

Dubai

Roya Medical Center,
Jumeirah 1, Al Wasl Road, Villa 198-A,
Dubai, UAE
https://royamedicalcenter.com/reproductive-immunology

Comment: "Royal Medical Center represents Braverman IVF & Reproductive Immunology. We treat the simplest to the most complex cases of infertility."

Bourn Hall Fertility Clinic,
Al Hudaiba Awards Buildings,
Block C, 7th Floor,
Jumeirah,
P.O. Box 113931,
Dubai, UAE
www.bournhall-clinic.ae

From website: "At Bourn Hall Fertility Clinic, we perform Reproductive Immunology. If an immune system abnormality is identified, treatment may be given in the form of steroid tablets, or with infusions of Intralipid, which is a mixture of fats and soya based protein, given intravenously. This may increase the chance of a successful pregnancy occurring in appropriate cases."

Egypt

Ganin Fertility Center,
Hosam Zaki, M.D.

RESOURCES

Salam Maadi Tower Beside As Salam Hospital,
Maadi Nile Cornish Cairo Egypt
www.ganin.com

From website: "When it comes to pregnancy; the immune system believes an embryo to be foreign matter. The immune system will attack the embryo, or the systems supporting it, and cause failure of implantation or a miscarriage."

Patient comment: "Provides testing for immune problems and immunotherapy. They also have a center in Illinois."

France

Hôpital Pierre Rouquès Les Bluets,
Dr Natalie Ledee,
4 Rue Lasson, 75571 PARIS CEDEX 12,
Tél. 0153364100
www.bluets.org

Comment: "Dr Nathalie Lédée is investigating the immune responses impli-cated in embryo implantation, the major factors limiting successful birth. She is working to provide personalized treatments to enhance fertility and the likelihood of a successful birth."

Germany

Dr C. Kling
Reproductive Immunologist,
Labor Fenner, Hamburg,
Germany
email: kling@immunologie.uni-kiel.de

Dr med Sylke Rechel-Fentz
Reproductive Immunologist,
Remlingstrasse 4,
D-67480 Edenkoben
www.immu-kinderwunsch.de

From website: "Our aim is to make doctors and patients aware of the topic of reproductive immunological issues. We can advise you also concomitantly to help achieve successful fertility treatment or in pregnancy. In addition to the "routine laboratory diagnostics", we also offer special examinations, such as DNA fragmentation in sperm, investigation of the activity of immunologically important cell populations or the determination of KIR and epitope types."

Wolfgang Würfel, M.D.
Weiterbildungen: Reproduktionsmedizin,
Kinderwunsch Centrum München Med. Versorgungszentrum
MVZ (Medizinisches Versorgungszentrum)
Ärzte dieses MVZ (13)
Lortzingstr. 26, 81241 München

RESOURCES

www.kinderwunsch-centrum-muenchen.de/ivf
Comment: Prof. Würfel works in the field of reproductive medicine, focusing on reproductive immunology and reproductive genetics. See his video: www.excemed.org/resources/role-immunologic-testing-after-failed-ivf-0.

Doctor comment: "It is high time that the extensive findings of reproductive immunology also find acceptance and wider consideration in reproductive medicine and obstetrics."

Dr Ingo Pfeiffer
Kölner Landstraße 205,
40591 Düsseldorf, Germany
Phone: +49 211 222444

Patient comment: "He prescribed Intralipid and performed the transfusion too."

Georgia

Chachava Clinic Reproductive Health Center,
Keti Gotsiridze, M.D.
Kostava Street. 38,
Tbilisi, Georgia
www.placidway.com
Greece

Ovum IVF,
Dr. Emanuel Economou,
383 L. Andrea Syggrou,
Athens, 17464 Greece
www.ovum-ivf.com

Serum IVF
Reproductive Immunology Centre,
Evinu 8,
Athens, Greece,
P.C. 11527
www.ivfserum.com

From website: "Studies continue to demonstrate that the complex communication between the implanting embryo and the mother's immune system is critical for pregnancy to succeed. Issues which cause miscarriages or repeat chemical pregnancies may also lead to recurrent implantation failure when they occur at the start of pregnancy. In these cases we make a thorough investigation of uterine, sperm, infection and where possible, genetic problems, but we will also try to find and address any immunological or blood clotting problems."

Lifeclinic IVF Clinic,
Dr Dimitris Papanikolaou,
166 Ippokratous Street,
Athens, TK 114 71
www.lifeclinic.gr

- 480 -

RESOURCES

Comment: "Life Clinic is led by Dr Dimitris Papanikolaou, a fertility special-ist, who until recently practiced reproductive medicine in two of the most successful fertility clinics in London. He has a special interest in immunological disorders in conception and recurrent miscarriages in early pregnancy."

Patient comment: "Called up this new clinic in Athens where the medical director is an ex-ARGC doctor. He said he will be conducting monitored cycles in much the same vein as the ARGC at obviously a cheaper price."

Lakentro Fertility Center,
Dr. Nikos Prapas,
Dr. Yannis Prapas,
4 Ag. Vasiliou St.
Postal Code: 54 250,
Thessaloniki
www.iakentro.com

From website: "Affiliated with Braverman IVF and Reproductive Immunology. Dr. Prapas and Dr. Prapas coordinate and perform all procedures at their state of the art facilities while the team at BRI offers diagnoses and treatments of immune related pregnancy complications. Patients from all over Europe have easy access to blood draws and have the ability to have medications ordered through their affiliation of doctors throughout Europe."

India

The Fertility Institutes (India)
Tel: 1-818-728-4600
www.fertility-docs.com

Website: "We work closely with the country's leading immunology experts, and offer full laboratory testing that includes preparation for and administration of paternal leukocyte immunization, aspirin/heparin/prednisone protocols as well as a variety of cutting edge methods to both improve pregnancy outcome associated with advanced fertility procedures, as well as to prevent pregnancy loss from occurring."

Juhi Fertility Center,
Dr Nirmala Agrawal,
10-5 -17, Masab Tank,
Hyderabad-500028
www.drnirmala.com

Patient comment. "Tests for immune problems and performs LIT."

Moolchand Fertility & IVF
Lajpat Nagar III (Near Moolchand Metro Station),
New Delhi, Delhi 110024, India
www.moolchandfertility.com

From website: "Our Reproductive Immunology Programme helps couples globally with recurrent IVF/ICSI failures and recurrent miscarriage. We test for Anti-Phospholipid Antibodies (APA), Anti-Cardiolipin Antibodies (ACA), Natural Killer Cells, Anti-Ovarian Antibodies (AOA), Anti-Sperm Antibodies (ASA), Lupus Anticoagulant

- 481 -

RESOURCES

(LAC), Anti-Nuclear Antibodies Screen (ANA), Anti-Microsomal Antibodies, Leukocyte Antibody Detection (LAD), HLA DQ ALPHA and BETA Embryo Toxic Factor (ETF), Sperm Penetration Assay (SPA), Acrosome Reaction (MCP, CD46), Chromosome Analysis, CD 3, CD 19, CD 16, CD 56 and TNF Alpha."

Dr Reita Ghosh
Reproductive Immunologist,
Double Helix, Plot No 6,
Vardhman Royal Plaza,
Gujranwala Town, Delhi 110009
www.doublehelix.co.in

From website: "Double Helix is a knowledge based laboratory where its scientific team is constantly abreast with the new advancements in reproductive immunology and is prompt to procreate the study which thus converts the scientific discovery into meaningful application."

Dr Raut's Women's Hospital,
Recurrent Miscarriage Specialists,
Karltopon Apartment,
Kalina Village Road,
Vakola, Santacruz East,
Mumbai, Maharashtra 400055, India
www.drraut.com

From website: "Immunological Reactions during pregnancy can play very important part in the causation of recurrent spontaneous abortion. Active Immunotherapy (Husband Lymphocyte Injection) can help to prevent RSA. Active Immunotherapy can be useful to reduce miscarriage rates in ART."

Indonesia

Universitas Indonesia Indonesia University,
Dr Ichramsjah A. Rahman,
Kampus UI Depok 16424, Indonesia
www.obgynfkuirscm.com

Patient comment: "Prof. Ichramsjah Rahman supports similar ideas about the connection between immune system and miscarriages as Dr Beer. Just like protocols in this book I went through monthly IVIG therapy etc."

Israel

Dr Howard Carp
Reproductive Immunologist,
Professor of Obstetrics and Gynaecology,
Tel Aviv University
email: carp@netvision.net.il

Comment "Dr Carp is an an expert reproductive immunologist and edited the 2014 book, "Recurrent Pregnancy Loss: Causes, Controversies, and Treatment."

Italy

Studio Semprini,
Dr Augusto Enrico Semprini,
Via Carlo Crivelli, 20,
20122 Milan, Italy
www.studiosemprini.com

Comment: Dr Semprini was trained by Dr. Beer.

IVI Italy
Piano 1 Interno 2,
Largo Ildebrando Pizzetti, 1
00197 Roma
https://ivi-fertility.com/clinics

Japan

Koji Aoki, M.D.
Reproductive Immunologist,
Nagoya City Johsai Hospital,
4-1 Kitahata-cho, Nakamura-j/ku
Nagoya 453-0815 Japan

Also at:
Toranomon Hospital,
Department of Ob/Gyn,
2-2-2 Toranonmon, Minato-ku,
Tokyo 105-8470, Japan
www.toranomon.gr.jp

Patient comment: "Ask for the doctors specializing in recurrent m/c. They do LIT using a different protocol than Dr Beer: 4 injections every 2 weeks."

University of Tokyo Hospital
Obstetrics and Gynecology,
7-3-1 Hongo, Bunkyo-ku,
Tokyo 113-8655, Japan
www.h.u-tokyo.ac.jp

From website: "Patients with immunological problems and those with thrombotic tendencies can benefit from treatment including IVIG, prednisolone, aspirin and heparin."

Jikei University Hospital
Department of Obstetrics and Gynecology,
3-19-18 Nishi-Shinbashi, Minato-ku,
Tokyo 105-8471, Japan
www.jikei.ac.jp.e.jd.hp.transer.com

RESOURCES

From website: "We perform anticoagulant therapy with aspirin-heparin and with husband lymphocyte, according to the condition of a patient for case to recurrent miscarriage and stillbirth, and the success rate is approximately 80%."

School of Medicine Niigata University
Department of Obstetrics and Gynecology,
1-757, Asahimachi-dori,
Niigata, 951-8510, Japan
www.med.niigata-u.ac.jp

Mexico

The Fertility Institutes
Guadalajara, Mexico,
Calzada Lázaro Cárdenas 4149,
Cuarto Piso, Esquina Av. Nino Obrero,
Jardín de San Ignacio, CP 45040,
Zapopan, Jalisco, México
www.fertility-docs.com

From website: "We offer complete couple tissue type compatibility testing through our association with a leading immunology laboratory. We work closely with the country's leading immunology experts, and offer full laboratory testing that includes preparation for and administration of paternal leukocyte immunization, aspirin/heparin/prednisone protocols as well as a variety of cutting edge methods to both improve pregnancy outcome associated with advanced fertility procedures, as well as to prevent pregnancy loss from occurring."

Instituto Vida,
Dr Garza Morales,
Alhelíes 51, Jardín,
87330 Matamoros,
Tamps., Mexico
www.institutovida.com

Comment: They have been using LIT since 1997.

Medica Fertil,
Dr Raphael Sanchez,
Colonia Alameda,
Calle Morelia 405,
Celaya, GTO 38050, Mexico
www.medicafertil.mx

IVI Anzures
11590 Colonia Nueva Anzures,
Delegación Miguel Hidalgo,
México D.F.
https://ivi-fertility.com/clinics

RESOURCES

Panama

IVI Panama
Calle 50 y 57 Obarrio (frente Seguros ASSA)
Ciudad de Panamá
https://ivi-fertility.com/clinics

Peru

Instituto de Ginecologia y Reproduccion,
Dr. Fabrizio Vizcarra,
Av. Manuel Olguín 1045,
Urb. El Derby,
Monterrico, Surco,
Lima, Perú
www.fabriziovizcarra.com

Philippines

Reproductive Immunology Centre,
Eduardo Lim, M.D.
Address1814 Medical Plaza Amorsolo Corner Dela Rosa St,
Makati City (near Manila)
Philippines 1229
Phone: 632 752 5254

Patient comment: "Dr Eduardo Lim trained with Dr Beer and follows his practices closely. The results from Eduardo Lim's clinic regarding LIT are very good so it is well worth the flight and the trouble. Performs both LIT and IVIG".

Center for Advanced Reproductive Medicine and Infertility (CARMI),
Cesar Joseph C. Gloria M.D.
Ground Floor, Medical Arts Building,
St. Luke's Medical Center-Global City,
32nd St. Bonifacio Global City,
Taguig City, Metro Manila 1112 Philippines
www.stlukescarmi.com

From website: "Our REI specialists are supported by experts from the related specialties who provide the required services on demand. Cesar Joseph C. Gloria had his residency in Internal Medicine at the State University of New York and pursued his fellowship in Allergy and Immunology in the same institution. He is board-certified with the Philippine Specialty Board of Internal Medicine, the Philippine Society of Allergy/Immunology, the American Board of Internal Medicine, and the American Board of Allergy and Immunology."

- 485 -

RESOURCES

Portugal

IVI Portugal,
H 1- 9ª, Avenida Infante Dom Henrique 333,
1800-282 Lisboa, Portugal

Also at:
Urbanização Casal de Gambelas,
Montenegro,
8005-226 Faro
https://ivi.pt/clinicas/lisboa

Russia

Center for Immunology & Reproduction,
Kashirskoye shosse 34a,
Moscow, Russia
www.cironline.ru

Saudi Arabia

Mouwasat Care Fertility,
Dr Elsamawal El Hakim,
Mouwasat Hospital Dammam
http://www.mouwasat.com

Comment: "Dr Elsamawal El Hakim specializes in male infertility, reproductive immunology and recurrent implantation failure. He previously worked as a Consultant in Reproductive Medicine at the ARGC UK."

Slovakia

GYN-FIV a.s.
Záhradnícka ulica č. 42
821 08 Bratislava
http://www.gyn-fiv.sk

From website: "Our Centre actively started to collaborate in the field of Reproductive Immunology with MUDr. Katarína Bergendiová, PhD. from the "ImunoVital" Centre in Bratislava and with MUDr. Dzurillová from the "Medicentre Dzurilla" in Nitra."

Singapore

Professor PC Wong
Head of the Department of Obstetrics & Gynaecology,
Yong Loo Lin School of Medicine,
National University of Singapore,
1E Kent Ridge Road Singapore,

Singapore 119228
www.nusmedicine.nus.edu.sg

Also at:
National University Hospital,
Emerald Clinic (Level 4),
Kent Ridge Wing,
5 Lower Kent Ridge Road,
Singapore 119074
www.nuhgynae.com.sg

Comment: "Professor Wong is extremely open-minded and incredibly helpful and willing to consult with reproductive immunologists in the United States."

Dr Sheila Vasoo
Reproductive Immunologist and Recurrent Miscarriage Specialist,
Mount Elizabeth Novena Specialist Centre,
38 Irrawaddy Rd, Singapore 329563
www.mountelizabeth.com

South Africa

Vitalab,
159 Rivonia Road, Morningside,
Johannesburg, South Africa
www.vitalab.com

Medfem Fertility Clinic,
Peter Place & Nursery Lane,
Bryanston, Sandton,
2060, South Africa
www.medfem.co.za

HART Cape Town Fertility Clinic,
Dr Klaus Wiswedel,
Christiaan Barnard Memorial Hospital,
Cape Town, South Africa
www.hartfertilitycapetown.co.za

Spain

Instituto Bernabeu Benidorm S.L.
Reproductive Immunology Unit,
Vía Emilio Ortuño, 21, 03501,
Benidorm, Spain
www.institutobernabeu.com

Centers also at: Madrid, Cartagena, Albacete, Elche and Alicante

RESOURCES

From website: "96% of our patients achieve a pregnancy over three courses of treatment. Europe's first ever pregnancy guarantee with 100% refund in case of unsuccessful result."

Diana Alecsandru, M.D.
Reproductive Immunogist,
IVI-RMA Global,
Avenida del talgo, 68
28023 Madrid
ivi.es/clinicas/madrid

Centers also at: Coruna, Malaga, San Sebastian, Pontevedra, Barcelona, Mallorca, Albacete, Bilbao, Santander, Zaragoza, Alicante, Valencia, Tenerife, Murcia and Valladolid

Dra. Amparo Oliver
Reproductive Immunologist,
Reproducción Asistida ORG,
Calle Profesor Beltrán Baguena 5,
Planta 7, Oficina 9
46009 Valencia, Spain
www.reproduccionasistida.org

Doctor comment: "The medical specialty of reproductive immunology can diagnose early autoimmune disease or signs of defects in immune regulation and thereby establish effective treatment options to achieve the goal of a healthy child."

Switzerland

Dr Hans-Rudolf Linder
Spitalgasse 36, 3011 Bern,
Switzerland
www.bernfamilie.ch

Patient comment: "I worked with Dr Rudolf Linder in Bern who was very open minded and supported all my treatments (IVIG, humira etc). I ended up having three live births under his care after a major struggle with secondary infertility and many chemical pregnancies."

Taiwan

Kohsiung Veteran's General Hospital,
No. 386, Dazhong 1st Road,
Zuoying District, Kaohsiung City,
Taiwan 813
www.vghks.gov.tw

Patient comment: "Performs LIT"

RESOURCES

Kuo So-nan Women's Hospital,
9-F, No. 21, sec. 2, Chunghsin Road,
Sanchung City, Taipei County,
Taiwan, R.O.C.
Phone: 886-2-29719511

Patient comment: "Performs LIT"

Turkey

Fertijin,
Dr Shafak and Dr Fevzi,
Nispetiye Avenue,
Bebek Yokusu Ramp,
Bebekdagi Street,
Istanbul, 34337, Turkey
www.fertijin.com.tr

*Patient comm*ent: "They do LIT. I believe Dr Shafak studied in America and therefore knows English."

Halit Firat Erden, M.D.
Obstetrician/Gynecologist,
Levazım Mahallesi,
Koru Sok. Zorlu Center No 2,
34340 Beşiktaş/İstanbul, Turkey
Phone: +90 533 191 11 11

United Kingdom

The Lister Fertility Clinic,
Dr Yau Thum,
Chelsea Bridge Rd,
London SW1W 8RH, UK
www.ivf.org.uk

From website: "If you have been counseled with regard to reproductive immunology testing and chosen to have the test performed, the results will inform us as to whether there may be an immune factor that may be affecting implant-tation."

Reproductive Health Group
Daresbury Park, Daresbury,
Cheshire, WA4 4GE
www.reproductivehealthgroup.co.uk

Comment: "Provides a full immune work up plus a full range of treatments for patients with unexplained infertility and recurrent loss. Testing of the immune system is also undertaken in the following cases: where there is a history of immune disorders, history of thyroid disease, or a previous pregnancy with placenta related complications such as pre-eclampsia, premature delivery or fetal growth restriction."

RESOURCES

Sims IVF Dublin
Clonskeagh Road,
Clonskeagh, D14 A312
www.sims.ie

From website: "We test whether you have antibodies that might hamper the conception and pregnancy process. We also test for Natural Killer (NK) cells, NK T-cells and general maternal cytokine profiles which are mediated by CD4 positive T-cells, all of which might have been overstimulated at some point. In vitro investigations employed at Sims IVF over the past 8 years reveal that intralipids have the ability to suppress NK cytotoxicity above and beyond that of IVIG, the previous agent employed."

Care Fertility
Beacon Court,
Sandyford,
Dublin 18
www.beaconcarefertility.ie

From website: "We can give you special tests which can identify if you are at risk of immune problems. These tests measure Natural Killer Cell activity."

The Priory Fertility Center
Priory Rd, Edgbaston,
B5 7UG, UK
www.bmihealthcare.co.uk

IVI Midland
3rd Floor Centre House,
Court Parade, Aldridge,
West Midlands,
WS9 8LT
www.midlandfertility.com

Comment: Fully onboard with all aspects of reproductive immunology for couples where pregnancy failure evades the normal parameters of diagnosis.

Glasgow Centre for Reproductive Medicine
21 Fifty Pitches Way,
Cardonald Business Park,
Glasgow, G51 4FD, UK
www.gcrm.co.uk

From website: "We offer corticosteroids, intralipids and clexane to selected patients with immune issues that underlie their infertility or recurrent miscarriage"

The Fertility & Gynaecology Academy,
Dr Amin Gorgy,
57a Wimpole Street,
London W1G 8YP,
www.fertility-academy.co.uk

From website: "The late Dr Alan E. Beer is widely credited to be a pioneer in the field of reproductive immunology. He believed it is not simply due to bad luck that some

- 490 -

RESOURCES

women fail to conceive or have repeated miscarriage. At The Fertility & Gynaecology Academy we have the experience to minimise recurrent miscarriage and IVF failure by investigating the immune system and offering immune therapy tailored to your individual situation. For an in-depth look at reproductive immunology we would recommend 'Is Your Body Baby Friendly?: Unexplained Infertility, Miscarriage and IVF Failure, Explained,' by Dr Alan E. Beer."

Centre for Reproductive Medicine Wales (CRMW),
Dr Amanda O'Leary,
Ely Meadows,
Rhodfa Marics,
Llantrisant, CF72 8XL
www.crgw.co.uk

Patient comment: "This clinic does various immune testing and treatments. They have worked very hard with me to avoid miscarrying again. They offer intralipid and other types of immune therapies."

Zita West Clinic,
Dr George Ndukwe,
37 Manchester St, London,
W1U 7LJ, United Kingdom
www.zitawest.com

Patient comment: "Dr Ndukwe trained with Alan Beer and is very familiar with reproductive immunology. He uses intralipid for IVF and is open to other immunotherapies. He also works with Zita West, an acupuncture and natural medicine specialist."

From website: "Pregnancy is the only situation where something completely foreign is allowed to stay in the body without being rejected. If something goes wrong with this immune mechanism, successful implantation could be hindered. That is why at the Zita West Clinic, we carry out tests to ensure that the woman has no immunological problems that could otherwise prevent a successful embryo implantation."

CARE Fertility,
Dr Adel Shaker,
Consultant Gynaecologist and Medical Director,
24-26 Glen Road,
Sheffield S7 1RA, UK
www.carefertility.com

From website: "We are now running the Reproductive Immunology (RI) programme. RI helps couples who have previously had recurrent IVF/ICSI treatment failures or recurrent miscarriages linked to abnormality in the woman's immune system, achieve a live birth."

Dr Hassan Shehata,
Recurrent Miscarriage Specialist,
New Life Clinic, 2 The Parade,
Epsom, Surrey,
KT18 5DH
www.miscarriageclinic.co.uk

RESOURCES

From website: "New scientific research that enables us to establish a link between recurrent miscarriage and the abnormal behaviour of the mother's immune system. We can do the diagnostic tests here in our clinic, and if the results are positive we can also offer you an extremely effective, safe and inexpensive treatment, after which the chances of a positive pregnancy outcome are increased to 80%. Treatments for infertility and recurrent miscarriage include Humira, Granulocyte-Colony Stimulating Factor, Prednisone and intralipid infusion."

Assisted Reproduction and Gynaecology Centre (ARGC),
Dr Mohammed Taranissi,
13 Upper Wimpole Street,
London, W1G 6LP, UK

Also at:
4420 Nash Court,
Oxford Business Park South,
Oxon, OX4 2RU
www.argc.co.uk

From website: "We were one of the first clinics in the UK to investigate the recurrent implantation failure of embryos and the immunology of implantation. This enables us to identify and offer treatment to couples suspected of suffering from this type of infertility. Our statistics from fresh IVF & ICSI cycles:

Age Groups	< 35 yrs	35-37 yrs	38-39 yrs	40-42 yrs
ARGC	80.2%	68.3%	50.0%	47.0%
UK Average	35.6%	31.9%	24.9%	18.5%"

Reproductive Health Group
Daresbury Park, Daresbury,
Cheshire, WA4 4GE
www.reproductivehealthgroup.co.uk

Also located at Manchester, Preston and London

From website: "Testing of the immune system is often undertaken in the following cases:
• Recurrent miscarriage (usually classed as 3 instances)
• Repeated failure of IVF (usually classed as 3 failed embryo transfers)
• Unexplained difficulties trying to achieve a pregnancy
• History of immune disorders
• History of thyroid disease
• Previous pregnancies where there have been placenta related complications such as pre-eclampsia, premature delivery or fetal growth restriction"

BMI The Blackheath Hospital,
Dr Christopher Steer,
Chelsfield Park Hospital,
Bucks Cross Road,
Chelsfield, Kent,
BR6 7RG, UK
www.infertilityinformation.co.uk

RESOURCES

The Lister Hospital Assisted Conception Unit,
Dr Yau Thum,
Chelsea Bridge Road,
London, SW1W 8RH, UK
www.thelisterhospital.com

Patient comment: "Dr Shehata and Dr Thum have published some research papers together on NK cells. Dr Thum is very knowledgeable on reproductive immunology and can help you overcome your fertility or miscarriage problem."

The Women's Natural Health Practice,
Dr Trevor Wing,
The Glasshouse,
River Lane, Richmond,
Surrey, TW10 7AG
www.womensnaturalhealthclinic.com

Comment: "This center has produced a very informative fact sheet about reproductive immunology and failed IVF:
www.naturalgynae.com/downloads/nav6_fact25.pdf

Venezuela

Centro Valenciano de Fertilidad y Esterilidad,
Antonio Sanoja, M.D.
Urb. La Viña. Calle Carabobo c/c Av. Carabobo.
Valencia, Edo. Carabobo, Venezuela
http://cevalfes.com.ve

Note: If you operate, work or attend a fertility center outside of the U.S.A that provides immune testing and immune therapy for infertility and recurrent loss, or if you wish to amend any of the information here, please contact jkantecki@gmail.com to be listed in the next re-print of this publication.

RESOURCES

Reproductive Immunology Laboratories

Rosalind Franklin University Clinical Immunology Laboratory,
3333 Green Bay Road,
North Chicago,
Illinois 60064
Phone: (847) 578-3444

MILab
246 E. Janata Blvd., Suite 260,
Lombard, Illinois 60148
U.S.A.
http://www.milab.us/index.html

ReproSource
300 Tradecenter Drive #6540,
Woburn, Massachusetts 01801
U.S.A.
http://reprosource.com

Reproductive Immunology Centre
Immunology Department
St Helier Hospital
Wrythe Lane, Carshalton
Surrey SM5 1AA, U.K.
http://www.ri-centre.co.uk

Journals and Societies

American Society for Reproductive Immunology (ASRI)
http://theasri.org

American Society for Reproductive Medicine (ASRM)
http://www.asrm.org

International Council on Infertility Information Dissemination (INCIID)
P.O. Box 6836
Arlington, Virginia 22206
U.S.A.
http://www.inciid.org

International Society for Immunology of Reproduction
http://www.isir.org.in/isir.htm

Journal of Reproductive Immunology
https://www.journals.elsevier.com/journal-of-reproductive-immunology

American Journal of Reproductive Immunology
https://onlinelibrary.wiley.com/journal/16000897

- 494 -

Articles about Reproductive Immunology

"Immunology May Be Key to Pregnancy Loss" (updated)
by Carolyn B. Coulam M.D. and Nancy Hemenway
http://inciid.org/immunology-key-to-pregnancy-loss-and-implantation-failure

"Shared Journey"
Reproductive Immunology page
http://www.sharedjourney.com/imm.html

"Intravenous Immunoglobulin for Treatment of Recurrent Pregnancy Loss"
Dr Coulam's controlled trial
https://www.ncbi.nlm.nih.gov/pubmed/8607936

Reproductive Immunology Discussion Sites:

INCIID Multiple Miscarriage/ Immune Issues discussion board
Moderated by Dr Carolyn Coulam
http://www.inciid.org/forum/forumdisplay.php?175-Miscarriage-Multiple-Miscarriage-and-or-Immune-Issues

Reproductive Immunology Resources
https://www.immunologysupport.com

Patient-to-Patient Support Sites:

Reproductive Immunology Support Group
Moderated by Jane Reed
https://groups.yahoo.com/neo/groups/immunologysupport/info

Alan E. Beer Medical Center Facebook page
https://www.facebook.com/BeerMedicalCenter

Fertile Thoughts Immune Issues board
http://www.fertilethoughts.com/forums/immune-issues

Fertility Friends Investigations and Immunology board
British community forum
http://www.fertilityfriends.co.uk/forum/index.php?board=52.0

Bub Hub: Reproductive Immunology forum
Australian community forum
https://www.bubhub.com.au/community/forums/forumdisplay.php?873-Reproductive-Immunology

- 495 -

RESOURCES

INDEX

INDEX

A

abortion, spontaneous. *See* miscarriage

aching joints. *See* joint pains

activated protein C resistance, 75, 333-334, 459

acne, 100, 118

acupuncture
electro-, 295,298
for fertility, xvi, 298-299, 442

adaptive immune response. *See* immune system

Addison's disease, 112, 446

age
effect on eggs, 130-134, 380-384
effect on fertility, 129-130, 378, 380

Alan E. Beer Medical Center for Reproductive Immunology 144, 156, 231
clinic address, 456
Facebook page, 497
future of the program, xii, 307

alcohol, 42, 100, 288, 290
inflammatory effect of, 286
TNF-alpha and, 430

allergens, 72, 102-103
definition of, 446

allergies, 102, 103, 237
definition of, 446
to heparin, 168

allergic sensitization, 102

alloimmunity, 63, 446

alopecia areata
and ANAs, 81, 388
and APAs, 71, 331
and premature ovarian failure, 112
definition of, 446

Alzheimer's disease, 119

American College of Obstetricians & Gynecologists (ACOG)
views on testing, xxviii, 45,
views on treatments, xxx, 40, 315

American Society for Reproductive Immunology (ASRI)
Antiphospholipid Antibody Committee of, 70
Dr Beer as a founder of, xii
Dr Clark, as President of, 191
views on reproductive immunology, 188, 190, 227, 318, 329, 408, 410

amniocentesis, 137

amniotic fluid
high cytokine levels in, 311, 344, 354
low levels of, 66, 136, 137, 158
meconium stained, 138

anatomical problems

cervical, 29, 30, 31, 48, 136, 311
uterine, iii, 29, 31, 45

anaphylaxis
as a Th2 allergic response, 102
definition of, 446

anemia, 66, 174

aneuploidy, 132, 133
definition of, 446
See also chromosomal abnormalities

antibiotics,
as a dietary contaminant, 276, 282
causing candida overgrowth, 99
immune calming effect of, 54, 99, 471

antibodies (immunoglobulins)
against hormones
overview of, 34-36, 42, 53-59, 107-128
to estrogen, 109, 362
to HCG, 111, 248, 363, 364
to progesterone, 32, 110, 362, 364
against neurotransmitters
low serotonin levels and, 106, 120, 126, 377
migraines and, 123
Raynaud's Syndrome and, 81, 124, 126, 127, 375-376
tests for, 44, 45
definition of, 446
See also antinuclear antibodies, antiphospholipid antibodies, antisperm antibodies, antithyroid antibodies, *and* blocking antibodies

anticoagulant therapy
arguments for use as a miscarriage treatment, 211, 212, 227
heparin, low molecular weight (Clexane, Fragmin, Arixtra) 169-170, 393, 394
heparin, regular molecular weight (Multiparin), 168, 393
personal experiences with, xix, xx, 237, 238, 241, 247, 250, 252, 253, 257
See also heparin

antidepressants. *See* selective serotonin reuptake inhibitors (SSRIs)

antigens. *See under* immune system

antinuclear antibodies
overview of, 79-81
debate over significance of, 195-197
definition of, 446
pathological evidence of, 156
testing for, 149, 196, 320, 336-339
treatments for, 165, 209, 227

antiovarian antibodies, 112, 113, 151, 361, 365, 371, 385, 402

antioxidants, 289, 292-294, 297, 434, 437, 440
See also flavonoids

antiphospholipid antibodies
anticardiolipin, 67, 71-72, 149-150

INDEX

anti-ethanolamine, 67, 68, 149-150, 159, 327, 330
 arguments for significance of, 192-194, 211, 329
 overview of, 68-73, 96, 107, 123
 definition of, 446
 testing for, 45, 136, 149-150, 155, 320, 327-333, 337-338
 treatments for, 161, 169-171, 208, 210, 393-394
antisperm antibodies
 arguments for significance of, 197-198, 320-321
 overview of, 83-85
 testing for, 44, 150
antithyroid antibodies
 data on, 314, 336, 348-349, 365, 401-402
 overview of, 32, 92-94, 96, 152, 158
 treatment for, 161, 194
 See also thyroid disease
anti-TNF therapy
 data supporting the use of, 383, 395-397
 Enbrel, Humira and Simponi, 172-174
 effect on success rates, 213, 214
 for endometriosis patients, 96-97
 healing effect on eggs, 133-134, 172-173
 opposition to the use of, 212
anxiety. *See* stress
apoptosis, 51, 212, 232, 345, 347, 363, 382, 392
 definition of, 447
APS. *See* Antiphospholipid Syndrome
aspartame, 275, 427-428
aspirin, 166, 170-171
 positive effect on pregnancy success rates, 196, 208-212, 390, 392, 393, 394
ASRI. *See* American Society for Reproductive Immunology
asthma, 100
 allergies and, 102-103, 110
 as a reaction to anticoagulants, 170
attention deficit disorder
 prevalence of, 139, 384, 385
 relationship to autoimmunity 139, 384 385
 risks from food additives, 275
toxic exposure and, 272, 426
autism, vii, 139
autoantibodies. *See* antibodies
autoimmune disease,
 association with reproductive failure, vii, 34, 40, 57-59, 68, 70, 79-81, 88,

192, 196, 208, 209, 313-315, 319-321, 329, 337, 338, 346, 349
 bacteria as an aggravator of, 97-100
 definition of, 447
 depression and, 120-122, 371-373
 diabetes and, 115-117
 diet and, 283, 288-294
 dioxins and, 264
 EMF radiation and, 270
 family history of, 71-72, 96, 385
 genetic risks for, 55, 318
 leptins and, 283
 obesity and, 113-115
 pesticides and, 267, 419
 solvents and, 269, 421
 tests for, 146-156
 women and, 92-96, 109, 139-141, 318

B

B cells, 30
 See also immune system
bacterial infection
 antiphospholipid antibodies and, 72
 antisperm antibodies and, 83
 autoimmunity and, 32-33, 55, 57, 68, 98, 126, 140, 338
 candida, 32, 99-100, 355-356
 chlamydia, 98,99,355
 gum disease, 32, 311
 gonorrhea, 99, 355
 pelvic inflammatory disease and, 97-101
 pre-term delivery and, 98, 354
 stillbirth and, 42
 tests for, 43, 44, 158, 173
Billingham, Dr Rupert
 as co-discoverer of LIT, 223, 224, 229
 timing of his death, 304
 studies, 167, 267, 393, 417
birth defects
 cleft palate/lip, 167, 267, 393, 417
 clubfoot, 269
 deafness, 269
 Down's syndrome, 30, 132, 242
 heart defects, 269
 neural tube defects (e.g., spina bifida), 77, 94, 137, 335, 350, 398
 toxins and, 269, 421
 See also chromosomal abnormalities *and* toxins, environmental
birth control pills
 risk factor for thrombosis, 72, 331
blastocyst
 adhesion to endometrium, 211
 definition of, 447
 development of, 61-62

- 499 -

INDEX

TNF blockers and development of, 174, 397
bleeding in pregnancy, 48, 90, 121, 373
  at implantation, 154
  See also subchorionic hemorrhage, *and* placental abruption
blighted ovum
  association with immune problems, 47, 147
  definition of, 447
  personal experiences with, 242, 254
blocking antibodies
  arguments for significance of, 200, 203, 230, 307
  overview of, 63-64
  definition of, 435
  LIT to boost low levels of, 163-164, 227, 324-325
  measurement of, 146, 158
blood clotting problems. *See* thrombophilia
blood pressure (high)
  dexamethasone and, 167
  EMF exposure and, 247, 426
  Graves disease and, 449
  HELLP syndrome and, 66, 72, 449
  hyperthyroidism and, 93
  obesity and, 113
  polycystic ovary syndrome and, 117, 118
  preeclampsia, 58, 319, 448, 452
  pregnancy-induced hypertension, 41, 66, 72
  stillbirth and, 42
  TNF blockers and, 173
  Type 2 diabetes and, 116, 367
blood tests. *See* immune testing
blood thinners. *See* anticoagulant therapy *or* heparin
Braverman, Dr Jeffrey
  Foreword by, vii-viii
  Braverman IVF & Reproductive Immunology, 144, 475, 479, 480, 483
    address details, 456, 467- 468

C

C-reactive protein, 114, 118, 359, 368, 370, 371
  definition of, 447
C-section. *See* Cesarean section
caffeine
  dehydration and, 295
  in patient history, 42-43
miscarriage and low birth weight and, 42, 285
cancer

breast
  association with obesity, 113, 114
  prevalence of, 262
  cervical abnormalities and, 30, 31
  inflammation and, 31, 311
  See also dysplasia
childhood, 269, 272, 421, 424, 425
diet and, 283, 284, 287, 292, 293
estrogen and, 109
faulty DNA repair and, 132, 381, 382
immune defense against, iii, 34, 50, 87, 88
immunotherapy and risk of, 140
pregnancy treated as a form of, xvii, 26, 51, 62, 63, 87, 89, 91, 237, 322
stress and, 106, 360, 373
testicular, 83, 263
toxic exposure and, 31, 262, 264, 266, 267, 269, 271, 272, 424
candida, *See* bacterial infection
Cardiolipin molecules, 67, 150
  definition of, 447
  See also anticardiolipin *under* antiphospholipid antibodies
cardiovascular disease. *See* heart disease
CD designations, 52-53, 316, 317
  CD3+ (Pan T-cells), 90, 147, 163, 199, 317, 318
  CD4+ (T-helper cells), 53, 90, 116, 147, 317, 319, 323, 324, 342
  CD8+ (T-cytotoxic suppressors), 62, 90, 116, 147, 317, 319, 323
  CD19+/5+ (B-1 cells), 85, 92, 107, 108, 111, 120, 122, 124, 147, 148, 151, 158, 314, 320, 348
  CD56+ cells (NK cells), 48, 163, 198, 199, 200, 206, 207, 319, 330, 341, 342, 356
  See also natural killer cells
  CD56+/CD16+ (peripheral blood NK cells), 147, 158, 199, 319, 330, 341, 342, 343, 345, 347, 348
  CD56+/CD16-(uterine NK cells), 88-89, 104, 111, 237
  CD57 cells (NK-like cells), 87-89, 104, 111, 237
  CD200, 227
  definition of, 447
Celexa. *See* selective serotonin reuptake inhibitors
cervix
  abnormal anatomy of the, 30, 31
  abnormal cells in the, 101
  bacterial infection of the, 97, 98, 99
  inflammation of the, 95
  See also cervical *under* cancer
Cesarean section, 122, 290
chemical pregnancy, 147, 341, 401
See also implantation failure
chicken pox, 32, 72

- 500 -

INDEX

chlamydia
  as a cause of ectopic pregnancy, 33,
    312
  as a trigger for immune problems, 32,
    47, 98-99, 355
  prevalence of, 33, 312, 354, 355
chromosomal abnormalities
  and age, xxviii, 129, 186, 130, 310,
    132, 381
  definition of, 132
  diet and, 287
  incidence of, 30, 310
  incidence in eggs of older women,
    132, 381
  incidence in embryos, 38, 313
  incidence in stillborn babies, 42
  miscarriages caused by, 29-30, 40,
    310
  testing for, 137, 156
  toxic exposure and, 30, 132, 261,
    263, 265, 269, 285, 286, 412, 414,
    415, 420, 429
  trisomy, 132
  See also birth defects
chromosomal analysis, 22, 23, 121, 138,
    366-367
chromosomally normal loss, viii, xxv,
    38, 40, 64, 69, 129, 144-145, 188,
    200, 315, 316, 325, 378
chromosomes
  definition of, 447
  structure of, 132
chronic fatigue syndrome 47, 125-127,
    376, 378
  aspartame linked to, 275, 427
  bacterial infection linked to, 98, 103,
    354
  depression associated with, 120
  endometriosis associated with, 96,
352
  Epstein Barr virus and, 448
cigarettes. *See* smoking
Clark, Professor David,
  career profile, 190-191
  on recurrent miscarriage, 40
  on reproductive immunology,
    201, 204, 205, 216, 222
  on "tender loving care," 216-217
  on testing for antinuclear antibodies,
    195
  on testing for antiphospholipid
    antibodies, 192
  on testing for antithyroid antibodies,
    194
  on testing NK cell levels, 199
  on the Ober Trial, 228-231

studies by, 310, 313, 315, 323, 358, 359,
    360, 386, 387, 395, 400, 405, 408, 409
Clexane. *See* low molecular weight *under*
    heparin *or* anticoagulant therapy
CMV. *See* cytomegalovirus
coagulation disorders. *See* thrombophilia
cocaine and infertility, 285, 429
coffee
  dehydration and, 289-290
  effects on immune system, 285, 429
Cohen, Jon
  as writer and journalist, 229
  contacting the FDA about LIT,
    229-230, 409
congenital defects. *See* birth defects
connective tissue disease, 55-56, 81, 269, 453
contraceptive pills. *See* birth control pills
contraceptive vaccine, 111, 364
corticosteroids, 165-167
  dexamethasone, 166-167
  prednisone and prednisolone, 165-166
  safety of, 165, 391
  side effects of, 167, 393
  success rates with, 209-210, 165, 391
Coulam, Dr Carolyn
  career profile, 193
  clinic address, 458, 463
  IVIG trials, 499
  moderator of INCIID Immune Issues
    discussion board, 499
  on lymphocyte immunization therapy, 203,
    230
  on recurrent miscarriage, 40, 499
  on testing for APAs, 194
Cox, Courteney
  her antiphospholipid antibody treatment,
    72
cramping, 176
  after embryo transfer or intrauterine
    insemination, 92
  during implantation failure, 92
Crohn's disease, 105,-106, 320, 359, 360
  and antinuclear antibodies, 81
  and antiphospholipid antibodies, 35, 73
  and activated NK cells, 89
  and infections, 100, 356
  and premature ovarian failure, 114
  and vitamin D deficiency, 177
  as a Th1-driven condition, 55, 58, 456
cytokines,
  about, 36-37, 52-53
  pro-coagulatory effect of, 60, 118, 150
  T-helper 1 (Th1) class of, 55, 57, 60,
    81, 90-92, 98, 199-201
  T-helper 2 (Th2) class of, 56, 64, 106
  See also cytokine ratios, interferons,
    interleukins, tumor necrosis factor alpha
    (TNF-alpha)

- 501 -

INDEX

cytokine assay, 39, 136, 151
cytokine ratios (Th1:Th2)
    as a predictor of reproductive failure,
    53, 58, 62, 89, 214, 216, 318, 319-
    321, 326, 345, 349, 385
    egg damage caused by high Th1
    levels, 90, 133, 174
    importance of, 31-32, 35
    regulation of
        using anti-TNF therapy, 136,
        172-174, 397
        using corticosteroids, 165, 397
        using LIT, 164
        using IVIG, 158
cytomegalovirus (CMV), 32, 164

D

D&C. *See* dilation and curettage
deep-vein thrombosis
    pregnancy risk and, 72, 333
    prevention of, 170
    thrombophilia and, 65, 66, 75
dental amalgam fillings, 81, 340-341
depression
    antibodies to serotonin and, 120-122,
    148
    association with autoimmunity, 47,
    93, 94, 104-106, 113, 114, 125, 126,
    127, 351-353, 360-361, 373-376
    diet and, 126, 287, 291, 293, 379,
    287, 434, 437
    EMF radiation and, 274, 428
    personal experiences of, xiii, xxiii,
    246, 247, 248, 257, 258, 283
    See also antidepressants
DES. *See* diethylstilbestrol
DHA (docosahexaenoic acid)
    in fish oil, 293, 438
diabetes
    autoimmune disease association, 32,
    56, 112, 369-370
    candida and, 99
    dietary risk factors for, 275, 283,
    284, 286, 429
    gestational, 114, 140, 168, 368,
    stillbirth, as a result of, 42
    toxic exposure and, 266, 270, 272,
    277, 424
    treatments for, 175-176
    type 1, 53, 55, 71, 93
    type 2, 114, 115,-119, 127, 140
diet
    anti-inflammatory foods, 288-289,
    296, 297
        The Plant Paradox, Dr Gundry S,
        283, 289, 295

flavonoids (antioxidants), 292-294
    immune aggravating foods, 281-284, 286-
    288, 433
    omega-3 fatty acids, 283, 288, 291-292,
    433, 434-437
    organic (benefits of), 277, 288, 290, 291,
    294, 297, 433
    protein, recommended amount, 289, 434
diethylstilbestrol (DES)
    association with reproductive
    abnormalities, 31
    association with immune problems, 31,
    311
dilation and curettage (D&C)
    cervical problems and, 31, 311
    definition of, 447
    personal experiences of, 240, 242, 245,
    248, 251, 252
    procedure versus natural miscarriage, 153
dioxins. *See under* toxins, environmental
DNA (Deoxyribonucleic Acid)
    analysis of, 151, 155, 196
    antibodies to, 35, 63, 79-82, 108
    chromosomes, relationship to, 29
    damage to, 116, 117
    definition of, 436
    diet, effects on, 266
    egg damage and, 133, 381, 382
    EMF radiation and damage to, 274, 423,
    425, 426
    fragmentation of, 116, 368
    genes for autoimmunity and, 124
    toxic exposure and damage to, 132, 133,
    263, 292, 310, 382, 414, 416, 423
DNA, antibodies to. *See* antinuclear
    antibodies
DQ alpha antigens
    compatibility between partners, (genetic
    matching), 50, 51, 61-64, 91, 324
    definition of, 449
    See also human leukocyte antigens *under*
    immune system
Down syndrome
    chromosomal defects and, 132
    frequency in Dr Beer's patients, 113
    toxic exposure and, 265, 415
drugs
    medical. *See under* treatments
    recreational, 42, 43, 76, 285, 286, 292,
    367, 429, 430
DVT. *See* deep-vein thrombosis
dysplasia, 101, 356, 357
    See also cervical *under* cancer

INDEX

E

eclampsia
definition of, 448
See also preeclampsia
E. coli, 32, 42
ectopic pregnancy
association with pelvic inflammatory disease, 97-99, 312, 355
chlamydia and, 33
increasing incidence of, 97, 353-354
eczema
candida and, 100
as an allergy symptom, 102
as a symptom of allergy to progesterone, 110, 357
eggs
age and, 129-134, 380-382
damaged/poor quality, 35, 112, 285, 286
improving quality of, 162, 173, 211, 214, 284, 289, 290, 380-384, 394, 441
low number retrieved in IVF, 47, 108
eggs, donor
failure with, 38, 39, 94, 151, 352
success with immunotherapy and, 129, 379
Electro Magnetic Field (EMF) radiation, *See under* toxins, environmental
embryo
as "foreign" to immune system, iii, iv, xxi, xxviii, 26, 35, 50, 61- 63, 79-81, 84, 85, 235
delayed development/poor quality, vii, 35, 96, 133
damaged by aggressive immune activity, 26, 30, 35, 58, 69, 96, 98, 107-108, 148, 149, 345, 347, 354
incidence of chromosomal abnormalities, 30, 38, 129, 310, 313
poor development in pregnancy, 34, 37, 58
protective immune response to, 89, 110, 111, 121, 172, 372
Enbrel. *See under* anti-TNF therapy
endocrine disruption, 262-264, 272, 276, 312, 413, 414, 415, 418, 425, 426
endometrial biopsy
definition of, 43
in a standard infertility work-up, 43-45
endometrium and endometrial development. *See under* uterine lining
endometriosis
anti-TNF therapy for, 97, 214

association with antiphospholipid antibodies, 34, 71, 96, 331
association with autoimmunity, vii, 47, 95-97, 122, 350-353, 383
association with reproductive problems, 95-97
definition of, 447
diagnosis of, 43
diet and, 176, 283, 291, 399, 435
poor egg quality and, 134
prevalence of, 262, 413
toxic exposure and, 262, 264, 266, 414, 415, 416
treatments for, 171, 176, 214, 298, 353
environmental factors. *See* toxins, environmental
Environmental Working Group,
report on pesticides in produce, 276, 427
report on toxins in umbilical cord blood, 271, 424
eosinophils. *See under* immune system
EPA. *See* U.S. Environmental Protection Agency
Epstein Barr virus
activation of immune system and the, 32
definition of, 447
estrogen
and coagulation disorders, 72
antibodies to, 57, 109-148, 362
definition of, 447
immune activating effect of, 72, 90, 92, 110, 114, 115, 300, 347, 363
low levels of, 109, 112
obesity and, 114
"pro-growth" effect of, 57, 92, 109
toxic exposure and imbalance of, 262, 264, 266, 267, 272, 276, 413, 415-418
vitamin D treatment for lack of 176, 297, 399, 441
See also estrogen *under* antibodies against hormones

F

factor V Leiden mutation, 34, 45, 73, 74-75, 152, 332-334
personal experience of, xxi
fatigue
as a side effect of medications, 167, 173
as a symptom of immune activation, 47-48, 90, 96, 103-104
as a symptom of thyroid disease, 93-94
See also chronic fatigue syndrome
Faulk, Dr W Page, 62, 225, 322, 407
FDA (U.S.). *See* U.S. Food and Drug Administration.
Fertility doctors,

- 503 -

INDEX

centers offering reproductive immunology (RI), 457-495
percentage using RI, 181, 399
those skeptical of RI, 38, 105, 144, 160-163, 240, 246
fetal demise. *See* miscarriage *and* stillbirth
fetal distress,
at delivery, 254
immune activation associated with, 137, 138
fibroids
effects on implantation, 31, 43, 311
prevalence of, 262, 264, 413
toxic exposure and, 264, 414-415
fibromyalgia, 109-110, 361-364
as a predictor of immune problems in pregnancy, 47, 120, 125-126, 127, 352, 376-378
association with endometriosis, 96, 352
toxic exposure and, 275, 427
See also chronic fatigue syndrome
Finch University of Health Sciences
as Dr Beer's former clinic location, xx
renamed Rosalind Franklin University of Medicine and Science, xii, xxi, 230
See also Rosalind Franklin University Center for Women's Health
fish oil. *See* omega-3 fatty acids
flares. *See* immune flares
flavonoids. *See* antioxidants
"flu-like" symptoms
after embryo transfer, 90
at implantation, 90
high cytokines levels and, 103, 126
side effect of anti-TNF therapy, 173
side effect of IVIG, 160
Folgard RX 2.2. *See* FaBB under vitamin supplements
folic acid
MTHFR mutation and lack of, 335, 398-399
supplements, 175
personal experiences with, xii, 76, 237, 241
follicle-stimulating hormone (FSH)
definition of, 448
function of, 107-108, 130, 379
cycle day 3 levels and, 108, 130, 361, 379
low progesterone and, 32
regulation of, 119, 298, 379
follicular fluid
TNF-alpha in, 133, 371, 382-383

toxins in, 262, 267, 292, 413, 418, 437
Food & Drug Administration. *See* U.S. Food and Drug Administration
free radicals, 132, 292-293, 437

G

Gamimune and Gammagard. *See under* intravenous immunoglobulin,
"gender-bending" chemicals. *See* endocrine disruption
genes, 449
See also DNA
genetic analysis. *See* karyotyping
genetic matching between partners, (DQ alpha matching), 26, 153-154, 448
genetic mutations
germline vs. somatic, 132
for inherited thrombophilia
factor V Leiden, 74-75, 332-334
MTHFR, 76, 77, 151-152, 175, 332-334, 451
Prothrombin 20210, 76, 334
heterozygous vs. homozygous, 151, 321, 335
toxic exposure and, 132, 263, 287, 382, 414
genital warts. *See* dysplasia
German measles, 32
gestational sac
abnormal size or shape, 90
Gleicher, Dr Norbert
contact information, 456, 468
on disagreements between reproductive immunologists, 221, 407
on endometriosis, 350, 353
on reproductive autoimmune failure, 193, 208, 320, 337
Glucophage. *See* metformin
glycodelin A (PP14)
definition of, 449
relationship to insulin, 118, 119, 370, 398
relationship to NK cells, 117, 368, 370
gonorrhea
about, 99, 355
association with losses, 33, 312
association with pelvic inflammatory disease, 98
Graves' disease
about, 93-94, 348
association with infection, 93, 98, 349-350, 354
definition of, 449
See also hyperthyroidism *under* thyroid disease
group B Streptococci
and stillbirth, 42

- 504 -

INDEX

gum disease
  association with APAs, 72
  association with preterm birth, 32,
    286, 311
  association with delayed pregnancy,
    286, 431
Gundry, Dr Steven
  The Plant Paradox, 283, 295-296
  on lectins, 284, 429

H

Harvard Medical School
  aspirin research, 170, 394
  egg rejuvenation research, 131, 380
Hashimoto's thyroiditis
  as a form of hypothyroidism, 94, 380
  association with infection, 98, 354
  definition of, 449
  personal experiences with, 237, 240,
    247
  See also hypothyroidism *under*
thyroid disease
hay fever
  as a Th2 allergic response, 102
HCG (human chorionic gonadotrophin),
  antibodies to, 35-36, 107-108, 111,
    363-364
  definition of, 450
  low/slowly rising levels, 36, 90
headache
  as a side effect of anti-TNF-alpha
    therapy, 173
  as a side effect of intralipid, 161
  as a side effect of IVIG, 160
  as a side effect of Viagra, 1172
  as a side effect of vitamin D therapy,
    176
  as a symptom of immune activation,
    103, 122-123, 124, 125, 148, 295,
    374-376
  See also migraines
heart attack
  inherited thrombophilia and, 73
  relationship to APAs, 63, 73
  relationship to PCOS, 118
heart disease
  cortisol levels and, 300
  depression and, 121
  EMF exposure and, 270, 422
  homocysteine levels and, 77
  immune activity and, 32, 47
  insulin resistance and, 116, 397
  lectins and, 281-284
  mitral valve prolapse and, 122
  obesity and, 116

HELLP syndrome. *See under* blood pressure
hematoma. *See* subchorionic hemorrhage
Hemenway, Nancy, 39, 314, 497
heparin
  definition of, 452
  dietary supplements with, 295, 300
  low molecular weight, 172-173, 396-397
  regular molecular weight, 171, 396
    Multiparin, 168
  personal experiences with, xix, xx, 240,
    241, 243,, 244, 250, 253, 255, 256, 260
  used with aspirin, 170, 212
  used with IVIG, 197, 331
  used with LIT, 230, 329
hepatitis
  association with APAs, 72
  association with premature ovarian failure,
    112
  IVIG screening for, 158
  LIT screening for, 163, 204
herpes virus, 100-101, 356
  as an immune activator, 32
  association with stillbirth, 42
heterozygous
  definition, 151, 449
high blood pressure. *See* blood pressure
Hill III, Dr Joseph. 'Immunotherapy for
    Recurrent Pregnancy Loss: 'Standard of
    Care or Buyer Beware' 190, 229, 230, 409
  as outspoken critic of LIT, 190
HIV
  association with APAs, 72
  IVIG screening for, 158, 160
  LIT screening for, 163
hives
  allergy to progesterone and, 103, 110
  as a side effect of heparin, 170
  as a side effect of vitamin D overdose,
    176
  as an immunological warning sign, 100,
    102
  CD19+/CD5+ and, 148
  personal experience of, 254
HLA. *See* human leukocyte antigens
HLA-G, 62, 63, 322-323
holistic therapy, 105, 279-300
homocysteine
  and MTHFR, 76-78, 151, 334-336
  treatment to reduce levels of, 175
hormones
  associated with autoimmune disease and
reproductive failure, 32, 38, 44, 107-111
  "gender bending," 264, 266, 272, 276
  immune system and, 35, 55, 56, 57, 58, 90,
    103, 127-128, 148
  obesity and, 114-117
  premature ovarian failure and, 112-113

See also antibodies against hormones, estrogen, follicle-stimulating hormone (FSH), HCG (human chorionic gonado-tropin), luteinizing hormone (LH), progesterone, serotonin *and* testosterone

hot flashes
  antibodies to estrogen and, 109
  premature ovarian failure and, 113

Howard, Dr Vyvyan, 276, 427

Hughes, Dr Graham, 71

Hughes' Syndrome. *See* Antiphospholipid Syndrome

human chorionic gonadotropin. *See* HCG

human leukocyte antigens (HLA). *See under* immune system

human papilloma virus (HPV), 101, 356-357

Humira. *See under* anti-TNF therapy

hypersensitivity. *See* allergies

hypertension
  and blood clotting disorders, 66
  and diabetes, 116, 367-368
  and immune dysfunction, 72, 94, 106, 120
  See also blood pressure (high)

hyperthyroidism. *See under* thyroid disease *and* Grave's disease

hypothyroidism. *See under* thyroid disease *and* Hashimoto's disease

hysterosalpingography (HSG), 43

hysteroscopy, 43, 45

I

IBD. *See* inflammatory bowel disease

ICSI. *See* intracytoplasmic sperm injection

immune flares
  after delivery, 56
  and SLE, 80
  natural treatment for, 290
  personal experience of, 240

immune system
  adaptive response, 50-53
  antigens
    antibodies and, 50, 52, 54, 62, 69, 83, 104, 261
  B cells, 52-59
  eosinophils
    definition of, 448
    role of, 102-103
  general overview of the, 49-59
  human leukocyte antigens (HLA), definition of, 450

genetic influence of, 55
  HLA-G as a "non-classical" form of, 63-64, 322-325
  role in general immune response, 50, 55
  role in pregnancy, 62, 200-201, 225, 321-322, 411
  innate response, 50, 52, 102, 311

lymphocytes
  definition of, 451
  roles of, 52-53
  test for antibodies to, 63

major histocompatibility complex
  definition of, 449
  role of, 50-51, 201, 321
  T cells, 50-53, 90, 92, 105, 118, 126, 147
  T regulatory cells, 62-63, 323-324
  See also, Th1 and Th2 immune response

macrophages
  function of, 50-51, 53
  in autoimmunity, 55, 104, 111
  in pregnancy, 58, 62, 95, 96, 323

mast cells, 102, 347

monocytes, 90, 156
  definition of, 452

neutrophils
  as a type of granulocyte, 449, 450
  definition of, 452
  inflammatory response and, 55, 90, 104
  Neupogen to increase levels of, 162
  population of, 50
  See also antibodies, CD designa-tions, cytokines, cytokine ratios, lymphocytes, *and* natural killer cells

immune testing
  antinuclear antibody test, 149
  antiovarian antibody test, 151
  antisperm antibody test, 150
  antiphospholipid antibody test, 149-150
  indications for, 44-45, 47-48
  leukocyte antibody detection assay, 146
  lupus anticoagulant antibody test, 150
  MTHFR test, 152
  NK cell assay, 148
  reproductive immunophenotype, 146-152
  Th1:Th2 cytokine assay, 151
  tissue analysis, 152-156

immune treatments. *See* treatments

immunoglobulins, 54, 152, 158, 192
  definition of, 450
  See also antibodies *and* IVIG

implantation failure
  acupuncture to treat, 298
  antibodies to hormones and, 107-111, 127-128, 362-364
  antibodies to neurotransmitters and, 120-122, 125

INDEX

APAs and, 192-193, 328-329
endometriosis and, 95-97, 134, 352
gum disease and, 286
immune problems and, 26, 32, 34,
36, 38, 40, 51, 57-58, 80, 83, 84, 89,
90, 91, 92-94, 104, 153-154, 195-
197, 341-348, 357
incidence of, 38, 40, 313
IVF failure and, 37-39
personal experience of, xii, xxi, 328,
243
thrombophilia and, 65-70, 104, 124,
155-156, 326
toxic exposure and, 33, 429-430
treatments to help prevent, 157-177,
202-204, 206-208, 211-213, 385,
399, 407-410
uterine fibroids and, 31, 311
International Council on Infertility
Information Dissemination (INCIID)
address of, 496
Coulam and Hemenway article for,
39, 314, 497
discussion boards, 497
infection. *See* bacterial infection *or* viral
infection
infertility
age-related, 132-133
allergies and, 102-103
ANAs and, 79-81
antisperm antibodies and, 83-85
causes of, general, 29-36
causes of, immune, 25, 28, 35-36, 39,
51-56, 57-59, 61-64
diabetes and, 115-119
distress associated with, 37-38
endometriosis and, 95-97
IBS and, 102-104
infections and, 97-101
inherited blood clotting disorders
and, 73-78
obesity and, 113-115
rate of, 38
recurrent IVF failure and, 37-39
secondary, 47
stress and, 105-106
tests to determine cause of, 146-153
thyroid disease and, 92-94
toxic exposure and, 31-32, 33-34
"unexplained," 38, 47, 61, 143
See also implantation failure
inflammatory bowel disease, 98, 104,
354, 357-358
See also irritable bowel syndrome
insulin-resistance
as an indicator of the need for
immune testing, 26-27, 47, 55, 116
PCOS and, 117-119, 369, 371

personal experience of, 237
treatment for, 118-119, 174, 397-398
See also diabetes
intracytoplasmic sperm injection (ICSI), 35,
83, 84, 221
interferons, 51, 53
definition of, 450
interferon-gamma (IFN-gamma), 57,
58, 89, 151
interleukins
description of, 51
Th2 cells and, 54
TNF-alpha and, 57, 40
See also cytokines
Intralipid
definition of, 450
use, administration and side effects, 160-
161, 388-389
intrauterine growth retardation
as an indicator of the need for immune
testing, 34, 66, 135, 137, 158
immune problems and, 214
risk associated with corticosteroids, 166-
167
thrombophilia and, 66
treatment with IVIG for, 158-159
intrauterine insemination, 67
personal experiences with, 235, 237, 251
intravenous immunoglobulin G (IVIG), 157-
160, 386-389
definition of, 450
Gamimune and Gammagard, differences
between, 159, 160
indications for use of, 136, 205-209, 216,
227
personal experiences with, 236-238, 240-
241, 243-244, 247-249, 250, 251, 252-253,
257
preconception use, 139, 173
studies to show validity of treatment with,
391, 395-396, 405, 406
use with anti-TNFa drugs, 134, 213-214
use with corticosteroids, 165
use with heparin, 194
use with LIT, 64, 326
in vitro fertilization (IVF)
association with APAs in failed cycles, 34,
69, 72, 193-194, 329
becoming pregnant without, vii, 113, 143,
182
chromosomal causes of failure with, 30,
144, 310
conventional approach to repeated failure
with, 42-46
criticism of immunotherapy with, 229, 409
definition of, 450
failure after (a) live-born child (ren), 91

INDEX

multiple failed cycles of, 37-39, 42-43, 99, 103, 312-314
natural ways to increase success of, 279-300, 441-443
older women and, 129-134, 378-381
pointless cycles of, 25, 27, 144, 182
poor ovarian stimulation and, 108, 129, 379
success rates with immunotherapy, 91, 347
toxic exposure effect on success of, 266, 267, 286, 418, 429
See also, infertility *and* implantation failure
irritable bowel syndrome (IBS), 103-104
See also Crohn's disease
IVF. *See* in vitro fertilization
IVF doctor. *See* fertility doctor
IVIG. *See* intravenous immunoglobulin G

J

Johnson, Professor Peter, 164
joint pains
ANAs and, 81
antibodies to serotonin and, 120
as a side effect of TNF-alpha therapy, 173
as a symptom of TNF-alpha activity, 55, 56, 103, 127, 136
CD19+/CD5+ cells and, 148
CD57 cells and, 87
food additives and, 275, 284, 427
personal experience of, 254
Journal of Reproductive Immunology
Dr Beer as former Editor-in-Chief of, xii
Dr Coulam as Managing Editor of, 191
Professor Johnson as Editor-in Chief of, 186
website address of, 496

K

Kantecki, Julia
personal story, xiii-xxi
karyotyping
as part of work-up, 45
definition of, 450
See also chromosomal analysis *and* chromosomes
kidney problems, 32
HELLP syndrome and, 72
IVIG treatment and risk of, 160
preeclampsia and, 41

Knox, Professor John, 272
Kwak-Kim, Dr Joanne
as a leading figure in the field of RI, 144
as founder of The Society for Immunotherapy and Investigation, 230
clinic address, 456, 462
personal experience as a patient of, xvii, xix, xx, xxii
studies by, 216, 315, 317, 318, 325, 385, 387, 399, 406

L

labor and delivery
immune problems and, 41, 48, 121, 344, 354
pre-term, vii, 33, 48, 66, 121
risks associated with "natural" birth, 137-138
stillbirth during, 42, 316
Ladd, Virginia, 72
laparoscopy, 43, 193
lectins. See under toxins, food related
Lerner, Dr Henry, xxviii, 310
leukocytes, definition of, 450
leukocyte antibody detection assay (LAD). See *under* immune testing
Lexapro. *See* selective serotonin reuptake inhibitors
LH. *See* luteinizing hormone
LIT. *See* lymphocyte immunization therapy
Liverpool Women's Hospital, xxiv
low birthweight
caffeine and, 285, 429
Dr Beer's approach to help prevent, 135, 137, 138
immune problems and, 34, 89, 211, 214, 343-344
IVIG to help prevent, 89, 158, 344
omega-3 to help prevent, 291, 436
toxic exposure and, 33, 264, 269, 270, 312, 414, 422
lupus. *See* systemic lupus erythematosus (SLE)
lupus anticoagulant
relationship to APS, 71
testing for antibodies to, 150, 192, 193, 196, 209
luteal phase
definition of, 451
in normal menstrual cycle, 107-108
luteal phase defect
and antibodies to hormones, 36, 108
personal experience of, 255-256
luteinizing hormone
antibodies to, 108
definition of, 451

- 508 -

INDEX

function of, 107-108
similarity to HCG, 111, 364
lymphatic drainage, 295, 299, 442-443
lymphatic system, 35, 79, 80, 299
lymphocytes, definition of, 451
  See also under immune system
lymphocyte immunization therapy (LIT)
  and the flawed Recurrent Miscarriage
  Study, 202, 224-232
  as a treatment for reproductive
  failure, 65, 163-164, 200, 203, 204,
  208-209
  availability throughout the rest of the
  world, 226, 407-408, 164, 207
  blocking antibody response from, 63-
  65
  combined with IVIG, 64
  critics of, 229-230, 409
  definition of, 451
  development of, 223-224
  Dr Beer's pioneering research on, 63,
  307, 325-326, 224
  FDA suspension of, 164, 216, 229,
  230
  personal experiences with, 241, 247,
  248, 251, 252-253, 255,
  safety of, 104, 204-205, 390
  success in trials, 202-203, 404-405
  to treat HLA compatibility, 65
  See also blocking antibodies

M

macrophages
  role in immune response, 50, 53, 55,
  62, 111, 323
  role in pregnancy, 57-58
  See also leukocytes and monocytes
major histocompatibility complex. *See*
  under immune system
mast cells, 102, 358
Matthias, Professor Gamal,
  Foreword by, iv-vi
  clinic address, 475
Medawar, Sir Peter, 223
menopause
  estrogen deficiency and, 103
  premature, 103, 112-113
  symptoms of, 113, 130
menstrual cycle
  endometriosis, effect on the, 95
  heavy periods, 94, 114
  irregular cycles, 109, 113, 118, 130
  lighter periods, 93
  premenstrual syndrome (PMS), 104,
  111, 238

toxic exposure, effect on the, 226, 268,
  416-417, 420
mercury. *See under* toxins, environmental
metformin, 115, 174, 397-398
  side effects of, 174
  to reduce miscarriage rate in PCOS, 118-
  119, 370
migraines
  antibodies to hormones and
  neurotransmitters and, 110, 120, 122-126,
  127,, 374-375
  association with inherited thrombophilia,
  71, 78, 375
  depression and, 106, 374
  high TNF-alpha levels and, 136
  personal experience of, 254
  toxic exposure and, 275, 427
  treatments for, 136
miscarriage
  antiphospholipid antibodies and, 71-73,
  96, 192-193
  antibodies to hormones and
  neurotransmitters and, 107-128, 360-367,
  371-378
  blood clotting problems and, 34, 59, 65-
  68, 155-156
  chromosomal causes of, xxviii, 29-30
  conventional approach to diagnosis of, 29-
  34, 44-46
  infection and, 97-103, 286, 353-357, 431
  in older women, 129, 379-380
  low glycodelin levels and, 118-119
  obesity and, 114
  occurrence of, xxviii, xxix, 30, 40, 310
  stress and, 105-106
  toxic exposure and, 31, 264, 269, 270, 274,
  285, 286, 414, 415, 417, 421, 422
  recurrent (miscarriage), xi, 39-40, 314-316
    blood clotting problems and, 59, 65-70,
    74-78, 326-336
    critics of immune treatments for, xxx,
    181-182, 187, 189-217, 399, 410
    genetic compatibility and, 61-64, 79-
    80, 200-201, 321-326
    immune hyperactivation and, xi, 26,
    34-36, 47-48, 51, 55-56, 84-85, 90, 92-
    94, 103-104, 195-200, 316-321, 336-
    339, 367-371, 382-384, 410-411
    personal experiences with, 182, 183,
    238, 240, 242, 243, 244, 247-248, 250,
    251-253, 254-257
    testing for, 135-136, 143-154
    treatments for, 129, 157-179, 188, 385-
    399
    "unexplained," vii-viii, xxix
mitral valve prolapse, 122
molar pregnancy, 84
  personal experience with, 240

- 509 -

INDEX

monocytes, 90, 156, 452
Mowbray, Professor James
  LIT trial at St Mary's Hospital, 202, 204
  on value of LIT, 225-226, 228-229, 407, 410
MTHFR mutation (C677T)
  association with miscarriage, 77
  definition of, 451
  elevated homocysteine levels and, 76-77
  homozygous vs. heterozygous, 77, 451
  personal experience with, xviii, 237
  prevalence of, 77, 335-336
  risk of neural tube defects and, 77, 335
  testing for, 151
  treatments for, 175
Multiparin. *See* heparin, regular
  molecular weight
multiple sclerosis
  association with immune problems, 53, 71, 119
  definition of, 451
  viral association, 56
Myalgic Encephalomyelitis (ME), 125-126
  See also chronic fatigue syndrome (CFS)
Myasthenia Gravis
  association with premature ovarian failure, 55, 112
  definition of, 452
mycoplasma. *See under* bacterial infections

N

natural killer cells (NK cells)
  antibodies to hormones and, 32, 107-111, 112, 120, 122, 123, 125
  antinuclear antibodies (ANAs) and, 79-80, 337
  antiphospholipid antibodies and, 70, 211-212
  cancer, defense against and, 26, 51, 88, 91
  definition of, 452
  diet, effects on, 283, 291, 434
  Dr Beer's observations and studies on, xi, 26, 38, 45, 65, 85, 88, 89, 90, 91, 107, 136, 341-343, 344, 361, 403, 404
  endometriosis, abnormal decrease in, 96, 352

general overview of, 35, 51-52, 87-88, 341-347
infection and, 98-101, 355-357
pregnancy, beneficial effects of, 57-58, 62, 88-89, 323
pregnancy, harmful effects of, 65, 88-90
suppression of by glycodelin, 117, 368
testing for (blood tests), 39, 45, 136, 147-150
Th1 immune response and, 55-56, 79-81, 88, 198-200
thyroid disease and, 50, 92-96, 347-348
tissue type compatibility as an aggravator of, 62, 200-204
treatments to suppress, 157, 158-167, 172-174, 204-209, 212-214, 298, 386-393, 395-397, 406-407
uterine, 35, 88, 89, 342, 343
uterine CD57 "NK-like" cells, 87-88, 104, 111
See also CD56+ cells (NK cells) *under* CD designations
Ndukwe, Dr George
  acknowledgement from Dr Beer, 304
  clinic address, 493
Neupogen® (filgrastim)
  use with intralipid, 161
  use and administration 162-163
neural tube defects. *See under* birth defects
neurotransmitters: endorphins, enkaphlins and serotonin, 119, 121, 372
  definition of, 452
  See also antibodies against neurotrans-mitters *under* antibodies, *and* serotonin
neutrophils
  as a type of granulocyte, 449, 450
  inflammatory response and, 55, 90, 104
  population of, 50
night sweats
  antibodies to serotonin associated with, 113, 120, 127
  anti-TNF-alpha treatment and, 173
NK cells. *See* natural killer cells
Nutrasweet. *See* aspartame

O

Ober, Dr Carole
  as author of Recurrent Miscarriage Study on LIT, 202, 226-230, 408
  association with author of Cochrane review on LIT, 229, 409
obesity
  and autoimmune disease, 113-115
  and depression, 121-122
  and diabetes, 115-117
  and PCOS, 117-119

- 510 -

INDEX

and reproductive problems, 113-119, 365-369
and thrombophilia, 72, 76
and toxic exposure, 272, 281
obsessive-compulsive disorder, 139, 384
obsessive thinking, 106, 140
omega-3 fatty acids
    anticoagulant effect of, 291-292, 433-437
    as a component of intralipid, 160
    fish oil, 291-292, 433-437
    immunomodulatory effect of, 287-288, 291-292, 433, 434-437
    pregnancy benefits of, 291, 436
    TNF-alpha and, 291, 434-435
oocytes
    definition of, 452
    See also eggs
oral contraceptives. S*ee* birth control pills
organic diet. *See under* diet, organic
osteoarthritis, 114, 293, 439
ovulation
    autoimmune disease and, 112, 305
    changes associated with:
        anti-TNF-alpha drugs, 174
        endometriosis, 96
        hormone imbalance, 32, 107-108, 110, 112
        obesity, 98
        PCOS, 102
        environmental factors, 248, 259
    drugs to regulate, 174, 398
    in a normal cycle, 107-108
    See also poor ovarian stimulation and, *under* in vitro fertilization

P

PCOS. *See* polycystic ovary syndrome
pelvic inflammatory disease, 47, 97-98, 353-354
phospholipids
    function and structure of, 67
    See also antiphospholipid antibodies *and* Antiphospholipid Syndrome
placenta
    calcification of, xxi, 137, 384
    development of normal, 57-58, 61-62, 89, 110, 117, 322, 342, 362
    development of defective, 69-70, 84,121, 136-137, 324
    effect of blood clotting problems on, 65, 66, 68, 70, 90,124-125, 192, 211, 217

inflammatory immune response against, 26, 30, 41-42, 58, 62, 80, 136, 172, 192, 318, 319, 337
Neupogen for growth of, 162
pathology of, 85, 143, 145, 152-156
substances crossing:
    corticosteroids, 165, 166, 391
    environmental toxins, 35, 267, 268, 271, 273, 276
    heparin versus low molecular weight heparin, 169-170
    TNF blockers, 174
placental abruption
    cocaine and, 285, 429
    definition of, 453
    See also subchorionic hemorrhages
PMS. *See* premenstrual syndrome
POF. *See* premature ovarian failure
polycystic ovary syndrome (PCOS), 114, 117-119, 215, 369-371
    definition of, 453
    treatment of, 174, 397-398
preeclampsia
    as a Th1-driven condition, 89
    as a result of inflammatory immune activity, iv, vii, 48, 58, 114, 214, 319, 343-344
    aspirin and heparin to help prevent, 171, 211,-212, 394
    association with obesity, 114, 366
    definition of, 453
    depression and, 121, 373
    HELLP syndrome and, 72, 449
    omega-3 fatty acids to help prevent, 291
    prevalence of, 41-42
    thrombophilia and, 65-66, 155, 326-327
    thyroid problems and, 94
pregnancy
    as a privileged immune state, 54, 57-58
    "chemical," 147, 341, 401
    difficulty achieving. *See* infertility
    labor and delivery problems, 35, 41-42, 48
    58, 66, 121, 137, 138, 316
pregnancy complications
    caused by immune aggravation, 34-36, 40
    See also birth defects, bleeding in pregnancy, blood pressure (high), chromosomal abnormalities, eclampsia, ectopic pregnancy, fetal distress, gestational *under* diabetes, hypertension, intrauterine growth retardation, low birthweight, miscarriage, preeclampsia, premature delivery, preterm labor, stillbirth, *and* subchorionic hemorrhage
preimplantation genetic diagnosis, 38
premature delivery. *See* labor and delivery problems *under* pregnancy
premature ovarian failure (POF)

- 511 -

INDEX

as an immune-related condition, 112-113, 151, 191,-192, 364-365, 385
association with antibodies to hormones, 127, 361-362
definition of, 453
premenstrual syndrome
association with antibodies to hormones and neurotransmitters, 120, 127
personal experience with, 245
prevalence of, 262
progesterone
antibodies to, 35, 103, 110, 357, 362,-363
definition of, 453
function of, 32, 57, 107, 108, 109
low levels of, 118, 128, 176
protein C and S deficiency, 34, 66-67, 75-76, 326-327, 333, 334
prothrombin 20210 mutation, 76, 334
Prozac. *See* selective serotonin reuptake inhibitors
psoriasis
as Th-1 driven condition, 47, 55
omega-3 benefits for, 291, 435
pulmonary embolism, 66, 72, 331

Q

quadruple screen testing, 140, 387
Quinlan, Annette, xxiv

R

rashes
as side effect of anti-TNF-alpha therapy, 154
as a side effect of intralipid, 164
as a side effect of LIT, 167
as a side effect of vitamin D overdose, 176
as a warning sign in pregnancy, 139
See also hives
Raynaud's syndrome, 47, 124-125, 375-376
ANAs and, 81
antibodies to hormones and neurotransmitters and, 126, 127
treatment for, 125, 376
recurrent miscarriage. *See* recurrent *under* miscarriage
Recurrent Miscarriage Study, 202-206, 392-393
Reed, Jane
acknowledgements by, 305
acknowlegement from Dr Beer, 303-304

as founder of the Yahoo Reproductive Immunology Support Group, xxiii, 497
data collected by, 64, 77, 325-326
personal story, 254-257
published studies by, 206, 213, 344, 353, 383, 394, 395, 396
Regan, Professor Lesley
as a "debunker of immune theories," 190
as an author of the RCOG 2003 Guidelines, 189, 310
on aspirin in IVF, 210
on Dr Joseph Hill, 229, 409
on LIT, 201-202
on "tender loving care," 212, 215
on testing for NK cell levels, 198-199
on treatment for recurrent miscarriage, xxx, 185, 186
on unexplained recurrent miscarriage, 181
personal experience of, 244
studies by, 315, 332, 333, 394, 400, 403, 406
Reiter's disease, 98, 354
definition of, 453
Reproductive Autoimmune Failure Syndrome, 70, 79, 196, 337
See also Gleicher, Dr Norbert
Reproductive Immunology Support Group. *See* Yahoo Reproductive Immunology Support Group
reproductive immunophenotype, 58, 146, 319, 347, 371
definition of, 453
retarded fetal growth. *See* intrauterine growth retardation
Rh blood type incompatibility, 42, 223
definition of, 453
rheumatoid arthritis
ANAs and 79
as a Th-1 driven condition, 53, 56
blood clotting problems and, 34,71
CD57 cells and, 87
decaffeinated coffee as an aggravator of, 285
estrogen-dominance and, 110, 363
lectins and, 284
obesity and, 114
omega-3 EFAs, for relief of symptoms of, 291, 435
remission of symptoms in pregnancy, 139
treatment with anti-TNF-alpha therapy, 172-173
thyroid antibodies and, 92-93
toxic exposure and, 269
treatment with IVIG, 157-158
unregulated activity of NK cells in, 55
rheumatoid factor
association with reproductive failure, 47, 196, 209

INDEX

definition of, 453
Ritalin, 139
Rodgers, Professor Ray, 131, 380, 381
Rosalind Franklin University Center for
Women's Health, xvii
    laboratory address, 196
    normal reference ranges from, 152
    success rates at after LIT suspension,
    230
Royal College of Obstetricians and
    Gynaecologists (RCOG)
    2003 Opinion Paper statements, 185-
    189
    opinions on miscarriage treatment,
    xxx, 310, 189, 400
    testing recommendations, 45

S

saline sonogram, 43
salmonella, 32
Sanow, Chris
    acknowlegement from Dr Beer, 303
Scher, Dr Jonathan
    as author of the book *Preventing
    Miscarriage: The Good News,* 240,
    241, 255
Sher Institute for Reproductive
Medicine, 144, 191
    clinic addresses, 456, 462, 465, 468,
    472
    use of intralipid, 161
    See also, Sher Dr Geoffrey
scleroderma
    ANAs, association with, 81
    APAs, association with, 71
    definition of, 453
    Raynaud's syndrome, association
    with, 124, 338, 376
Scott, Dr Jim
    as author of the Cochrane review on
    LIT, 202, 229, 409
secondary infertility. *See under*
    infertility
selective serotonin reuptake inhibitors
    (SSRIs): Celexa, Zoloft, Prozac,
    Lexapro, etc.
    how they work, 122
serotonin
    CFS, fibromyalgia and, 125-126, 377
    definition of, 453
    depression and, 120
    effect on blood vessels and uterine
    lining, 58, 119-120, 121, 372, 374
    effect on implantation, 121, 372
    influence of diet on levels of, 287,
    289, 431, 434

migraines and, 122-123
obesity and, 121-122
Raynaud's syndrome and, 124-125
sensitivity to stress and, 105, 106, 121,
    358, 373
symptoms of low levels in reproduction,
    121-122
tests that indicate low levels of, 128, 148
TNF-alpha and its relationship to, 105,
    123, 358, 372
treatments to increase levels of, 122, 123,
    125, 375, 376
See also antibodies against
    neurotransmitters *under* antibodies, *and*
    selective serotonin reuptake inhibitors
Shehata, Dr Hassan, xxv, 114
Sher, Dr Geoffrey
    as the medical director of SIRM, 144
    IVIG study by, 161, 194, 212
    views on reproductive immunology, 182,
    212
    studies by, 323, 330, 393, 395
Sher Institute of Reproductive Medicine
    (SIRM)
    clinic addresses, 456, 462, 465, 466, 468,
    472, 493,
sleep disorders, 106
    antibodies to neurotransmitters and, 81,
    120, 125, 127
Sjögren's syndrome
    ANAs, association with, 81, 337
    APAs, association with, 71
    bacterial infection and, 98
    definition of, 453
smoking
    as a cause of reproductive aging, 285, 286,
    429-430
    free radical production and, 292
    increased risk of miscarriage and, 42
    inflammatory effect of, 285, 430
    thrombophilia, risk factor for, 72, 76
sperm
    absence of live/abnormal, 83, 150, 261,
    263, 264
    low counts of, 85, 263, 264, 266, 267, 268,
    272, 285, 286, 339, 414, 415, 418, 419,
    431
    molar pregnancy and, 84
    ways to improve the quality of, 289, 290,
    291
    vasectomy reversal, effects on, 85, 339
    See also antisperm antibodies *under*
    antibodies, *and* intracytoplasmic sperm
    injection
SSRIs. *See* selective serotonin reuptake
    inhibitors
steroids. *See* corticosteroids
St. Mary's Hospital London, xxx, 189

- 513 -

PCOS study from, 216, 406
personal experience of from a former
nurse, 244
Professor Mowbray's LIT research
at, 202, 204, 225
Professor Regan's APA study at, 216
Professor Regan's NK study at, 198-
199, 403
stillbirth
causes of, 41-42
frequency of, 41, 316
inflammatory immune response and,
58, 104, 138, 287, 358, 431
preeclampsia and, 58
studies on, 316-317
thrombophilia and, 66
toxic exposure and, 267, 417-418
Strachan, Gillian, xxiv-xxv
stress
associated with:
autoimmunity, 104, 105-106, 121,
122, 124, 358-360
cortisol levels, 285, 300, 443
herpes, 100-101
IVF failure, 37-38, 312-313
mind-body therapy to help relieve,
217, 299-300, 443
reproductive problems, 42-43, 105-
106
thrombophilia, 76, 77, 106, 335
Stricker, Dr Raphael
as successor to Dr Beer, xii, 144
on IVIG research, 205-206, 207, 386
stroke
and PCOS, 118
and thrombophilia, 47, 66, 68, 71, 75,
78, 327
Antiphospholipid Syndrome and, 68-
70, 71
as an indicator of the need for
immune testing, 47, 66, 106
personal experiences of, 250
subchorionic hemorrhage (or
subchorionic hematoma)
association with autoimmunity, 90,
136, 137, 346-347
association with thrombophilia, 66,
327
definition of, 454
IVIG to help prevent, 158
See also bleeding in pregnancy
supplements. See vitamin supplements
syphilis, 33, 42, 72, 312
systemic lupus erythematosus (SLE)
association with
ANAs, 80, 337-338
APAs, 34, 70, 329
ATAs, 95, 349

increased miscarriage rate, 80, 337
viral infection, 93, 350

T

Taranissi, Dr Mohamed, 144 acknowlegement
from Dr Beer, 304
clinic address, 494
personal experience as a patient of, 244
T cells. See under immune system
"tender loving care" (TLC)
as a treatment for miscarriage, 105, 165,
189, 212, 215-216
testicular cancer, 85, 263
testicular dysgenesis syndrome, 272, 424
testosterone
definition, 454
high levels in PCOS, 118, 369
toxic exposure and low levels of, 264, 265,
267, 416, 418
tests for immune problems. See immune
testing
Th1 immune response
aging and, 129
anti-TNF agents to regulate, 172-173,
212-213, 395
Crohn's disease and, 103-104, 357
corticosteroids to regulate, 390
diabetes and, 116, 367
in autoimmune disease, 53, 56, 88
in normal reproduction, 53, 54, 56, 57,
62, 63, 79
in reproductive failure, 53, 88-91, 198,
200, 203, 316-318, 319, 324, 343-344
IVIG to regulate, 158, 386
LIT to regulate, 163
omega 3 fish oil to regulate, 291, 436
stress and, 106, 358, 360
toxic exposure and, 265, 415
thyroid disease and, 94, 350
Th1:Th2 cytokine ratio
test to determine, 151-152
Th2 response
in pregnancy, 62, 105
thrombophilia (and thrombosis)
acquired, (APA-related), 34, 71, 330-331,
446
arguments for significance of, 211-212,
217
definition of, 454
pathological evidence of in pregnancy
tissue, 155
testing for, 74, 152, 155, 332
treatments for, 169-170, 175, 393-394
See also antiphospholipid antibodies
dehydration and, 290
diet and, 289, 293, 438

INDEX

health problems associated with:
maternal disorders, 66, 72, 140
migraines, 123, 375
miscarriage and infertility, iii, 34,
65-66, 78, 124, 326-327, 331-336
preeclampsia, 66
Raynaud's syndrome, 124, 375
subchorionic hemorrhage, 66
inherited (genetic conditions)
factor V Leiden mutation, 34, 74-
75, 332-334
MTHFR mutation, 76-77, 334-
336
protein C and S deficiency, 34,
75, 334
prothrombin 20210 mutation, 76,
334
smoking and, 285
thyroid disease
arguments against the significance of,
186, 192, 194, 401
association with increased NK cell
activity, 32, 55, 92, 94, 348, 350
association with reproductive failure,
26, 47, 94, 216, 348, 401-403, 406
general overview of, 92-95, 347-350
hyperthyroidism, 93-94
Hashimoto's thyroiditis
association with infection, 32
definition of, 449
personal experiences with,
240, 243
hypothyroidism, 76, 78
Graves' disease
association with infection, 93-
94, 349
association with premature
ovarian failure, 112, 349
definition of, 449
implantation failure and, 32 infertility
and, 26, 56, 94, 349
miscarriage and, 26, 56, 94, 347
tests for, 44, 95, 158
toxic exposure and, 266, 268, 419
treatments for, 56, 94, 157-158, 160-
161, 195
See also antithyroid antibodies
thyroiditis. *See* thyroid disease
thrombocytopenia, 66, 393
thrombophlebitis, 66
tissue analysis, iv, 30, 43, 44, 45, 85,
144, 145, 152-154
See also endometrial biopsy
tissue factor, 75
TLC. *See* "tender loving care"
TNF-alpha. *See* tumor necrosis alpha
toxins, environmental,

and autoimmune disease, 35, 68, 100, 126,
377
and chromosomal damage, 132
and reproductive problems, 261, 263, 271-
273, 411-428
alkylphenols, 262-265, 415
Bisphenol A (BPA), 81, 265, 338-339,
413, 415-416
benzene, 269, 420-421
dioxins, 240, 400
reproductive problems and, 35, 264,
414
Electro Magnetic Field (EMF) radiation,
270, 274, 422-423, 425-427
mercury
about, 263-264, 414
autoantibody production and, 81, 296,
338-339, 440
chelators of, 296, 440-441
hazardous blood levels of, 263-263
in fish, 264, 291
PBDEs (fire retardants), 268
pesticides
association with CFS, 110
average annual consumption of, 262,
412
petrofluorochemicals (PFCs), 268, 420
phthalates, 265-266
solvents, 269, 421-422
toxins, food-related
aspartame, 275, 427-428
See also aspartame and *under* migraines
lectins, 281
monosodium glutamate (MSG), 275-277,
427
See also immune aggravating foods *under*
diet
toxoplasma gondii, 32, 311
treatments (for immune-mediated
reproductive failure), 157-180
See also anti-TNF-alpha therapy,
corticosteroids, heparin, intralipid,
intravenous gamma globulin (IVIG),
lymphocyte immunization therapy (LIT),
Neupogen, Viagra and vitamin D
trisomy
association with advancing age, 133
description of, 30, 132
personal experience with, 242
See also chromosomal abnormalities *and*
Down's syndrome
trophoblast
definition of, 455
function of, 61-62
pathology to reveal inadequate invasion of,
153-154, 156
tubal blockages. *See* ectopic pregnancy *and*
pelvic inflammatory disease

- 515 -

INDEX

tumor necrosis factor alpha (TNF alpha)
  defense against cancer, 5, 87
  definition of, 455
  endometriosis and, 97, 134, 354, 384
  as a danger to pregnancy, 5, 89-90,
    100, 114, 214, 346-347, 356, 366
  testing for, 151-152
Turner syndrome
  and premature ovarian failure, 132
  as a chromosomal abnormality, 116
  definition of, 455

U

U.S. Center for Disease Control and
  Prevention
  on prevalence of diabetes, 116, 367
U.S. Environmental Protection Agency
  (EPA):
  on toxic fetal exposure, 265, 271,
    423, 424
ulcerative colitis, 104, 358
ultrasound
  Dr Beer's protocol in pregnancy,
    135-137
  to detect pelvic problems, 45, 117
University of Chicago Hospitals
  Dr Ober's LIT study at, 226, 227
uNKs. *See under* natural killer cells,
  uterine
U.S. Food and Drug Administration
  (FDA)
  Jon Cohen contacting the, 229-264
  on mercury contamination, 263-264
  on safety classication of anti-TNF-
    alpha blockers, 174, 396-397
  on suspension of LIT, 204, 216, 226,
    229, 231, 232
uterus
  anatomical problems, iii, 29, 31, 43-
    44, 311
uterine lining (endometrium)
  arguments against testing for uNK
    cell levels, 198-199
  definition of, 449
  normal monthly development of, 110,
    121, 372-373
  poor blood flow to, 66, 118, 124-125,
    153, 154, 211, 326, 370,
  poor development caused by:
    antibodies to hormones and
      neurotransmitters, 35-36, 107-
      108, 117, 119, 120, 121, 128, 262
    abnormal immune activity, 89, 90,
      98, 104, 111, 115, 346
    PCOS, 102, 353, 363, 368

treatments to improve blood
  flow/thickness/immune tolerance of:
  intralipid, 160-161
  metformin, 174, 398
  Neupogen, 162
  omega 3 fish oil, 291, 436-437
  Viagra, 171-172, 395
  See also endometriosis, fibroids,
    implantation failure, placental abruption

V

vaginal Viagra (Sildenafil Citratate), 171-172,
  395,
vasectomy
  antisperm antibodies as result of, 85, 339
viral infection
  as a trigger for autoimmune diseases, 55,
    56, 72, 81, 126, 338, 378
  Grave's disease, 93, 350
  tests for, 44
  See also Epstein Barr virus
Vitamin D therapy, 175-176, 399
vitamin supplements
  FaBB, 175
  preconception use, 290, 297, 441-442
  use with corticosteroids, 148
  use with metformin, 174
  vitamin B6, 77, 175
  vitamin B12, 77, 174, 175, 335
  vitamin D, 175-176
vitiligo
  as a Th1-driven condition, 53
  definition of, 455
  relationship to premature ovarian
    failure, 112

W

West, Zita
  clinic address, 494
  clinic success rate, 280, 429
  natural immunotherapy program, 279-300
  on acupuncture, 298, 442-443
  on detoxification, 295-296
  on foods to avoid, 286-288
  on foods to include, 288-294
  on gluten, 284-285, 442
  on lectins, 281, 283-284, 429
  on mind-body therapy, 300, 443
  on probiotics, 282, 293, 295
Winger, Dr Edward
  his role in Dr Beer's program, 231
  studies in association with Reed J and/or
    Stricker R, 206, 207, 213, 231, 326, 344,
    354, 383, 394, 395, 396

- 516 -

INDEX

Y

Yahoo Reproductive Immunology
   Support Group
   data collected by, 336
   moderated by Jane Reed, 257, 303
   web address, 257, 498
   See also Reed, Jane

Z

Zoloft. *See* selective serotonin reuptake
   inhibitors
zona pellucida
   definition of, 455
   hardening of, 134
   normal function of, 61
   See also eggs
Zouves, Dr Christo
   acknowlegement by Dr Beer, 304
   clinic address, 458, 460
   forward by, iii
   personal experiences from patients
   of, 238, 239, 252, 253